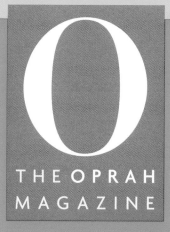

Live Your Best Life

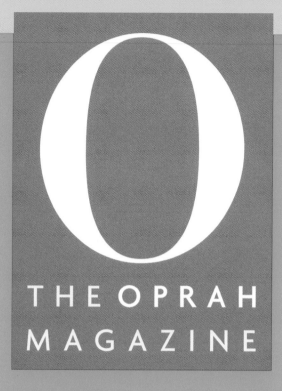

O — THE OPRAH MAGAZINE

Live Your Best Life

A Treasury of Wisdom, Wit, Advice,
Interviews, and Inspiration from
O, The Oprah Magazine

Oxmoor House®

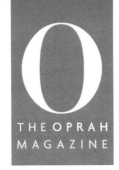

THE OPRAH
MAGAZINE

Contents

Here We Go by Oprah 6

YOUR Personal Best 8

First things first: Living your best life starts with being your best self—feeling good, looking good, finding a sense of balance and purpose. Take care of yourself and the rest will follow.

DIET & EXERCISE 10

HEALTH & BEAUTY 39

BALANCE 53

HAPPINESS 67

CONFIDENCE 81

DREAMING BIG 95

SPIRITUALITY 103

Relationships 118

The people in your life sustain you, revive you, comfort you, and may even keep you healthy. They can also drive you completely crazy. Here's help.

DATING 120

COUPLES 131

MARRIAGE 157

SEX 175

TALKING & LISTENING 187

FAMILY 201

ON BEING A PARENT 219

FRIENDS 239

Living IN THE World 250

The final piece of a well-lived life is the difference you make in the world. There's no shortage of ways to give back—or stories to inspire you.

EVERYDAY HEROES 252

GIVING BACK 279

MAKE A CONNECTION 309

ABOUT THE CONTRIBUTORS 328

PHOTOGRAPHY & ART CREDITS 330

INDEX 332

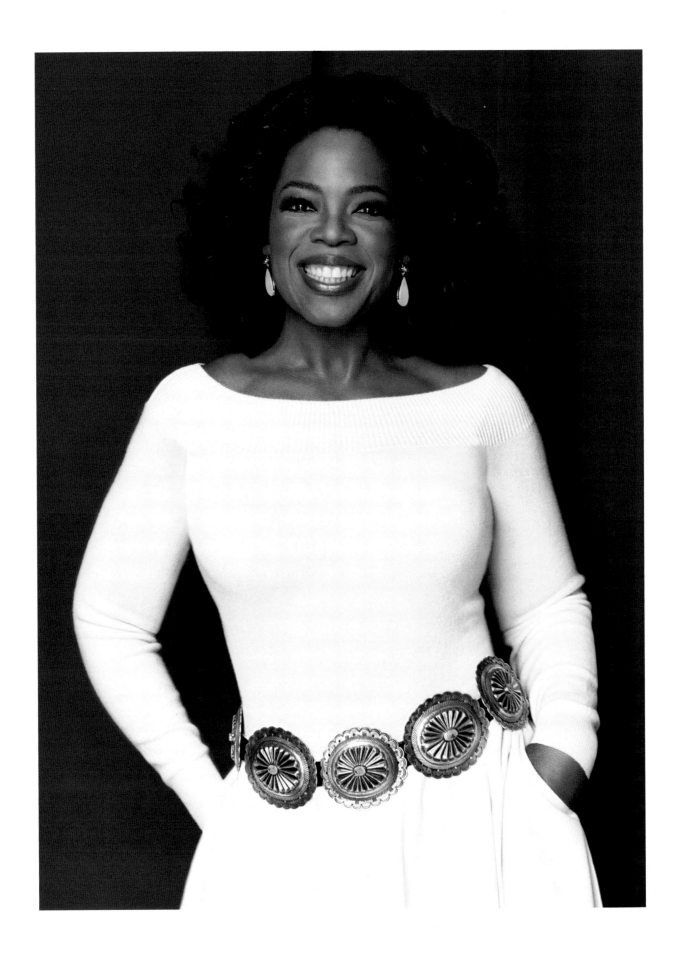

Here We Go

You have in your hands the first annual volume of *Live Your Best Life,* with more than 100 articles culled from the pages of *O, The Oprah Magazine*. Our idea was to do the rip-and-save for you—and pull it all together in a book you can turn to whenever you want inspiration, advice, or a shot of comic relief (see "Extreme Breakups," page 152, and "How Not to Turn Into Your Mother," page 205).

I wanted to put something in this goodie bag for everyone. Our "Your Personal Best" section has you covered if you're working toward a peace treaty with your bathroom scale (or magnifying mirror), as well as a wealth of info on health, confidence, money, and the pursuit of happiness. "Relationships" takes you from meeting your match ("Personal Ads: The Dos, The Don'ts, The Absolute Musts," page 124) to living with his annoying habits ("Every Little Thing He Does Is Stupid," page 143) to finding your mutual bliss ("Sex Is Sublime," page 181). We've also got sanity-saving strategies for dealing with family and friends. Our third section, "Living in the World," includes conversations with three of my favorite people: Senator Barack Obama (the speech he delivered at 2004's Democratic convention made the hair on the back of my neck stand up), rock star/activist Bono (he's fighting to save an entire continent from AIDS), and singer/songwriter Alicia Keys (her future is so bright, it burns my eyes). And there's no shortage of everyday heroes, whose courage and inspiring ideas (from getting cancer patients to laugh to helping girls lift themselves out of poverty) redefine what is possible for one woman to do.

We aim to delight. That's why we've made these pages so lush and colorful and so much fun to thumb through. My wish for you is the same as my wish for myself: to keep growing, learning, and getting better. I hope this book helps you move even closer to your best self.

Oprah

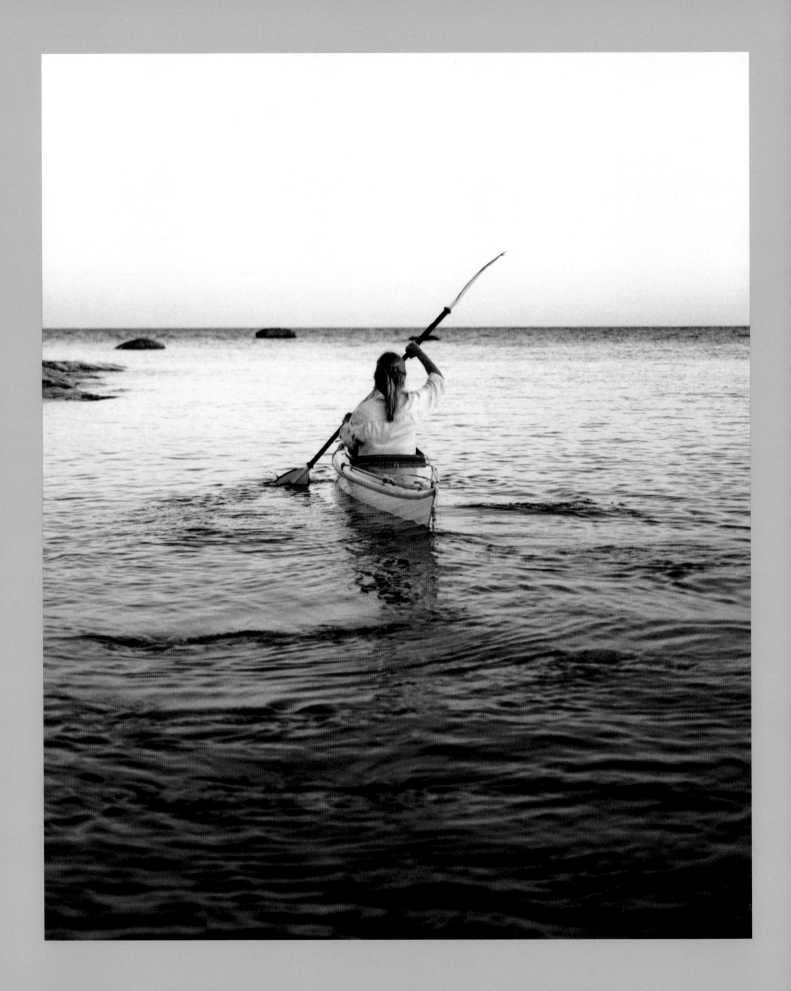

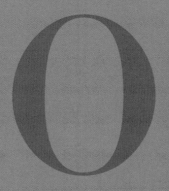

YOUR
Personal Best

First things first: Living your best life starts with being your best self—
feeling good, looking good, finding a sense of balance and purpose.
Take care of yourself and the rest will follow.

Diet & Exercise 10

Health & Beauty 39

Balance 53

Happiness 67

Confidence 81

Dreaming Big 95

Spirituality 103

O

Diet & Exercise

Dr. Phil: "Even if you've failed at every diet, you can succeed now"

PHILLIP C. McGRAW, PhD, on what he's learned after a year of trying to jump-start America's weight loss revolution.

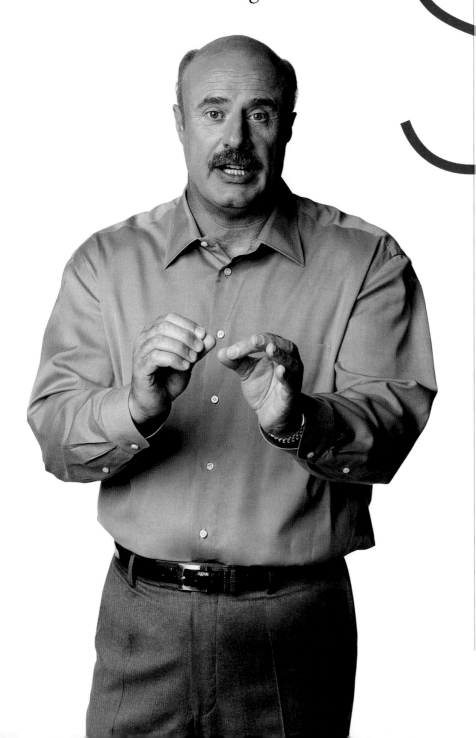

SINCE I STARTED WRITING MY book *The Ultimate Weight Solution* and working with overweight people, including the 13 Weight Loss Challengers on my show, I have learned volumes about what it takes to have a real shot at losing weight and maintaining that loss. You don't need me to tell you there's no magic diet pill to make your body (and your life) perfect or that the "30 pounds in 30 days—without any exercise!" ad you read is nothing more than wishful thinking. People know the truth when they hear it, but sometimes it can be hard to hear against the roar of empty promises the multibillion-dollar diet industry throws at them. The fact is that losing weight and keeping it off isn't easy, but it is absolutely doable.

Whether you're 25 or 400 pounds overweight, it's not too late to change the way you live, feel, think, and look. Your goals are within reach—if you go about achieving them the right way. What have I learned after spending a year trying to help America get real about weight? Plenty. Some of it I knew for sure, as Oprah would say, and some of it was brought home by the struggles of real people in the real world with real challenges.

THE OBSTACLES

The truth is that food is a tremendous coping mechanism for many people. You have probably used food to deal with emotional demands—whether to ease the pain of loneliness, anxiety, worry, or depression—or to celebrate life events. Food is powerful because it gives people a perception of relief, and if you remove that security and fail to put something else in its place, a vacuum is created. People naturally return to what they know best, which is using food for inappropriate reasons and in inappropriate ways. When you stop medicating feelings with food—which is an absolute must in order to get healthy—you need to have other ways to deal with emotions. Instead of turning to a pint of ice cream on lonely or stressful nights, make a commitment to treat psychological problems with psychological solutions, and substitute exercise, relaxation, and rational thinking for that caloric quick fix.

Overcoming the momentum of a long history of emotional eating is a huge challenge. The good news is that you don't need a heart attack or other life-threatening event to motivate you to change your behavior. If you haven't gotten the wake-up call yet, I'm giving it to you: The time is now, and it's not too late. Get out of your comfort zone and do something different. When you do, you'll generate a new history that predicts a new future.

FOR MANY PEOPLE, FOOD IS AN addiction. Addictions are not cured; they're managed one day at a time. Days add up to weeks, weeks add up to months, and before you know it, you have a new lifestyle and a new self-image. Fifty years of living the same way do not make it impossible to start living differently. Even if you've failed at every diet you've tried, you're capable of succeeding now.

Everyone has a personal truth—what she believes about herself when no one else is looking or listening. If you have failed with your weight loss efforts time and time again, you may be left with a personal truth that says, "I simply don't deserve to be anything other than fat and unhealthy." One of my greatest challenges has been convincing people that they can exercise control in their lives, and that they deserve to be healthy and happy.

A major hurdle that always seems to trip people up is thinking that they just need a little more willpower. It isn't about gritting your teeth, bearing down, and finding the strength deep within to carry you through the day. Willpower is fueled by emotion and is amazingly fickle. Motivation will wax and wane. Sure, you can rely on these things when you're pumped up and excited, like in the first few weeks of a New Year's resolution. The trick is to set up your life and program your world in such a way that you make progress and get closer to your goal even when you don't feel like it. When your willpower is nowhere to be found, you need to have your emotions, logic, environment, behavior, food plan, exercise, and social support system in place to keep you moving in the right direction.

BEST PRACTICES

Different methods work for different people. But there are certain actions common to almost every person who achieves weight loss goals. These steps work because they have to do with lifestyle and programming, not unreliable willpower.

Clean up your environment.

Think about it: If you go through your house and remove everything that is counterproductive to the program—such as impulse foods, prepackaged foods, snacks high in sugar or fat—you'll be less prone to eat those foods. You're more likely to eat a cookie at 11 P.M. if it's sitting on your kitchen counter than if you first have to get dressed and drive to the store to buy that cookie. It's a simple environmental control, but it makes a huge difference. You can also make superficial changes to remind yourself that it's not too late to start again—rearranging your furniture, getting a new haircut, or waking up at a different time. While these actions seem to have nothing to do with weight management, they can help you feel different and reinforce that it's a new day.

Move it to lose it.

Exercise is crucial. You can't lose weight and keep it off without awakening your body and your metabolism. If you get off the couch with some regularity and increase your energy output, you will dramatically alter your body's efficiency.

Timing is everything.

Most people who slip up while trying to lose weight do it during a narrow window of time and place. Audit your day and determine when you tend to make the most destructive eating decisions. Arrange to do something else during that time, something incompatible with eating. If you usually snack in the kitchen when you get home from work, come in a different door, take a shower first, or, better yet, use that time to exercise.

Mix it up.

The problems with diets are too numerous to list here, but certainly one of them is the tendency for people to rebel against a plan that's too restrictive. You don't need to give up ice cream forever, run from carbohydrates, or count every calorie. Instead eat a variety of healthy foods—fruits and vegetables, lean proteins, good fats, and, yes, some starches—in manageable portions. It's about being flexible, creating a plan that works with your life, and practicing moderation across the board.

Don't go it alone.

If you want to lose weight and keep it off, you need the people in your life to be supportive. Educate your loved ones about the changes you are making, what your needs are, and how family and friends can help. Break free from those who weigh you down (pun intended). And don't be afraid to make new friends—people with similar values who don't feel threatened by your changes and won't urge you to eat.

OF COURSE, THERE WILL BE HARD times when you make the wrong choices or when you're stuck in a rut. You need to behave your way to success. I knew I was undertaking a major task when I said that I wanted to start a movement in America, but I am seeing it happen. Millions are turning away from misleading diets, learning to get real about why they eat what they eat, and changing their lifestyles. I hope you are among them—starting now. ●

Making Peace
with Your Body...

The world tells you to love yourself as you are... but prefers you thin. So you not only hate your body but hate yourself for hating your body. **MICHELLE BURFORD** got fed up, found a revolutionary new bottom line, and shed 64 pounds along the way.

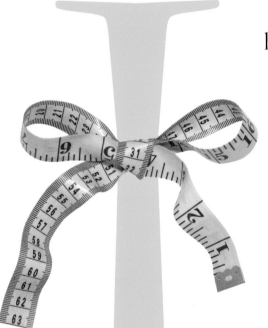

I'M NO FOE OF THE FAT WOMAN— I'm just a reformed binge-aholic weary of the pat advice I get from well-meaning people: *Love yourself as you are. Let go of your body hatred and "embrace" the cottage cheese on your thighs. Tell yourself every morning that you're a goddess.* Trouble is that while I can tell myself whatever I want, the world around me says something far different. In every diet commercial, on every lingerie billboard, in every whispered hallway conversation, I see and hear what few dare say forthrightly: That you're indeed judged by the span of your hips. That there's a tipping point that takes you from acceptably chubby to uncontrollably overweight. That *plus-size* and *full-figured* are just euphemisms for *big* and *fat*. And no matter how many overweight women I hear claiming that they've come to terms with their extra pounds, I know my mood rises and falls with the number on my scale every morning. I also know the one question I've lived with for too long: In a culture that worships cantaloupe-size boobs and a taut behind, isn't body dissatisfaction 100 percent guaranteed?

I say yes. And after 20 years of contending with the ticker tape of negativity that streams through most every woman's brain each day, I'm finally ready to tell myself the truth about it—and to take responsibility for ending the hell ride. "The pat answers we hear about loving our bodies are just a gut-level reaction to the messages of self-hatred that seem so inescapable in our world," says Cynthia Eller, author of the canny and witty book *Am I a Woman?* "How are we really supposed to love ourselves when even a model touted as 'the new curvy woman' is just ten pounds heavier than the stick figures usually shown? You can't help knowing that neither woman represents you. Even women at a healthy body weight sense that anything less than perfection must be fixed. We really do want to accept our bodies, but deep down we also know that the insane deprivation we subject ourselves to in the name of this unattainable perfection is at odds with real self-love."

Which is why, instead of hosting even one more moanfest with my girlfriends about how the obese are, at best, tolerated, I've adopted what I call a Former Fat Girl's Manifesto: That though my body isn't nearly what it could be, I'm doing all right if I can keep it from what it used to be. That if I can manage to waste only one afternoon on self-loathing for every 23 of self-loving, then I've still won my fight. That on those days when I do ward off a double-cheeseburger binge, I shouldn't berate myself for instead craving Manolo Blahniks. That maybe the most any of us can expect of ourselves isn't perfection but progress—even when it's as small as picking off three of the five pepperonis on a pizza slice before inhaling the rest.

During this cease-fire I've called with my body, I haven't exactly surrendered the handgun I've so often drawn to scare my weight into submission. The truth is that I may never. But if, during my farewell to (Jell-O) arms, I manage to keep my weapon lowered at my hip even one time more often, I've resolved that I'll call that good enough. ●

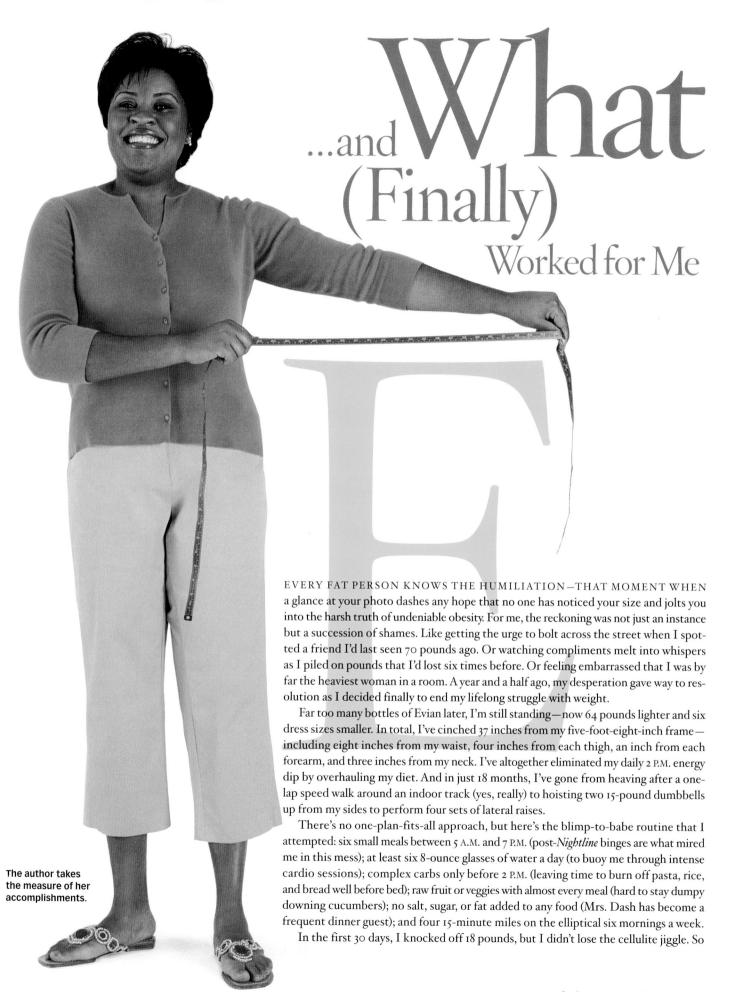

...and **What** (Finally) Worked for Me

The author takes the measure of her accomplishments.

EVERY FAT PERSON KNOWS THE HUMILIATION—THAT MOMENT WHEN a glance at your photo dashes any hope that no one has noticed your size and jolts you into the harsh truth of undeniable obesity. For me, the reckoning was not just an instance but a succession of shames. Like getting the urge to bolt across the street when I spotted a friend I'd last seen 70 pounds ago. Or watching compliments melt into whispers as I piled on pounds that I'd lost six times before. Or feeling embarrassed that I was by far the heaviest woman in a room. A year and a half ago, my desperation gave way to resolution as I decided finally to end my lifelong struggle with weight.

Far too many bottles of Evian later, I'm still standing—now 64 pounds lighter and six dress sizes smaller. In total, I've cinched 37 inches from my five-foot-eight-inch frame—including eight inches from my waist, four inches from each thigh, an inch from each forearm, and three inches from my neck. I've altogether eliminated my daily 2 P.M. energy dip by overhauling my diet. And in just 18 months, I've gone from heaving after a one-lap speed walk around an indoor track (yes, really) to hoisting two 15-pound dumbbells up from my sides to perform four sets of lateral raises.

There's no one-plan-fits-all approach, but here's the blimp-to-babe routine that I attempted: six small meals between 5 A.M. and 7 P.M. (post-*Nightline* binges are what mired me in this mess); at least six 8-ounce glasses of water a day (to buoy me through intense cardio sessions); complex carbs only before 2 P.M. (leaving time to burn off pasta, rice, and bread well before bed); raw fruit or veggies with almost every meal (hard to stay dumpy downing cucumbers); no salt, sugar, or fat added to any food (Mrs. Dash has become a frequent dinner guest); and four 15-minute miles on the elliptical six mornings a week.

In the first 30 days, I knocked off 18 pounds, but I didn't lose the cellulite jiggle. So

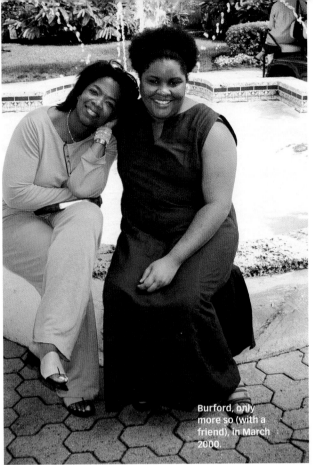

Burford, only more so (with a friend), in March 2000.

the following month, I hired a trainer at my gym to guide me through an hour of weight training three days a week. A few weeks later, on my trainer's advice, I switched from a long, slow jog (which does burn fat, he claims, but doesn't deliver the speedy results of a more intense workout) to a 40-minute run that keeps my heart rate at 70 percent of its maximum. To save my knees, I then traded in the treadmill for an elliptical machine. Finally, I bought a food scale that revealed just how heaping my "three-ounce" helpings of salmon had been.

Four months into my revised routine, I'd tightened my abs and arms and lost another 30 pounds—and with every pound shed, there entered a doubt: What would keep me from regaining the weight? Why would this time be different? I followed that question all the way back to a page in my seventh-grade yearbook, to a sentence scrawled in faded pen from a male classmate whose face I can't recall but whose words still sting: "To Michelle—the gigantic black girl who sat in front of me all year." The day I read that, I was 11 and already 25 pounds overweight. Even after I'd squirreled away that yearbook in an attempt to forget it, I spent the rest of junior high imagining that my friends were snickering at my figure.

Nine months ago, I realized for the first time that, in the 19 years since I tried to bury my classmate's cruelty, his words have quietly stalked me through every New Year's resolution, through every promise to lose weight that I've ever made and broken. In part, I hadn't shed the pounds permanently because I substituted one silly boy's assessment for my own: I'd never sustained a weight loss because I didn't truly believe that a "gigantic black girl" could. Which is why, each time that slight and its attendant skepticism have surfaced over the past year, I've practiced replacing them with my own plotline: me, 30, and thin at last.

At the end of last summer, I tripped into a teensy relapse—okay, a titanic re-

gression. I let a lengthy to-do list truncate my gym time for an entire month. Week one without weight lifting: no noticeable difference. Week two: catatonic after lunch and dodging my trainer's voice mails. Week three: exhausted upon wake-up and hauling eight extra pounds on my thighs. Week four: digging for photo proof that I once did mount a stair climber. About six weeks before I had to squeeze into a periwinkle chiffon bridesmaid dress—the kind you might need a forklift to zip up—I finally crawled my way back to the New York Sports Club to peel off those same eight pounds and lose four more.

If offered a choice between a root canal and six sets of push-ups, I'd leap into that dentist's chair—I hate to exercise that much. And though I'd relish the joy of squeezing back into my size-6 button-flies, the truth is that I'd love to replace my Evian with Häagen-Dazs and skip the daily sweat sessions altogether. But aside from persevering, my only other option is to live out my life miserably obese. And since I accept that my only two choices are to be fat or to fight it, I'd much rather be prying myself out of bed to meet my trainer at 6 A.M. than hastening the death of my spirit, one spoonful of ice cream at a time.

This summer, as I inch toward my goal weight, the questions I challenge myself with are what they've always been: Will I give up a half hour of sleep for a stint on the stair climber? Am I willing to push myself to do one last set of chin-ups even when I'm exhausted? Will I stop complaining that there's no time to shop for my six meals a day and start making preparation a priority? Have I decided I'll do whatever it takes to have the healthy body I say I want to build?

These daily attempts at courage—and not just the acquisition of a fitter figure—are what, I hope, have permanently changed me. And this time around, losing the weight has become about forgiving myself for failing time and time again—and simply rising up to start over no matter how many times I do. ●

Michelle's Menus

HERE'S A SAMPLE OF MY SIX DAILY MINI-MEALS: 5 A.M. Before the gym, a cup of dry granola. After the gym, a banana, some celery, and an egg white. (I count pre- and post-gym as just one food hit.) 8:30 A.M. Container of nonfat yogurt and half a Snickers bar (I sin daily but early). NOON Six ounces of grilled mahimahi, a tomato, and a cup of roasted potatoes (plus some raw carrots if I'm still hungry). 2 P.M. A fistful of grapes, four ounces of low-fat Swiss cheese spread, and seven whole wheat crackers (my last carb fix for the day). 4 P.M. A can of plain tuna in water and a cup of steamed kale (it's a daily fight to get in enough veggies). 6:30 OR 7 P.M. Four ounces of grilled chicken, salad without dressing, and a peach. REST OF THE NIGHT Nothing or as much Crystal Light drink mix as I can hold.

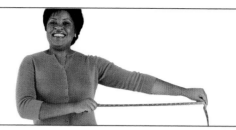

MICHELLE BURFORD unveils the mottoes that guided her from thick to thin.

Words to Lose By

A binge is like a banquet in a graveyard.

When I've been tempted to overeat, a reminder that I'm slowly killing myself is often enough to make me throw down that fork.

Lose weight like you date.

Try more than one approach at a time—hire a trainer, drop the salt, find an accountability partner, keep a journal of your progress. And start saying the hard things (beginning with the word *no*) instead of downing the Twinkies.

Take it to the Net.

In the first month of my weight loss attempt, I signed on to both Yahoo and oprah.com and found hundreds of online support groups. My e-mail buddy has been my lifeline—a mother of four in Tallahassee whose real name I don't even know has extended encouragement and advice, exchanged weigh-in results, and shared difficulties and triumphs with me.

Failing to plan is planning to fail.

If you're exhausted and cranky after work and your fridge is filled with fattening food, you're probably going to do the easiest thing (I would) and reach for what's nearest. That's why I now do all my grocery shopping on Sundays, then plan my week's meals. Takes me a couple of hours—but then during the week all I have to do is grab and go.

Stay ahead—go to bed.

It's tough to order chow mein at midnight when you've been asleep since 9:30. Instead of reaching for the Godiva, climb into bed early when you feel an evening craving coming on. If I do have to stay up and I decide to give in to the longing, I have a rule that I must drink three full glasses of water before hitting the sheets—sometimes I won't binge simply because I hate guzzling all that water.

Yes, pout—then pounce.

When this war with my weight has knocked me to my knees, I allow myself only one song on the "poor me" soundtrack before I jump to my feet again. Turn that whine into a win! Victors are really just temporary quitters who then regroup with a vengeance.

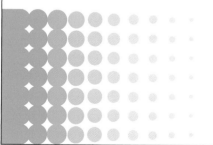

Give Us This Day Our Daily Motto

Instead of padlocking the fridge, why not bite off a little weight loss inspiration? Tape these nuggets of wisdom where you can see them—in your wallet, on your mirror, on your computer screen....

Get great at the wait.
Be patient—the ability to persevere is what separates whiners from winners.

Nothing tastes as good as being thin feels.

A U-turn beats no turn.
It's never too late to stop a binge: Six Oreos are better than six Oreos plus a piece of pie.

Give what you need.
Find a partner you can support when she's feeling weak—and let her do the same for you.

Think: What would I be feeling if I weren't eating?

Front-load to prevent buttload.
Stacking most of your calories toward the front end of the day usually means you'll be carrying a lot less junk in your trunk.

WHEN THE GOING GETS

a habit isn't a constant struggle is a liar. What you need could be a pep talk (listen
(like naltrexone for alcohol abuse) or a try-everything strategy (which seems to

Goal Interrupted

Bob Greene gets on the phone with three women who fell off the weight loss program.

Shedding Post-smoking Weight

Rita Cruse, 53, contacted *O* with a combination of pride and frustration. Six months before, she'd quit smoking—one of her toughest challenges ever—but had immediately faced a seemingly inexorable weight gain. "I've hired a personal trainer," she wrote, "I go to a gym six days a week, I eat well, and I have never been this heavy."

"Quitting smoking is a huge victory," Greene assures her on the phone, "the single best thing you could do for your health, and far more important than losing a few pounds." But, he also tells her, because of the way cigarettes affect your body, it can take a year to get weight control back to normal.

"Forget about the scale," Greene says. "Pay more attention to how your clothes feel." He also advises her to increase her walking pace. "You need to regain lung capacity and the ability to process oxygen. I want you breathing pretty hard, huffing and puffing, able to talk only in sound bites while you're working out."

He tells Cruse she'll soon see the results of her efforts. "It's like the universe telling you, Rita, you smoked for so many years, you're going to have to pay the price and invest at least one year back into yourself."

When Food Is Your Best Friend

Despite working out four days a week, Cynthia Richards has recently topped out at her highest weight ever. The 47-year-old tells Greene that she began turning to food as her "best friend" when she was 10 and her mother became seriously ill. "Now I'll be good for a couple of weeks and then everything starts adding up—work, travel, family commitments—and food becomes the solace again," she confesses. Food is a replacement for something—she knows that much but can't articulate what that is.

Greene advises Richards to keep a journal and to use it at the very moment she starts overeating. "That moment is the closest you're

Science's Best New Strategies...

Smoking. On their own, individual treatments don't pack a great punch, but together they're turning into a knockout. You can double your chances of quitting if you combine nicotine replacement and support groups or go on the prescription drug bupropion (Zyban). If you're worried about getting hooked on the patch, gum, lozenge, or inhaler, relax. Nicotine replacement doesn't appear harmful: In one five-year study of almost 6,000 people who used the gum, no serious side effects or increased risk of cardiovascular problems were reported. And for all serial quitters, science shows that the more attempts you make, the more likely you are to ultimately succeed. Translation: Try everything, and keep on trying.

Drinking. The big news here is the drug naltrexone (ReVia and Depade). The more science uncovers about the brain's response to addiction and habit, the more pharmaceutical treatment makes sense. For people with drinking problems, "craving increases after they take the first drink—naltrexone blocks that," says Joseph R. Volpicelli, MD, who first researched the drug as an alcohol dependence treatment at the University of Pennsylvania. Taken in combination with psychotherapy, naltrexone reduces the risk of a binge by about 50 percent. Although the drug is typically used with abstinence as the goal, Volpicelli says it's also helpful for those who want to moderate their drinking. (For moderation support groups, check out moderation.org.)

Overeating. Preliminary research has found that binge eaters who filled out questionnaires about their food habits, then discussed the answers with a researcher in a short, nonjudgmental interview, almost tripled their odds of quitting at the end of four months. "It's a very warm, empathetic style of interaction," says the study investigator, Erin Dunn, a psychology resident at the University of Washington. What this means is that a sympathetic friend—or counselor—who will help you think through the pros and cons of changing your eating patterns can make all the difference. Sandra Weinberg, a New York City psychotherapist who works with eating disorder patients, points out that the people closest to you can sometimes make you feel judged, but finding someone impartial to talk to is "really helpful because the muscle of opposition doesn't move in right away to prevent consideration of change." —*Maia Szalavitz*

TOUGH

...the tough get help. And anyone who says changing in as Bob Greene remotivates three fitness dropouts). It could be a pill work for smoking). The point is, if you've fallen, we've got ways for you to get up.

going to get to understanding what it is you're replacing with food," he explains. "Is it self-validation, is it someone else in your life? See if you can put your finger on it and figure out what else you could be doing besides eating to make that feeling of emptiness go away."

Greene urges Richards not to beat herself up when she does have that second or third portion. "It's simply a missed opportunity to shed some light on what you can change in your life." Understanding is key, he tells her: "Once you identify what in your life is making you eat when you're not hungry, you actually have the power to change it."

When Eating Blocks Pain

Shortly after Susan Reneé Bergo submitted her weight loss contract, she was blindsided by the most devastating news a parent can receive. Her 23-year-old son had been killed in a car accident. For a time, everything fell to pieces as she coped with her grief. She wrote to *O,* "As for my 'success' story, there is none. I failed."

Bergo, 57, wanted to offer encouragement to others. "There must be hundreds of women out there," she wrote, "who had the finest intentions and then life circumstances thrust them right back in the grip of eating for comfort, boredom, loneliness, and despair."

"Food's natural purpose is to comfort us, and we shouldn't try to do away with that," Greene tells her when they speak. "But we can limit its impact." What really matters, Greene reminds her, has little to do with weight—it's about feeling fulfilled. And Bergo's challenge is to resurrect the things from her life that give it meaning and to turn toward them rather than toward food. "Tomorrow do something to make each of those areas of your life—work, friends, family, spirituality—better." He suggests: Once she's focusing on that bigger picture, she can write a list of things to do—other than eating—to get through the painful moments. "Food is like a drug," Greene says. "It gets you past that moment of discomfort. But the irony is that you were meant to feel whatever it is."
—*Michelle Stacey*

Are You Ready to Change?
And what to do if you're not quite there.

As you settle into your daily KitKat bar, the thought hovers, *Give it up, wimp.* That you're planning to quit junk food might be stating things too boldly; someday you'd like to clean up your diet and lose the weight. But—with excuses growing like a conga line—today, clearly, is not going to be that day.

You beat yourself up for being weak, but your inaction doesn't necessarily mean failure. When it comes to making a change, most people pass through a series of predictable phases starting with precontemplation, according to research by James Prochaska, PhD, professor of clinical and health psychology at the University of Rhode Island and coauthor of *Changing for Good.* Answering these questions, he says, can help you see where you are on the readiness continuum. For each phase, he offers the best strategies to move you along.

Questions

1. Do you plan to address your problem this month?
2. Do you intend to address it in the next six months?
3. Have you taken significant action toward solving it in the past six months?

Scoring

No to all questions: Precontemplation
No to all but number 2: Contemplation
No to only number 3: Preparation
Yes to number 3: Action

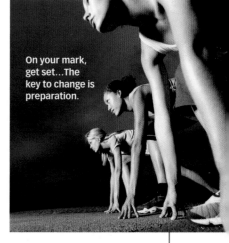

On your mark, get set...The key to change is preparation.

Solutions

PRECONTEMPLATION: You can't deal with your habit right now.
Strategies: Learn about the benefits of changing (try not to dwell on what you have to give up). Read about people who have broken the same habit and what they got out of it.
CONTEMPLATION: You want to change but aren't quite ready to act.
Strategies: Envision yourself having quit the habit. Focus on the disadvantages of continuing the behavior and the advantages of changing it (say, the $3,000 a year you spend on cigarettes versus the Caribbean vacation you could afford if you stopped).
PREPARATION: You're ready to take a step.
Strategies: Go public. Tell your friends, spouse, coworkers when you plan to quit smoking, for example (the announcement will make it harder to back out). Allow yourself the freedom of trying different methods—support groups, medication, therapy—so that if you can't stand one option, you know there are other routes available.
ACTION: It's time to make a move.
Strategies: Join a self-help group, see a counselor, get a prescription for Zyban (smoking), sign up for a treatment program. Tell the important people in your life that you need support and may not be at your best for a while. Make this change your top priority, and be as easy on yourself as you would if you were undergoing major surgery. —*Maia Szalavitz*

KEEPING IT O

Everyone can lose weight…temporarily. The catch is, almost everyone—we're 20 percent? What do they know that the yo-yo-ers don't? Since 1993 a team of scientists their weight loss year after year. Four of them are here to tell you exactly

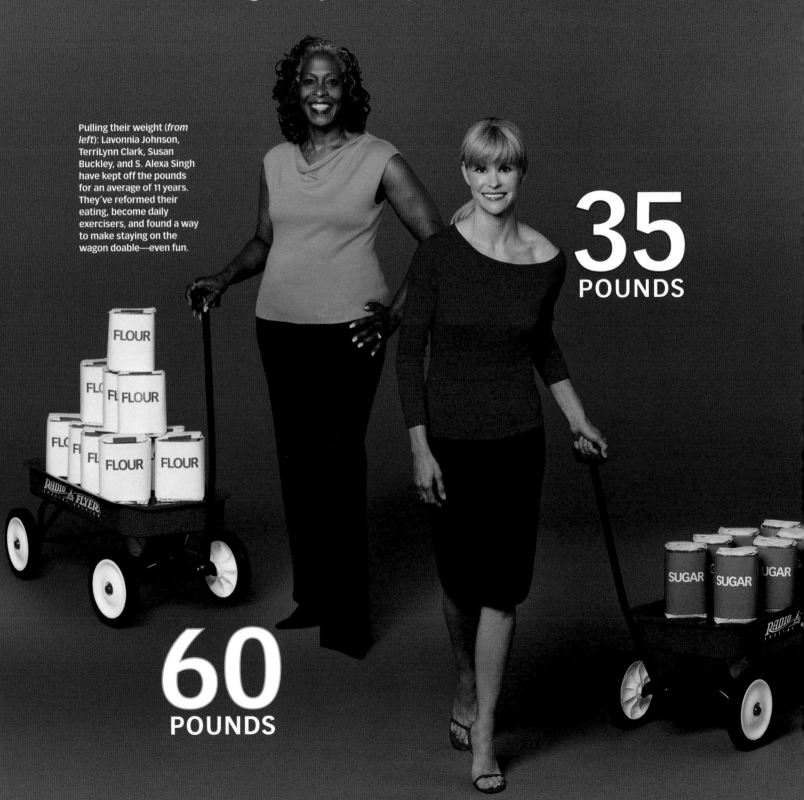

Pulling their weight (*from left*): Lavonnia Johnson, TerriLynn Clark, Susan Buckley, and S. Alexa Singh have kept off the pounds for an average of 11 years. They've reformed their eating, become daily exercisers, and found a way to make staying on the wagon doable—even fun.

35 POUNDS

60 POUNDS

FF-FOREVER

talking 80 percent—gains it right back. But what about the other, successful has tracked more than 3,000 dieters who've managed to defy the odds and maintain how to do it. SAMANTHA DUNN reports.

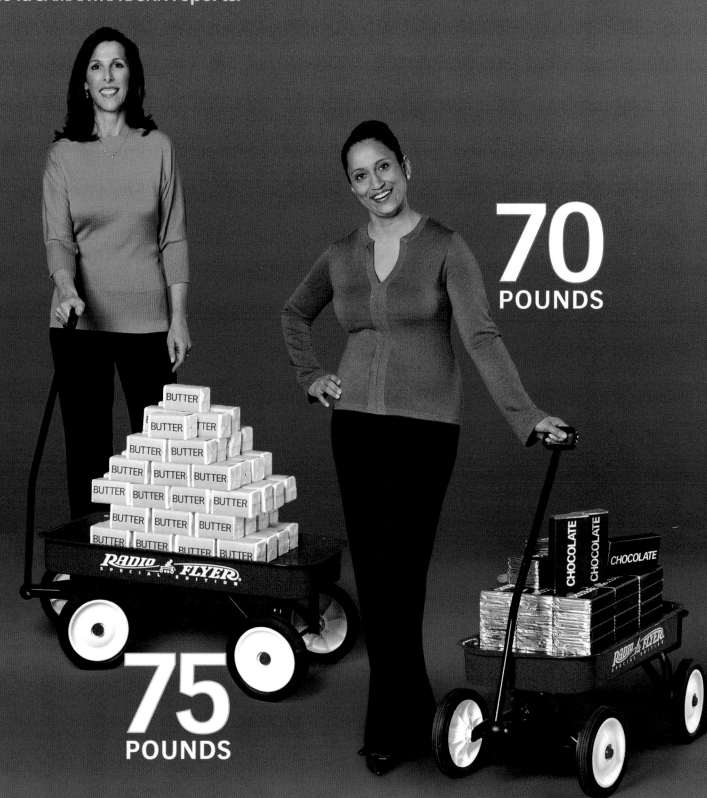

70 POUNDS

75 POUNDS

SUSAN BUCKLEY DARTS THROUGH the aisles of her local Whole Foods Market in Highlands Ranch, Colorado, as confidently as if she were walking through the rooms of her own house. The store is well-worn terrain for this 47-year-old registered dietitian, who's shopping for an evening get-together with friends and family. A bag of organic tortilla chips catches her eye, and she flips it to the label side—as she does with literally every item she touches—computing serving size, fat, and other nutrient content. "Two grams of protein per serving. Not bad," she says as she nods in approval. These chips will make it to her table. "Now all we need is salsa...."

This sort of food savvy didn't always come naturally to Buckley, although it's hard to believe, looking at her shapely 136-pound, 5'6" frame. Buckley grew up in a home where a typical meal was macaroni and cheese with fish sticks; her mother weighed close to 300 pounds despite the weight loss gimmicks she constantly tried. Chubby as a kid, when Buckley hit puberty at age 12 the family doctor prescribed a diet. "That," she says, "was the first of every single diet in the world."

After years of yo-yoing

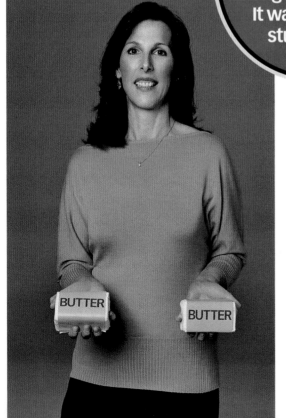

between 118 to 180 pounds, Buckley finally topped the scales at 205 with the birth of her second daughter.

"I was getting in the shower one day, and I looked in the mirror. I had one of those stomachs that kind of folds over on itself. I went, 'I am so sick of being here,'" she says. "I had a 5-year-old and a newborn, and I just felt like crying because I didn't want them to watch me struggle with my weight the way I'd watched my mother struggle with hers. I knew I had to do something, but since I was nursing I could not go on another crazy diet. It's one thing to make that decision for yourself; it's another when you're a nursing mother."

So, for the first time, she joined Weight Watchers and attended for three months until she felt she could stick to a program on her own. She also bought a cross-country-ski machine that she used when the baby was napping. In a little more than a year she was down to her goal weight of 135. Yet the extraordinary thing about Buckley is not that she lost 70 pounds or that her success inspired her to become a professional dietitian but that 11 years later, she is still keeping it off. "I call myself a long-time loser," she says, "and am proud of it."

> "Learning to take care of my body instead of being at war with it changed everything. It was powerful stuff." —Susan Buckley

SINCE 1993 RESEARCHERS WITH the National Weight Control Registry have tracked the progress of some 3,000 people like Buckley to find out what it takes to lose weight—not for two weeks or two months but for good. "Everyone was saying how 95 percent of dieters fail. We thought, *Why not study the 5 percent who succeed?*" says James O. Hill, PhD, director of the Center for Human Nutrition at the University of Colorado, who cofounded the registry with Rena Wing, PhD, director of the Weight Control and Diabetes Research Center at Brown University. Hill is one of the country's leading obesity

researchers and is on a crusade to change the shape of America. A member of the National Institutes of Health (NIH) panel that developed U.S. guidelines for prevention and treatment of obesity and chair of the first World Health Organization Consultation on Obesity, Hill has published more than 200 scientific articles and co-authored *The Step Diet Book: Count Steps, Not Calories, to Lose Weight and Keep It Off Forever* (Workman), which comes with a pedometer. "The whole key to dealing with obesity is learning to keep weight off," says Hill.

Today the National Weight Control Registry is the largest database of information on people who have achieved this uncommon victory. To join, one must be 18 or older and have maintained a weight loss of 30 pounds or more for at least a year. (Call 800-606-NWCR for information on enrollment.) Participants are asked to fill out questionnaires periodically; some (who agree to it) are the subject of "ethnographies"—studies conducted by researchers who move in with them for a while, poke around their fridge, watch them work out, and record their daily habits and attitudes. "The information we have gathered from these people in the registry is the best hope we have of learning how to help others keep weight off," Hill says. And he believes that because of skyrocketing obesity—and all the attendant health problems like diabetes and heart disease—Americans are in critical need of this information. "If we don't turn the tide in the next few years, I think we're lost," he warns.

If the registry is any indication, there is reason for hope. First of all, Hill says, according to all their research, the often-cited, dismal 5 percent success rate for dieters appears in reality to be a more odds-friendly 20 percent. Also, the average registry participant has lost about 60 pounds and maintained it for at least five years. Approximately half lost the weight on their own without any formal program or help.

"What I am beginning to learn," says Hill, "is that there are a whole bunch of ways to lose weight, but not a lot of ways to maintain the loss. Maintaining is much more of a formula." While a wide variety of diets—from Atkins to liquid fasts—helps participants take off the pounds, the winning strategy for keeping the weight off is a low-calorie, low-fat meal plan with lots of fruits and vegetables: 24 percent fat, 56 percent carbohydrates, and 19 percent protein. The maintenance formula also entails being more aware of what you're eating, keeping tabs on how much you weigh, and, perhaps most of all, getting regular physical activity. Beyond that, however, lies an intangible element Hill says is crucial: Everybody who manages to keep pounds off has found a way to link positive behaviors with some other aspect of her life—exercising as a time for connecting with friends, for example, or eating healthfully to set a good example for the kids. Any long-term behavior change is formidable, but if it makes you feel better emotionally, physically, and/or spiritually, you are more likely to stick with it. "This is the most important new discovery we have made in quite some time," Hill stresses.

Spend any time with long-term losers and you'll find them talking not about what they've lost but about what they have gained. Buckley, who now does four miles a day on a treadmill, three times a week, along with three sessions at the gym, observes, "For me the experience of nourishing my body, of taking care of it instead of being at war with it, changed everything. I learned you could treat your body well and give it exercise and make it feel good. You could feel emotionally nurtured by that, too. It was powerful stuff."

"If I've had a bad day, I leave it in the pool. Swimming helps take away all the pain and stress." —Lavonnia Johnson

LAVONNIA JOHNSON IS A CASE-worker for Congresswoman Eleanor Holmes Norton in Washington, D.C.—and

KEEPING IT OFF FOREVER
The 10 Rules

1. Always eat breakfast. Try to get more of your food early in the day and less at night. Nearly 90 percent of the National Weight Control Registry participants report eating breakfast at least four days a week.

2. Move. Everybody knows that regular, sustained exercise is a must, but the incidental movements in life also add up. Chuck the remote. Make two trips to the laundry room instead of one. Park in a distant corner of the lot. Going to the gym twice a week won't cure a lifestyle that is sedentary in every other way. The good news: No fancy trainers are required. Walking is the most common exercise among registry participants, and they average 11,000 to 12,000 steps—roughly five and a half to six miles—every day.

3. Read labels. "We are portion-control challenged in this country," Susan Buckley says. Be guided by the number of serving sizes listed on a package. (A Coke has 100 calories per eight-ounce serving, but a 20-ounce bottle contains two and a half servings, or 250 calories; a snack-size bag of 150-calorie-per-serving Cheez Doodles is, believe it or not, two servings.)

4. Keep track. How often are you working out? What and when did you eat today? "I toss my food journals when I'm done, but they keep me aware and conscious," says TerriLynn Clark. Also, weigh yourself on a regular basis—most registry participants get on the scale at least once a week.

5. Plan for the rough patches. James O. Hill, director of the Center for Human Nutrition, says stressful times—and they'll come—can trigger you to go back to old habits, especially in the first six to 12 months after a weight loss, before the new habits take hold. So have a strategy in place (call friends, take yoga—anything but food) and write it down.

6. Start small after a slip. If your weight creeps up, don't do anything drastic. Cut dessert, skip wine with dinner, take another walk around the block. "Unless you take baby steps, it can be very frustrating," S. Alexa Singh advises.

7. The more consistent, the better. Researchers compared participants who basically followed the same diet every day with those who ate more on weekends and holidays than during the week. People in the first group were one and a half times more likely to maintain their weight within five pounds over a year.

8. Make special occasions count. "Before you walk in the door of a restaurant," Buckley says, "think, *Is this just a meal I don't want to cook at home, or is it a special occasion?* If it's the latter, go ahead and indulge, because such moments come only once in a while. Otherwise, you need to think about portions and what you order."

9. Don't wait to get a life. "I hear people say, 'When I lose weight, I'm going to do this or that' or 'When I lose weight I am going to start living,'" Buckley says. Start doing now what you dream you will do. The rest will follow.

10. Know it will get easier. The longer you keep the weight off, research shows, the less effort it takes.

—S.D.

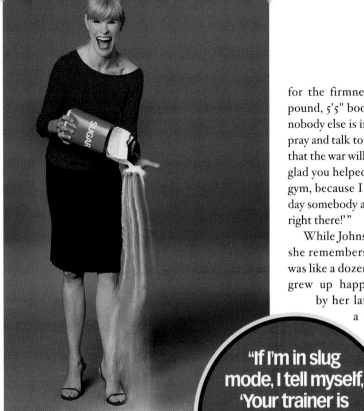

for the firmness and tone of her 170-pound, 5'5" body. "I'm so thankful when nobody else is in the pool, because then I pray and talk to God. I pray for the world, that the war will stop, and I say, 'God, I am glad you helped me get back here to the gym, because I was having such a rotten day somebody almost made me slap them right there!'"

While Johnson says this with a smile, she remembers all too vividly what life was like a dozen years ago. Although she grew up happily in North Carolina, by her late 30s she found herself a divorced single mother struggling to raise three children, depressed, and getting "drunk as a skunk" too often. The day her youngest son was born, her mother passed away; some years later her ex-husband died of AIDS. "I cried for years and years, and as I cried I gained weight," says Johnson, who once hovered near the 230-pound mark.

Being told she was too heavy to continue as a research subject for an NIH

> ### "If I'm in slug mode, I tell myself, 'Your trainer is downstairs and she'll be angry if you don't go meet her.'"
> —TerriLynn Clark

if you're going somewhere with her, be prepared to walk. Johnson routinely goes to work/church/the grocery store on foot, come heat or high water. In her vernacular, something that's "close" could mean a few city blocks away, but if she tells you something is "not far," you'd better be wearing good walking shoes.

Just this would be enough exercise for some, but for Johnson, 53, walking is only an extra. Twice a day, morning and evening, you'll find her at the gym (conveniently located eight blocks from both work and home), swimming and water jogging in the pool for a total of about three and a half hours. With the number of friends she has made in the decade since joining her gym, she says she has to split her workout just to keep in contact with all of them. "I've met so many wonderful people," she says. "It lets me know I'm not on the boat all by myself. All these other people are out there saving their lives, too."

Beyond the social element, her time at the pool is also an expression of her spirituality, a kind of daily baptism. "If I've had a bad day, I leave it in that water. It helps take away all the pain and stress," says Johnson, who also credits water resistance

years ago she started swimming regularly even before she changed her eating choices from fried food to fresh vegetables, fruits, and lean meat like turkey.

Without knowing it, Johnson was implementing a key element that would allow her to be a successful loser. Hill explains: "One of the big things dieters aren't aware of is that when you lose weight, your metabolism goes down, meaning the number of calories you burn each day goes down. You can't restrict calories forever, but there's a simple answer to that—build up physical activity before and during weight loss, so that by the time you reach your goal you're doing enough extra activity to make up for your drop in metabolism."

Johnson sometimes brings her 8-year-old grandson to the pool so he can develop good exercise habits early. And at her office—where she stocks her desk with cans of tuna and sardines and popcorn for quick energy boosts—she acts as the semi-official cheerleader for eating well, keeping a scale by the door for anyone who enters. Even her participation in the National Weight Control Registry, which she's been a part of since 1998, gives her motivation to continue the behaviors that help her stay fit. "When you keep yourself in check and healthy, you can help other people," she says. "And when I help somebody else, I am helping myself, too."

Small lifestyle changes repeated consistently seem to create the biggest ripple effect over time.

study for which she'd volunteered was a turning point. "A doctor in the study told me, 'You want to see your kids graduate from school? You want to see your grandchildren born? If you want to see those things, you have to lose weight. If not, you're going to die an early death,'" Johnson recalls. That doctor encouraged her to do some kind of activity she liked, so 12

TERRILYNN CLARK, 39, WAS THIN, growing up as an active kid in Michigan, and today she's a 5'7", 120-pound homemaker and mother of two living in Gainesville, Georgia. Between then and now, however, was a 35-pound weight gain and many attempts to take it off. "There was a whole lot of trial and error, the starving, the not eating anything at all," says Clark, who has kept her weight steady for the past 17 years.

The motivation to get control of her body came indirectly. In her early 20s, Clark was still living at home with her parents and had a series of dead-end jobs. But the graduation of her best friend from college lit a spark. "Seeing what she accomplished really had a profound effect on me, in the sense that I realized there was nothing I, too, couldn't do," Clark remembers.

Clark began merely by eating smaller portions of her normal meals and exercising with simple calisthenics and bike riding. It took her one year to lose the weight and ingrain habits she now maintains daily: Each morning she gets up before her two daughters and does aerobics or strength training or works out with an exercise DVD (her favorites are by Kathy Smith and Karen Voight). To have a meal with Clark is to watch portion control in action—at a Mexican restaurant she orders the chicken quesadilla plate and eats about a third of the dish. No complicated order, no request for dressing on the side. "I believe in being moderate with everything," she says, "not cutting out all carbs, for instance, or even all junk food. You have to have balance. Just like the four legs holding up a chair, if one is shorter, the chair is more likely to fall over."

Clark is the poster girl for another key principle: Small lifestyle changes repeated consistently seem to create the biggest ripple effect over time, says Hill.

As an at-home mother with two children, ages 2 and 6, in rural Georgia, Clark

> When you keep
> yourself in check
> and healthy,
> you can help
> other people.

doesn't have a wide social circle from which to draw for inspiration. It's those habits she developed while losing that keep her on track—plus a few little mind games she plays with herself. "I enjoy exercise even more now that I have children because it's time for myself, but some days I really don't feel like it," she admits. "If I get in that slug mode, I say to myself, 'Okay, your personal

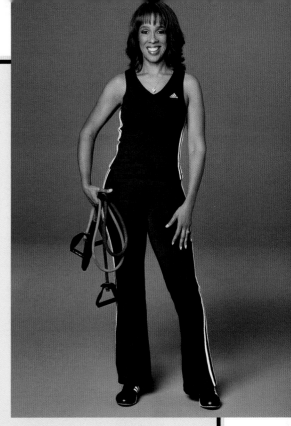

...AND THEN THERE'S GAYLE

Midway through a business lunch at a fancy, celebrity-packed restaurant in New York, Gayle King's eyes—trained so expertly to read a teleprompter without letting on—have locked into focus. The object is a large white cake across the room. And while she works her way through scallops, vegetables, and bread, making conversation, it's clear that her mind is far away, fully engaged in trying to spearfish that cake off the cart—which is rolling away to where Joel Grey is having his birthday—and onto her plate.

Dessert? Bread? Most women on weight patrol are picking at arugula salads. But to *O*'s editor at large, a good lunch is a terrible thing to waste; she just won't eat much dinner.

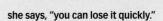

Two years ago, Gayle dropped 20 pounds during a three-month makeover with trainer Jim Karas. He put her on a daily at-home exercise program of aerobics, with a heavy emphasis on free weights and resistance bands (which Gayle swears by), and helped her get her diet under control. She has not only kept the weight off, she has lost another 4 pounds—4.1, to be exact (which her scale is)—and has dwindled from a size 14–16 down to a 10, sometimes even an 8.

Gayle credits Karas with two pieces of wisdom that made the difference this time: First, he told her, maintenance is just as much work as, if not more than, losing the weight ("I'd never heard that before," she says), and second, she would not have to deprive herself.

In the new world according to Gayle—who stands 5'10" and weighs 150.5—staying sleek is about being calculating. "I deny myself nothing," she says. "Some people don't eat pasta or bread or sweets *ever*. I love those foods too much. So for the most part, I eat healthy, but if I go to a party or on vacation, I'm going to enjoy it; then I work extra hard to get back to where I was." Extra hard might mean going a few days without bread or dessert, or bumping up her exercise to two sessions a day. "I've learned that when you gain weight quickly,"

she says, "you can lose it quickly."

Another trick that has worked is lowering her crisis weight ("the number where you buckle down") from 155 to 152. "If I'm above 152, I just don't go to the office birthday party," she says, "because I know I can't resist the cupcakes." And she's a new member of the breakfast club—"I used to skip it, but Jim told me, 'Big mistake.'" As a rule, nothing enters her mouth without serious evaluation. She used to eat bread just because it was there; now it's got to be worthy of blowing the calories. And while Krispy Kremes are still her "heroin," when she decides to indulge, she limits herself to two per sitting.

The other factor is exercise—an hour a day, six days a week—basically the routine Karas gave her. Not that she loves it, because she doesn't, but "to look the way I want to look," she says, "it's a necessity." She confesses to weighing herself about once a day, "even though they say you shouldn't. The scale is addictive, and if I have a big event coming up, it helps me see how much wiggle room I have."

Back at lunch, she does manage to score some of Grey's vanilla-icing cake for the table and relishes every last crumb of her slice—an accomplishment, she says. "Back in the day, I would've had two." —*Liz Brody* trainer is downstairs and she is going to be really angry if you don't go down there and meet her!'"

Despite her discipline, Clark occasionally indulges a nagging sweet tooth, and every once in a while stands up that personal trainer. How does she keep a slip from turning into a landslide? "Forgiveness is the biggest thing," says Clark, a member of the registry since 1996. "I have candy, then feel a little guilty. But I wake up the next day and tell myself, 'You know what—yesterday was yesterday, and it's okay, you're going to be fine.' A lot of people will have one bad day and then just continue that bad day."

S. ALEXA SINGH, 44, SITS IN THE coffee shop in the bookstore near her home in Westminster, Colorado, a quart-size sports bottle full of water next to her and the self-help best-seller *Who Moved My Cheese?* in her hand. It's a fitting place to find her because what she learned from books enabled Singh to transform herself from a 5'5", nearly 200-pound depressed person, who had trouble just getting out of a car, into a successful MBA student with a 125-pound runner's physique.

> When you gain weight, don't panic. Just eat 75 percent of what you normally would at dinner.

Born in India, Singh married an American and began living a completely different life in this country. "He's a big guy, and I was eating the kinds of food he would eat—pizza, burgers, and the like," she recalls. American habits slowly took root, like sitting on the couch watching television and driving around a parking lot looking for the space closest to the entrance.

"Sizes kept going up and new clothes kept coming. I didn't even realize I had gotten that fat," she remembers. "Then one day, I ended up in the emergency room with chest pains. I was 34 at that point. I have a son, and I wanted to be alive for him." It was for her son that she started to lose weight, illustrating another important principle: When health rather than attractiveness is the motivation, the results are more likely to stick.

Singh had always been a good student—even earning an engineering degree in India at a time when few women went into that field—so to start getting healthy, she went where good students go: to the public library, checking out books on nutrition and fitness. "I started reading about eating less and exercising. I read about the food pyramid and I started counting servings based on that," says Singh, who quickly sketches the pyramid breakdown of grains, fruits, vegetables, dairy, meat, and sweets on a napkin. After having lost some 70 pounds—and keeping them off for seven years—by following these principles, she finds them more than second nature.

Singh joined a gym, but exercise didn't come so easily. "I could not even walk because of the stress on my knees. I remember walking 12 steps on the track and bursting into tears, thinking, *I can't.* But I started one step at a time, and now I can run six miles and not even know it," she says, smiling. She runs at least four times a week and uses a treadmill or goes hiking on other days when her schedule isn't too demanding.

Singh began in early 1994, and by 1997 she had reached her goal weight. The process, she says, made her know her body so well that now she can plan for a five- or even ten-pound weight gain—say, around the holidays—and not worry. "I know exactly what to do to take it off," she says. "I just cut back on the extras that I've allowed myself and get back to my regular eating," which is basically fruits, vegetables, whole grains, milk, and lean protein—"very boring," she concedes.

Hill points this out as another important feature of maintenance: When your weight goes up a little, don't panic or do big things. Go back to eating about 75 percent of what you normally would at dinner, and if you don't start losing, do that at lunch too. "Success is about having a strategy," he says.

Other things changed for Singh once she lost weight. For the first time in a long time, she set goals, like going back to school for an MBA, which she received in May 2004, and then looking for a job. "My son got me started, but what kept me going was the weight loss," she says. "Mastery over your body makes a difference; I can sense that. I used to be like the little engine that could, and it took my weight loss for me to remember that. It was a very valuable gift to myself." ●

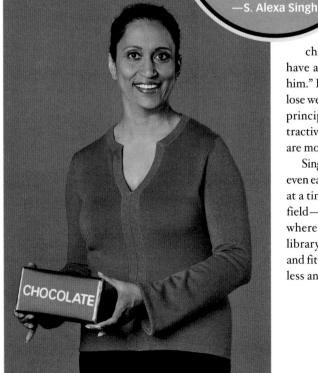

"At first I walked 12 steps on the track and burst into tears. Now I can run six miles and not even know it."
—S. Alexa Singh

CHOCOLATE

The Plateau: What to do when you hit the weight loss wall—seven ways to get over it.

BY DAVID L. KATZ, MD

ONE OF THE MOST COMMON FRUS-trations in weight loss is when all progress halts despite the fact that you are diligently following your plan. Such plateaus are predictable and explainable. Basal metabolic rate (BMR)—the energy required to keep the heart pumping, lungs expanding, kidneys filtering, and all other vital bodily functions going when the body is at rest—accounts for 60 to 70 percent of the calories you burn and depends, for the most part, on body mass. When weight loss occurs, body mass goes down; so does BMR.

Consider an example: You weigh 162 pounds and eat 1,900 calories a day. To lose a pound a week, you've got to cut between 500 and 600 calories per day. So you restrict yourself to 1,400 calories, and the weight comes off. But suddenly, after week six, the scale refuses to budge. This is because with the weight loss, your BMR has also declined (say, from 0.95 to 0.75 calories per minute), and where your body used to burn 1,368 calories per day, now it's using only 1,080. At this weight, there's also less of you to move around, so you burn fewer calories working out and waste fewer calories as heat. All in all, your daily calorie expenditure is now pretty close to what you're taking in. You've hit a new—and probably very annoying—equilibrium. Now that you know why it happens, here's what to do:

1. Hang in there. You may feel stuck, but you're probably still losing weight—just not enough to register on the scale. But even dropping a third of a pound per week means that in a year, you'll be down a whole 17 pounds.

2. Avoid fuzzy math. It's common to overestimate calories burned and underestimate calories eaten. Look for places where calories may hide—dressings, spreads, sauces, croutons, and condiments. Are you tasting a lot while cooking? Finishing what the kids leave on their plates? Absentmindedly grabbing handfuls of nuts, chips, or candy? You might try keeping a detailed food diary. Remember that for each pound you want to lose, you need to cut at least 3,500 calories—and if you don't want to eat less, to lose the same pound you'll have to add about ten extra hours of brisk walking or the equivalent.

3. Put up some resistance. Increasing physical activity is particularly useful for moving beyond a plateau because exercise both uses calories and builds muscle. The more muscle you have, the higher your BMR, which is why working out with light weights or doing some kind of resistance training can be especially helpful. In fact, increasing your muscle mass as you lose body fat can compensate for the decline in BMR induced by weight loss.

4. Up your protein quotient. There is some evidence that shifting fat and carbohydrate calories to protein calories may help preserve BMR during weight loss. But don't overdo it—20 percent of daily calories from protein is as high as you should go.

5. Shake it up. Many fitness gurus claim that surprising your body with a change in diet, workout, or both can jostle you out of a weight loss rut. The science is pretty thin here, but the advice is reasonable because variety can keep you interested. Instead of constant dieting, you might try alternating calorie-cutting days, for example, with less-restrictive maintenance days. Switch to a new type of exercise. Alternate aerobic workouts with light weight training. A change may be just what you need to get the progress rolling again.

6. Recharge your drive. If your motivation is flagging, write down all the reasons you originally wanted, and still want, to lose weight. Look at the list every day. Also let friends and family know what you're up to, and ask for their support.

7. Reconsider the skin you're in. A plateau is an opportunity to reassess whether further weight loss is worth all the work it will take—and to reconsider whether you may, in truth, now be at a perfectly healthy weight and don't need to go any lower. If you do choose to stop where you are, turn your focus toward maintaining what you've achieved and keeping your body in good shape. Remember, eating well and being physically active are good for you. Do a little of both every day, and you will be a total success. ●

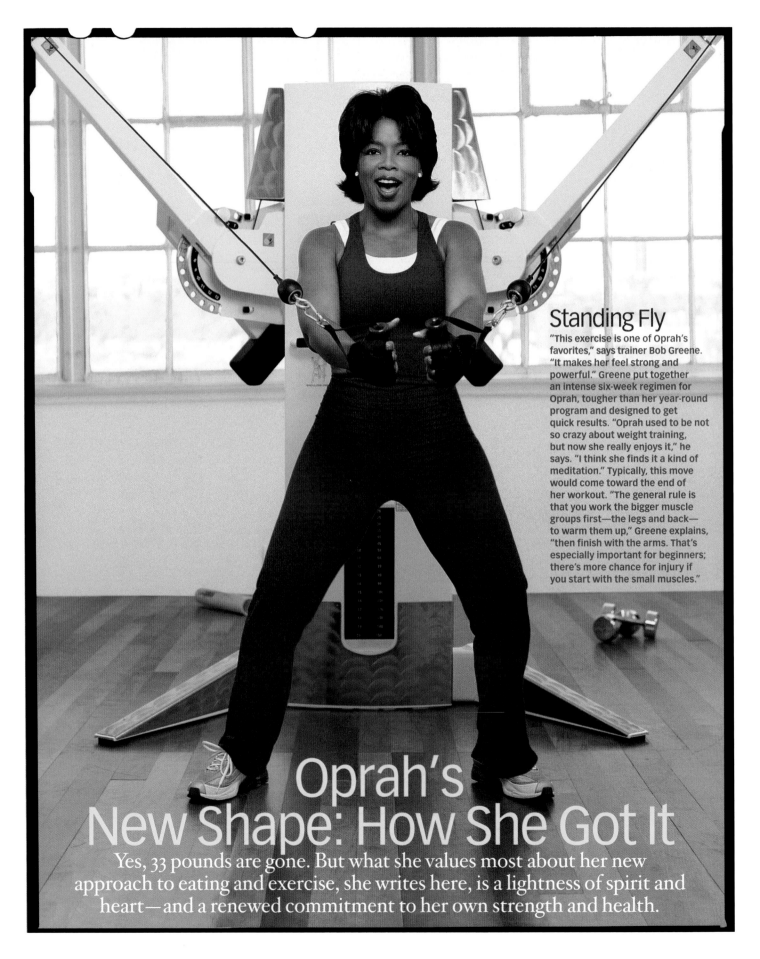

Standing Fly

"This exercise is one of Oprah's favorites," says trainer Bob Greene. **"It makes her feel strong and powerful."** Greene put together an intense six-week regimen for Oprah, tougher than her year-round program and designed to get quick results. **"Oprah used to be not so crazy about weight training, but now she really enjoys it,"** he says. **"I think she finds it a kind of meditation."** Typically, this move would come toward the end of her workout. **"The general rule is that you work the bigger muscle groups first—the legs and back—to warm them up,"** Greene explains, **"then finish with the arms. That's especially important for beginners; there's more chance for injury if you start with the small muscles."**

Oprah's New Shape: How She Got It

Yes, 33 pounds are gone. But what she values most about her new approach to eating and exercise, she writes here, is a lightness of spirit and heart—and a renewed commitment to her own strength and health.

I'VE BEEN STRUGGLING WITH MY weight since I was 22. I'm now almost 49 [at the time of this writing] and ready for the battle to be over. I've lost and gained too many times to count. I've used food to relieve stress, for comfort, and to momentarily stand in for joy.

In 2001, when I was having chest palpitations, I really started to understand that too much weight is too hard on your heart. I took my own advice and made the connection: There is no true love of self if you're abusing your health.

In the past, every time I'd started a weight loss regimen, it was out of vanity. But I'm not a vain person by nature—so it was difficult to maintain a healthy weight just to stay a certain size (preferably 8).

In 1988 the nation watched while I starved myself (using Optifast) for four months so I could fit into a pair of jeans. I got down to 145 pounds—and stayed there for one day before the regaining began. I reached my highest weight in 1992, wobbling around at 237 pounds.

I couldn't stand to look in a mirror or look strangers in the eye—I was that disappointed in myself. So I started working out with Bob Greene, who from the beginning told me that my issues were not about weight. Weight was the symptom of a much bigger problem: my unwillingness to fully love, support, and give to myself on a daily basis what I so freely give to others.

We worked out together for a year. I lost the weight. Ran a marathon, and, give or take ten pounds, kept it off for four years. Then came my beef trial and my devastating disappointment over the box office response to *Beloved*. I emotionally ate my way back to around 200 pounds. That was my weight in August 2001 when I walked into my doctor's office complaining of heart palpitations. My blood pressure was 180/90. My doctor gave me a grave look and said, "You need to lose weight." Tell me something I don't know, I thought smugly. I didn't take her advice seriously. After all, I'd been heavier and had never felt my heart racing. I'd had perfect blood pressure—110/70—for years, even at my heaviest.

I hadn't accounted for getting older and the effect of compounded weight on my

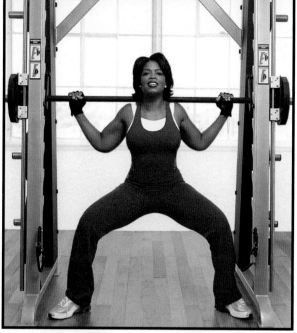

Squat

"Squats are very efficient," Greene notes. "They work not only the buttocks but also the quadriceps— the muscles at the front of the thighs—and, as you go down slowly, resisting gravity, the hamstrings, at the back of the thighs." Oprah is using a Smith press, a contraption that supports the weight if you lose your grip. Tips from Greene: Don't sit too low; that puts pressure on the knees. Keeping the toes pointed outward also helps protect the knees.

Incline Press

"Don't fall for the myth that you can increase breast size by doing presses; you can't," Greene says. "The breasts are made up of glands, not muscles. But you can train all the chest muscles supporting the breasts. You tone the muscles of the chest with exercises like this, and that makes everything look perky."

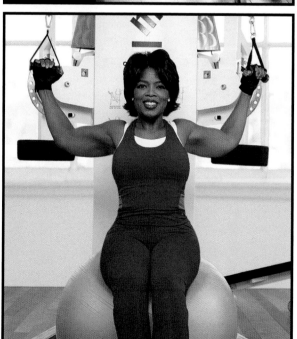

Lat Pull

Shaping your upper body with weight training does two great things, Greene points out: "It's good for your posture—and when you add tone and shape to your shoulders and lats, your waist and hips look trimmer."

29

heart, combined with hormonal changes. I kept going from doctor to doctor, trying to figure out why I couldn't sleep. I remember waking up many a night, my heart pounding, thinking, *I've done a lot of good work, I have a lot of beautiful things—which means nothing in this moment. I'm building a new house I may never get to see because I have a heart problem.*

Then I ran across Dr. Christiane Northrup's book *The Wisdom of Menopause*, which suggested eliminating refined carbohydrates—sugar and all the white foods that immediately convert to sugar in the body. I cut out white rice, white pasta, and white breads. I reduced my salt intake. My blood pressure dropped. My heart stopped racing. I could sleep through the night, so I had more strength to work out.

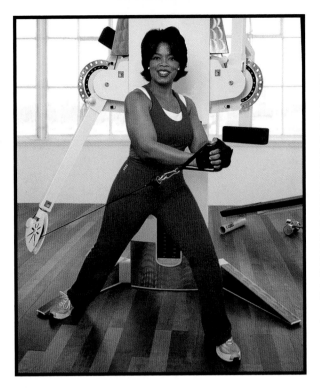

Rotary Torso

Here's a direct route to the oblique muscles. "They're the stabilizers of your torso," Greene says. "Strong obliques ensure good posture, and they allow the rest of your workout to be more effective." Oprah is enthusiastic about this move. "The thing about each one of these exercises," she says, "is that the more you do them, the better you get. It's quite an accomplishment to see and feel your body getting stronger. You'll start to notice a difference after about three weeks."

OPRAH'S BOOT CAMP Trainer BOB GREENE shows no mercy.

When Oprah asked me to design a six-week boot camp program of exercise and healthy eating, her goal wasn't only to look stunning for the Emmy Awards. She also wanted to jump-start a rededication to health, strength, and self-nurturing. Oprah signed a contract with herself—a powerful motivator, most people find—committing to consistent exercise, healthful food choices, and a daily cutoff time for eating. Since your metabolism slows as you approach bedtime, the later you eat, the harder it is to burn calories. I also suggested that during boot camp she give up alcohol, since it slows the metabolism. Oprah launched this program just three weeks before Emmy night. [Editor's note: Before you try an intense exercise program, consult a trainer and your doctor.]

CARDIOVASCULAR WORKOUTS
Six mornings a week: Forty-five minutes of aerobic exercise, including at least two of the following: Power walking on a graded treadmill (up to 10 percent), jogging, elliptical exercise, stair stepping, or rowing.
Four or five evenings a week (before dinner): A 20-minute workout using one of the above exercises. These sessions gave Oprah a chance to reflect on her progress toward her goals.
Once a week: On a day with no strength training, Oprah replaced her usual aerobic exercise with a 75-minute run.

STRENGTH TRAINING
Four or five times a week: Thirty to 40 minutes of strength training, usually two days in a row, followed by a day off. Oprah preferred to train before her aerobic workout. Her warm-up: a 15-minute power walk.
Day One
▪ Squats: Three sets of ten using 50 pounds of weight. Remember: This is a customized program; these weights may not be appropriate for everyone. (Works the buttocks, quadriceps, and hamstrings.)
▪ Leg extensions: Three sets of ten using 60 pounds. (Quadriceps.)
▪ Leg curls: Three sets of ten using 60 pounds. (Hamstrings.)

▪ Chest presses: Three sets of ten using 50 pounds. (Chest.)
▪ Incline presses: Three sets of ten using 40 pounds at a 45-degree angle. (Upper chest.)
▪ Lat pulls: Three sets of ten using 50 pounds. (Upper back.)
▪ Seated pull-downs: Three sets of ten using 50 pounds. (Biceps, chest, and shoulders.)
▪ Standing flies: Three sets of ten using 20 pounds. (Chest.)
▪ Seated rows: Three sets of ten using 50 pounds. (Back and shoulders.)
▪ Back extensions: Three sets of ten on a back-extension device or a Roman chair. (Lower back.)
Day Two
▪ Shoulder presses: Three sets of ten using ten-pound dumbbells. (Shoulders and upper back.)
▪ Lateral raises: Three sets of ten using ten-pound dumbbells. (Shoulders.)
▪ Frontal raises: Three sets of ten using ten-pound dumbbells. (Shoulders and arms.)
▪ "Thumbs down" raises: Three sets of ten using five-pound dumbbells. (Shoulders—rotator cuff—and arms.)

▪ Standing cable-cross curls: Three sets of ten using 20 pounds. (Biceps.)
▪ Rotary torso: Three sets of ten on each side using 20 pounds. (Abs—obliques.)
▪ Back extensions: Three sets of ten. (Lower back.)

ABDOMINAL WORK
Every Day
▪ Incline crunches: Three sets of 30 at three increasingly difficult inclines.

STRETCHING
After every workout, Oprah did stretches for her whole body, although 80 percent of them focused on her legs.

The Emmy Awards fell halfway through boot camp, and there were many toasts in Oprah's honor after she won the Bob Hope Humanitarian Award. She declined even a sip of Champagne, because that was part of her commitment. But I think she was feeling bubbly enough already.

> ## You've got to love yourself and do the work to sustain your most powerful engine: good health.

And I lost ten pounds almost immediately. At that point, I wasn't trying to lose weight—I was trying not to die.

I talked with Bob, who suggested I take this special time in my life (approaching the Big M) to "nail it for good. You know that two of the most drastic effects of aging are the loss of muscle and bone—and strength training is one of the best ways to counter both of them."

I'd done weight training with him before but hadn't been consistent, because I'd never really cared about building or preserving muscle. I just wanted to fit into a size 8.

But I finally got serious about weight-resistance training, and I've watched my body reshape itself. I alternate upper and lower body work at least five times a week. Sometimes I do two back-to-back days of full body, followed by a day off to recoup, and repeat that cycle for a couple of weeks. I also do about 30 minutes of aerobics each day.

I've learned that you can look to other people and programs for inspiration to jump-start yourself, but you have to develop a plan that will work for *your* life. There are no shortcuts or secrets, no magic patches or pills. If you're reading this article, you've probably dieted and exercised enough to know the truth.

You've got to love yourself and do the work it takes to sustain your most powerful engine: good health. Without it nothing else matters.

I've gotten a clean bill of health from my doctors—no cardio problems—but I'm still striving every day toward a healthier me. The side effect: I've now lost 33 pounds. I'm on no particular diet—I just eat smaller portions, and I still watch the refined carbohydrates. I favor fish, chicken, fruit, vegetables, and lots of soups. And I don't eat after 7:30 P.M. Not even a grape.

I feel great. I'm sleeping well. I'm loving myself. ●

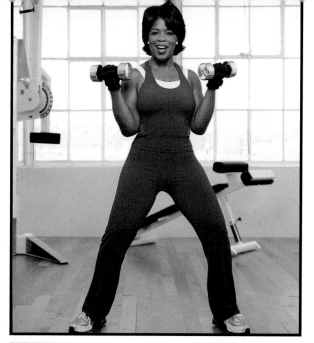

Biceps Curl

"A lot of people overdo one exercise," Greene says. "It's important to remember to balance your training, working the muscles on both sides of a joint. Don't work the biceps without working the triceps; don't work the quadriceps without working the hamstrings."

Triceps Extension

"Everybody has a gorgeous set of triceps and abs," Greene says. "The trouble is that in some people, they're hidden under body fat." You can do triceps extensions all day long, Greene says, but nothing's going to happen unless you also lose body fat. "There's no such thing as spot reducing," he says. "You can't tell your body to draw energy only from the fat on your arms and nowhere else. Great results come from trimming fat as you train muscles."

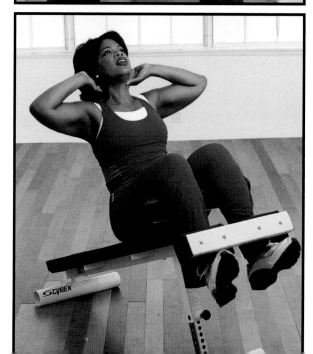

Incline Crunch

"Oprah hated these when she started doing them ten years ago," Greene recalls. "But now she can do them at the toughest incline. She has perfect form. Notice that she's got her chin up; the mistake that most people make is rolling their chin down to their chest, which creates the risk of neck injury." Abdominal muscles respond well to daily training, according to Greene. "When they're done properly," he says, "crunches can help align the spine."

Stroll in the park
(with headphones).
Dance to that
old-time rock 'n' roll.
Climb not every
mountain, but just
one. Pamela Peeke,
MD, helps three
women find their
inner get-up-and-go.
BY MICHELLE STACEY

I Hate to Exercise, but I Love to...

THERE IS AN ABSOLUTE EPIDEMIC IN THIS COUNTRY (PLEASE, DON'T sit down for this news) of inactivity. Sixty percent of American adults work out only occasionally, and 25 percent don't do it at all, according to the U.S. surgeon general's office. The number one reason people give for not exercising is lack of time. But if fitness were fun, wouldn't you somehow squeeze it in?

Underneath your body's lassitude, it really does want to move; your job is finding the activity that makes motion irresistible. That's one thing Pamela Peeke, MD, author of *Fight Fat After 40*, is expert at. In her clinical practice, Peeke counsels women on how to make exercise a joy, with an emphasis on thinking outside the box. "There's a small group of natural athletes who exercise for performance," says Peeke, "and another small group of women who keep at it for appearance. For everyone else—the ones who say they hate going to the gym—there's always a hidden motivation you can tap into somewhere, but you have to forage to find it."

Peeke agreed to let us in on three "hard cases" to see how she works through the layers of resistance to find the one reason (or three or six) for moving that will get each woman out the door. In her method may lie your answer: skiing, pole vaulting, kayaking, trapeze flying, or who knows, maybe even the dreaded gym.

THE DANCER
Hillary Buckholtz, 23, student
5'11", 180 pounds

A hundred pounds heavier when she first met with Peeke, Buckholtz was a morbidly obese 13-year-old. "I was overwhelmed by my weight, depressed, shamed," she says. "I'd seen between 10 and 20 doctors, and nothing had worked." Peeke would

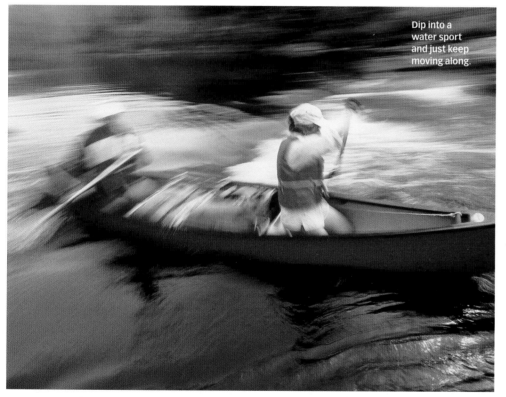

Dip into a water sport and just keep moving along.

take her new patient on walks near the office as she figured out an eating and lifestyle plan for her. "It made a huge impression on me," says Buckholtz, who was at the time completely sedentary, even phobic about exercise; any exertion took her breath away and made her ache. "The walks taught me to enjoy nature for the first time, and Pam would be waving and saying hello to friends. I've never forgotten it."

Now Buckholtz walks at least an hour a

day, always with headphones playing her favorite music. Music, it turned out, was the key, especially accompanying the exercise Buckholtz loves most: dancing, anytime, anywhere. "I'm not very coordinated, so dance class didn't really seem like an option," she says, "but I dance with my friends at concerts, around the house, up and down the stairs, almost anywhere." She had been too self-conscious to indulge in such silliness until Peeke kept asking her, "When do you feel active and good? Think about it."

"I saw a lively spirit who loves music and moving with it," Peeke says. "I encouraged her to get out those CDs and to rock and roll whenever she felt like it." Buckholtz, now over her fear of gyms, supplements her dancing and walking with two strength-training sessions a week. "It helps to have a routine, to do it even if I'm not feeling motivated," she says. Dance classes may not be far behind.

THE MOUNTAINEER
Wendy Easton, 33, office manager
5'2", 140 pounds

"I hated exercising, even as a kid," says Easton. "I was small, skinny, totally unathletic. I never played any sports. I used to

joke that I joined the navy just to get out of gym class." The joke may have been on her during boot camp, "but once that was over you weren't required to work out," she says, "and I later failed two navy physicals." Her inactivity eventually became a real millstone as she put on 35 pounds during her four years in the military and then another 20 over the next four years. "I went to Weight Watchers, lost some weight, gained it back, all the time never exercising," says Easton. The turning point came when she took a job in Peeke's office last January. "Dr. Peeke asked me, 'What do you do for exercise?' " she recounts. "And I said, 'Well, I walk to the car. I walk up three flights to my apartment. That's about it.' " Peeke had a new mission: Get Easton moving.

"Nothing seemed to work," says Peeke. "As far as Wendy was concerned, only health freaks walk or go to the health club." ("I'm pretty stubborn," Easton admits.) Finally, in March, Peeke found the right carrot to dangle: a staff trip to Aspen to climb a 14,000-foot peak at the end of the summer. You can come, she told Easton, but only if you get in shape for it.

It was the right message at the right time. Easton was the kind of reluctant exerciser who needed a very concrete goal—a mountain summit—and she was also at a point in her life when she was open to suggestion. So for the first time ever, she joined a gym, telling her trainer she wanted to get into condition for a mountain climb. "I was never one for much discomfort," she says, "but the climb gave me the motivation to start. It was the trigger." Striding on the treadmill or the elliptical trainer, she now thinks of mountains, and of a better balance in her life. And she has started looking forward to her workouts. "However things turn out in Aspen," Easton says, "I now know that this is something I need to do for a lifetime, both to control my weight and to feel healthier."

THE HOCKEY PLAYER
Mary Trow, 49, attorney
5'3", 120 pounds

Trow initially went to Peeke in an early-40s panic. "I was slightly overweight, and definitely sedentary," she says. "I had never really exercised, and I realized that if I didn't do something, my future was not

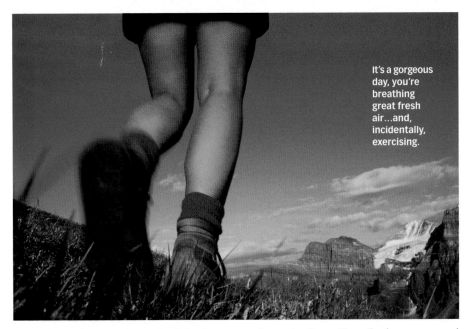

It's a gorgeous day, you're breathing great fresh air...and, incidentally, exercising.

going to be very attractive." So she met with Peeke, feeling motivated but a little wary: "My hallmark," Trow says now, "was 'It's not supposed to hurt!'"

She started walking, then running, and while the activities didn't exactly hurt, they were boring. "I really did hate exercising at that point," says Trow. Peeke encouraged her to push herself, to expand her ideas of what exercise could include. After one of those sessions, Trow saw an ad for a women's ice hockey league and, with her new physical confidence, went to check it out.

She is now a dedicated hockey player in what she calls the old-ladies' league (it actually includes women from ages 15 to 55), and her physical universe has been transformed. "This is the first time in my life I've been a committed athlete, and I never thought I'd be here," says Trow. Rather than considering her body merely something to be looked at, she makes demands on it, uses it, pushes it to new levels of accomplishment. And to improve her game, she now lifts weights twice a week and either Rollerblades or runs five days a week. "You can get incredible pleasure from training your body to do something physical," she says.

Peeke explains that Trow needed an activity to get her mind far away from the stress of running her own legal firm. "Hockey was the ultimate release for her, and the other exercise she does is no longer perfunctory upkeep for midlife girth control but a means to an end." ●

But I **Love** to...

The women you're about to meet were allergic to the gym, but they've each become so passionate about an activity, they've forgotten they're exercising.

TRAPEZE FLYING

Denese Senno, 42, travel agent

"As a kid in gym class, I was the last one picked for the team. I have always thought of myself as unathletic and uncoordinated. But when I saw a picture of a trapeze class, I clipped it and saved it in my wallet. Years later I got on my first trapeze. I was really scared and begged the instructors to let me come down. But I did it, and it was fun! Now I exercise so I can be strong and flexible enough to take classes at the Trapeze School in New York City, where there's a little saying that goes, 'Forget fear. Worry about the addiction.' It's grueling, but what can I say? I'm flying—and there's nothing like that feeling."

ICE HOCKEY

Frann Warren, 46, marketing consultant

"A bunch of us who spent years watching our kids play hockey thought it looked pretty fun, so we decided to give it a try. We lined up a coach and formed a women's team called the Motherpuckers. It's a fabulous workout: We come off the ice dripping wet, our legs strong and our muscles tight. At first it was all about getting over the fear of making fools of ourselves. Now we make sure our families come to watch us play."

KAYAKING

Anna Newman, 42, fourth-grade teacher

"The first time I kayaked, I went around the southern tip of Manhattan at dusk. And even though the next time I kayaked, I capsized in the Hudson River, I was hooked on the sport. Aside from providing great exercise—my arms have gotten so strong—it feels really wonderful, like being off in the islands."

SOFTBALL

Felicia Amatuzzo, 35, stay-at-home mother of three

"I'm the captain of my team, which is composed mostly of family and close friends. Our games, sometimes three a week, are not only exercise but also a way to get out and be social. My daughter has made me promise that I'll keep playing so that when she's old enough she can join my team."

BIKING

Renee Johnson, 48, retired homemaker

"I bought a bike a few years ago and fell in love with it. I now have three friends with whom I cycle across Iowa every summer. We've also done other major bike trips, like Lance Armstrong's Ride for the Roses in Texas. We train by doing 'Wednesday-night salad rides,' where we bike for 25 miles, eat a salad, and cycle home. The first time I rode across Iowa, it felt like the biggest accomplishment of my life."

MARATHON WALKING

Betty Lawson, 61, telecommunications consultant

"I walked my first marathon—the New York—in 1999, two years after being treated for breast cancer. I did it with a few friends, and we were so intimidated. But there were all these people cheering for us. It was exhilarating. Now I've done six marathons, some of them as part of Fred's Team, which raises money for cancer research, so that's icing on the cake. Life has been pretty crazy in the last few years, and this provides a real piece of sanity." —M.S.

You say you'd love to get more exercise, but you don't have time? That's what these five women thought—until we put them in the hands of professional organizer Julie Morgenstern and fitness coach Karen Voight. At the three-month mark, we checked in.

BY AMY DICKINSON

No Time for Exercise

"CREAKY KNEES."

"The dog ate my sneakers."

"The kids have taken over the treadmill to stage hamster races."

People find all sorts of reasons to avoid exercise, but the most common excuse is that we just don't have the time. With this in mind, *O* challenged any reader too busy for fitness to send in a typical day's schedule. Then we selected a few of the most harried and put each in touch with organization maven Julie Morgenstern and workout authority Karen Voight. Watch how our experts achieve mission impossible—divining time where none seems available and coming up with innovative ways for the frantic to stay fit.

Terie Theis, age 36

"I spend so much time on work, house, and husband that I have no idea who I am anymore, other than what I am to others."

As a trial attorney and marketing director for her law firm in San Diego, Theis has burned through several secretaries with her demanding workload. She and her attorney husband work long hours, often on weekends. "I take care of everything having to do with our home—the banking, bill paying, etc.—as part of my control-freak nature," Theis says. "I spend so much time on work, house, and husband that I have no idea who I am anymore, other than what I am to others." Her goal is to get back to the "hot body" she used to have before she hit 30 and the pounds started creeping up.

Julie's advice: Theis is a classic type A personality and she needs a structured program. Theis concedes that the best strategy for her would be to schedule her exercise the way she schedules her clients—say, three evenings a week, when she might otherwise try to squeeze in more work. She should also let her husband be more involved in running their home so they both have time on the weekends—perhaps to work out together.

Karen's advice: With Theis's high drive, she would benefit from a workout that exhausts her. After some discussion, Karen comes up with the idea of training to run in the P.F. Chang's Rock 'n' Roll half marathon for the Leukemia & Lymphoma Society three months away. "It satisfies that feeling of 'I'm putting in a hundred percent,'" Theis says. "And on Saturdays, you have to get to the practice session at 6:30 A.M. If I were doing it just for me, I'd roll over and hit the alarm clock. But because charity is involved, there's another reason for me to get up." Karen agrees with Julie about the importance of scheduling exercise and also recommends that Theis commit to a personal trainer at least once a week—an idea the lawyer plans to follow up on.

Three months later…"I've been so turned on to fitness," Theis says, "I'm now a type A about exercise." Karen's marathon idea was a winner. Theis joined a running group and aced the half

marathon in Phoenix (so what if she had no time to shower before jumping on the plane for her next appointment). She also started using Karen's stretching and yoga tapes, which come in handy when she gets home at 9 or 10 at night and still has energy to squeeze in a balancing workout. Taking Julie's advice, Theis started permitting herself to leave the office "at a decent hour" two days a week to meet a personal trainer at the gym she recently joined. As for the chores, they have not exactly been delegated ("My husband started his own firm in July, and our cats don't do dishes"). But Theis has learned to accept when things aren't done

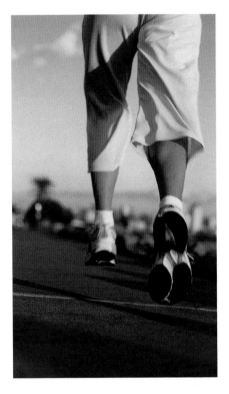

perfectly and has made small adjustments—for example, exercising instead of making dinner and asking her husband to bring home takeout. "Bottom line," says the fitness convert, "the bed doesn't know when it's not made and the dishes don't know when they aren't done, but my body does know when I have not exercised."

Jennifer Duden, age 30

"I want to devote what little weekend time I have to tending the yard, napping, and recharging for the next week."

Even though Duden doesn't have children, her job in St. Louis Park, Minnesota—head office manager for a performing arts school—and the demands of a husband, house chores, a dog, and yard work all push her to capacity. After working until 6 P.M., Duden picks up her husband, and they spend their evenings buying groceries, doing housework, making dinner, and playing outside with Sammie, their Border collie. Since Duden works every Saturday until 2 P.M., she says, "I want to devote what little weekend time I have to tending the yard, napping, and recharging for the next week."

Julie's advice: Evenings are probably the best place for Duden to steal time for workouts. One idea is to trade off the meal preparation duties: Her husband, for example, could take responsibility for the dinner prep while she exercises; then after dinner, she'd clean up. And in Sammie, Duden may have the perfect built-in companion for her workouts—especially since Border collies need so much activity.

Karen's advice: Using Sammie is a great idea, "but if you're just throwing a ball, only the dog's getting exercise." Karen suggests Duden walk the dog for 20 minutes three days a week. Eventually, she might try walking one block and running the next. When the Minnesota winters get too cold to stay outside, workout videos are a good option.

Three months later…Duden was relieved, after talking to Julie and Karen, to discover that she didn't have to devote a daunting hour a day to exercise. She has been walking Sammie regularly—coaxing herself out the door by telling herself it'll only be for ten minutes, "but I usually get into it and go for at least 20." The extra activity has helped Duden feel noticeably more relaxed. For the months when the windchill heads below zero, she's thinking about buying a treadmill.

Carolyn Carter, age 43

"Sometimes I don't even have the energy to work, let alone exercise."

Carter's life is beyond busy. With a husband, three children, a full-time job in the information technology field, and a freelance graphic design business on the side, the Detroit resident starts her days at 5:30

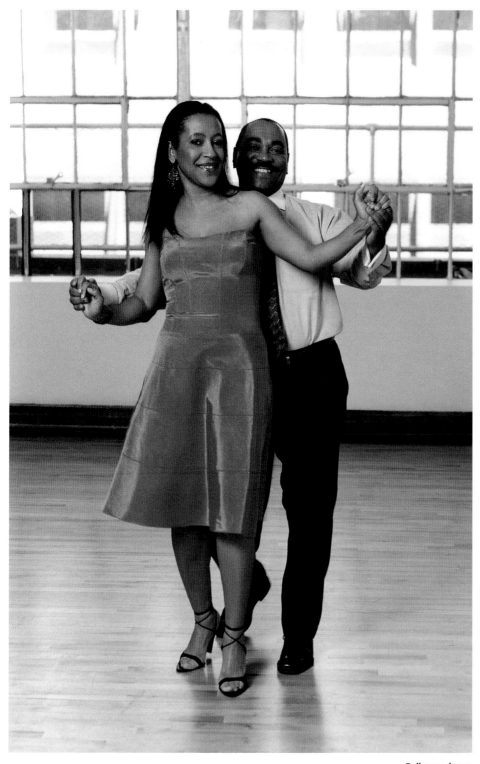

Ballroom dance classes allow Carolyn Carter to sneak in a workout while spending cha-cha time with husband Mark.

A.M. and proceeds at a manic pace until she falls into bed, exhausted, sometimes as late as 1 A.M. Driven to advance her career, Carter takes classes after-hours. She also teaches computer classes two nights a week at her church. "Sometimes I don't even have the energy to work," she says, "let alone exercise." Her only nod to fitness has been to sign up for ballroom dance lessons one night a week with her husband as a way for them to spend some time together.

Julie's advice: "Carolyn's schedule is like an overstuffed closet—activities are shoved in with no rhyme or reason, and, like a messy closet, her life needs to be neatened up." After a lengthy discussion, the two determine that Carter must home in on her own priorities and start saying no to any activity that doesn't further them. Carter agrees and decides that her long-standing commitment to teach computer classes will have to go. Knowing that the contents of Carter's "life closet" will just expand to fill the space created by having two weeknights free, Julie suggests that Carter immediately replace teaching classes with taking classes—something fun and active in addition to ballroom dancing.

Karen's advice: At 43 Carter should pay attention to gaining strength. And toning up doesn't have to cost her any extra time. A step or a pair of five-pound weights would mean that while she's waiting for the coffee to brew, she could do two minutes of curls, squats, or steps-ups; then, as the oatmeal cooks, two more minutes, and so on. (A liter bottle of water also provides a heavy enough weight for a nice biceps curl.) "I need something I can do right when I roll out of bed," Carter says. Karen warmly offers to send her workout tapes— *Burn & Firm* (cardio/weight circuit training) and *B.L.T. (Butt, Legs & Tummy) on a Ball*—as well as a balance ball, but is stern: "I don't want to send the tapes and then not have you use them."

Three months later…Carter has taken the ball and bounced with it, losing six pounds in the process. She started doing a ball workout with Karen's video three times a week and—although she never went for Karen's kitchen workout—has embraced the idea of slipping in a little fitness here and there while doing everything else.

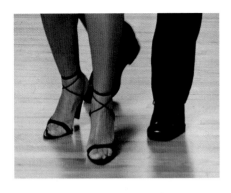

"Having four flights of stairs in my house allows me to get some exercise into my schedule," says Carter, who also continues her ballroom class once or twice a week, walks when she can, and (drumroll) has just joined a gym with her husband. "Exercise has changed my life," she says. "I realize I cannot take care of my family if I am not at my best. I won't have Beyoncé's body, but I bet you I can do the bootylicious with the best of them!"

Layni Craver, age 46

"I tend to spend the weekend days trying to sleep and trying to convince myself to do the cleaning, grocery shopping, and other chores."

Craver, a nurse, lives in Davenport, Iowa, with her husband and 15-year-old son. During the week, she runs a busy ob-gyn office; on weekends she takes two overnight shifts at a local hospital to help make ends meet. "I tend to spend the weekend days trying to sleep and trying to convince myself to do the cleaning, grocery shopping, and other chores," she says. "If my husband didn't do the laundry, we'd all be wearing bedsheet togas." Craver used to keep in shape by biking the seven-mile commute to and from her day job, and she loved it. But when the office shut down its shower facility, she put away her bicycle. Since then, her weight has gone from 170 pounds up to 200, and she's unable even to walk up a flight of stairs without getting winded. "I'm a nurse," she says, "and I know better than to keep up this unhealthy lifestyle."

Julie's advice: There must be a way around the shower obstacle. After going over Craver's intense schedule, Julie helps her develop a plan in which she takes her bike to work in the car and cycles home at least two nights a week. On those evenings, her husband would then drive her back to retrieve her car from the office. It would also be great if Craver could find a way to fit in ten-minute bursts of exercise at work.

Karen's advice: Good plan, but after learning that Craver suffers occasional back spasms and stiff joints—the toll, perhaps, from all that bike riding—Karen advises a walking program with deep stretching. Craver worries that she won't do it, "because it bores me to tears." How about listening to a book on tape, Karen asks. "Books on tape usually last 36 minutes per side," she says. "They're broken into segments, so you're motivated to keep walking because you want to hear the end of the segment." Stretching, according to Karen, should be done after the walk.

Three months later…Ah, the real world. Life has taken a 180-degree turn and thwarted Craver's best intentions. After consulting with Julie and Karen, she quit her nursing job and landed in a completely new industry (software). She has a high-pressure position that requires her to live in another city during the week and travel constantly. "Julie had some excellent time management suggestions that would likely have worked had my life remained as it was," Craver says. "And the personal attention from Karen really inspired me, despite the end result." She has used the videos Karen sent for stretching, and she's been thinking a lot about Karen's insistence on the importance of valuing one's own needs so that others will value us. "Something tells me," Craver says, "that this idea is going to end up being the key to getting exercise back into my life."

Debra Peel, age 48

"My cell phone typically starts ringing at 7 in the morning, as clients and colleagues begin to check in."

Peel's job as a private investigator in Panama City, Florida, makes her schedule erratic, always unpredictable, and at times out of control. "My cell phone typically starts ringing at about 7 in the morning, as clients and colleagues begin to check in with me," she says. Long hours spent sitting during surveillance jobs mean that she's sedentary for much of her work time. Her husband, a sheriff, pulls a regular shift, but the couple take care of their young grandsons every weekend to give a break to their daughter, who is battling a serious illness. All these factors have contributed to Peel's gaining about 85 pounds to weigh in at 235. Exercise is critical not only to get her body under control, she says, but "as a stress reliever as well."

Julie's advice: It would be great for Peel to "put herself first" by starting each day with an exercise routine. During their conversation, Julie convinces the overextended sleuth that she needs to treat herself like a valued client and turn off the cell phone until a reasonable hour. Another idea: Peel is chained to an old hairstyle that takes too much time to maintain every morning; by getting an easier cut, she could free up some valuable minutes.

Karen's advice: Molding away in a spare bedroom is a treadmill that Peel used to enjoy using—perhaps she could dust it off and start walking again. Peel agrees this is a good idea…that is, until Karen prescribes 20 minutes at a stretch. "Okay, five minutes," Karen says. "Five minutes is just fine. Listen to upbeat music and you'll increase your pace." If Peel invests in a set of five-pound weights, Karen adds, she could start a 15-minute body sculpting program at home.

Three months later…Peel has reacquainted herself with the treadmill. Having decided not to take calls until 8 A.M. ("treating myself like my number one client, as Julie advised"), she walks for five to 20 minutes three times a week before eating breakfast, listening to music as she strides. Post-it notes all over the house urge "walk, walk, walk," but by now they're hardly necessary. Peel, and everyone else, can see the rewards: She has lost 25 pounds and dropped from a size 22 to a 16. "I feel so different," she says. "I have more energy, a bounce where I was dragging. I feel like I've been given a new lease on life." •

Health & Beauty

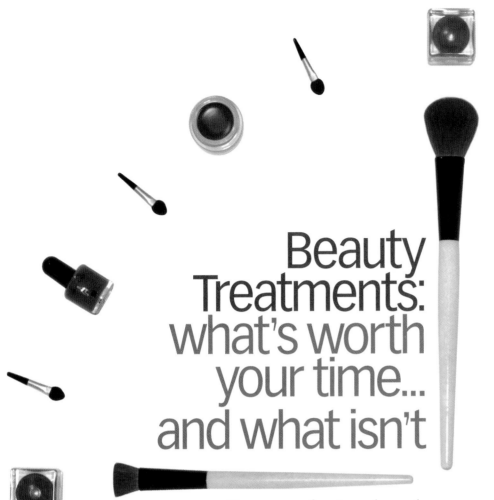

Beauty Treatments:
what's worth your time... and what isn't

From professional teeth whitening to a daily splash of toner, the things we do for beauty don't just cost money, they take a chunk out of our day. **BETH JANES** subjects five popular options to a rigorous cost-benefit analysis.

I ONCE SPENT 90 MINUTES NAPPING, WRAPPED IN a blanket that delivered gentle electrical currents to my clay-and-seaweed-coated "problem" areas. Post shockfest, the aesthetician, tape measure in hand, tried to convince me that I'd lost an inch all around. The only thing I'd actually lost: consciousness.

Though you can almost always find some kind of payoff from a treatment (a refreshing nap, for instance), when free hours are scarce, what matters is *results*.

Professional teeth whitening

Involves either power bleaching (a light or heat source helps gel penetrate your tooth enamel) or whitening gel in custom-made trays you wear at night.
Time investment: Power bleaching requires one to three visits, 30 to 90 minutes each. Trays require two to five

5 MINUTE MAKEUP

Alarm didn't go off? No problem—at least when it comes to doing your face. All you need are five minutes and these four products, says celebrity makeup artist Regina Harris.

1. Tinted moisturizer or a foundation in stick formula, which has more pigment so you need less. You can blend it with your fingers, and it doubles as a spot concealer. Black Up Stick Foundation Cream comes in a wide range of shades.

2. Mascara, to help brighten and emphasize your eyes. Choose one based on your specific needs—volume, curl, lengthening, or a multitasker like Cover Girl Triple Mascara. If lashes are straight, it's worth taking the time to curl them because you'll look more awake, says Harris.

3. Blush in cream and stick formulas, like I-Iman Makeup Double-Duty, because you can blend them quickly with your fingers for a natural flush and use them to brighten your eyelids.

4. Sheer lipcolor or gloss for natural-looking color and shine. Don't bother with liner, dark or matte colors, stains, or long-wearing liquid lipsticks; all require a slow, steady hand.

visits, 30 to 60 minutes each (the dentist makes an impression of your teeth, fits the trays, and checks your progress at separate appointments), plus filling, cleaning, and wearing them each night for two to three weeks.

Cost: $500 to $1,500 for power bleaching; $400 to $800 for trays and gel.

Worth it?

Yes, if…

■ **Your stains are yellowish and your teeth were whiter when you were younger.** These cases show the best results, says Marc Lowenberg, DDS, of Lowenberg & Lituchy, cosmetic dentists in New York City.

■ **You have reasonable expectations.** Your teeth probably won't get white as snow, says Lowenberg, but professional bleaching can brighten them enough to make a noticeable difference in your appearance.

■ **You want a quick fix.** Power bleaching can whiten in just one visit, but keep in mind that the trays tend to get teeth whiter because the bleaching gel stays on longer than during in-office treatment.

No, if…

■ **Your teeth have been stained by antibiotics like tetracycline;** they won't whiten.

■ **You drink a lot of coffee, tea, cola, or red wine, or you smoke.** A professional cleaning, whitening toothpaste, floss, and at-home whiteners (and discontinuing the offending behavior) usually lift these stains, says Lowenberg.

■ **Your budget won't allow for it.** Over-the-counter whiteners like Crest Whitestrips or paint-on products (which have a binding ingredient that increases staying power) such as Colgate Simply White Clear Whitening Gel do work well, though they're not as strong as the gel professionals use, says Lowenberg.

Bottom line: Ask your dentist. He or she can help you determine if your teeth will respond well to bleaching and if a professional treatment or an over-the-counter whitener will give you the results you want.

Laser hair removal

The Food and Drug Administration considers the treatment, which received clearance in 1995, a "permanent reduction," not removal. Still, Melanie Grossman, MD, a cosmetic and laser surgeon in New York City, says that she's seen many patients whose hair has not grown back. Research shows there's a low incidence of side effects, and new lasers can now safely treat all skin tones, including very dark, with little risk of scarring.

Time investment: Five to seven monthly treatments, 15 to 20 minutes each (depending on the size of the area being treated).

Cost: $300 to $1,000 per treatment.

Worth it?

Yes, if…

■ **You can afford it.**

■ **You regularly struggle with razor burn, waxing and shaving irritation, or ingrown hairs.**

No, if…

■ **You can't tolerate mild and temporary discomfort** (like a rubber band being snapped against your skin).

■ **You can't make a commitment for the necessary monthly appointments.**

Bottom line: Weigh the time and money devoted to shaving or waxing (and fighting ingrowns) over a year versus the time and money you'll spend on laser treatments.

Toners

These claim to remove residue, dirt, and oil, balance the pH of your skin, exfoliate, and help treat acne.
Time investment: A few minutes a day.
Cost: $5 to $30.
Worth it?

Yes, if…
■ **You have acne or extremely oily skin.** A toner containing salicylic acid will remove excess oil and penetrate pores to fight acne, says Leslie Baumann, MD, director of cosmetic dermatology at the University of Miami.

No, if…
■ **You have normal or dry skin.** Toners often contain alcohol and other drying agents, and any "grime" you see on a used cotton ball after you wash your face is probably your skin's natural (and harmless) oils.
■ **You wash with face cleanser, not soap.** Today's cleansers don't leave a residue on your skin the way soaps do, says Baumann.
■ **You use a creamy cleanser,** because these washes leave moisturizers on your skin, which might feel like residue. If you don't have dry skin, switch to a less moisturizing cleanser and forget the toner.
Bottom line: Unless you have acne or oily skin, skip it.

Spa facials

Often these include cleansing, steam, mask, and massage (and sometimes extraction).
Time investment: 60 to 90 minutes.
Cost: $60 to $150.
Worth it?

Yes, if…
■ **You have normal skin** and you just want to relax.
■ **You want a temporary glow.**

No, if…
■ **You have sensitive or acne-prone skin.** The products used during a facial (which may have higher percentages of active ingredients than what you normally use) can cause redness or an allergic reaction. Facial massage may also aggravate hair follicles and lead to a breakout, says Baumann. "I don't recommend letting an aesthetician not trained by a dermatologist perform extraction," she says.
■ **You're looking for a dramatic change in your skin.** The products are not on your skin long enough to make a real difference, says Baumann.
Bottom line: Facials feel good, but they don't do anything to improve the quality of your skin long-term.

Salon hair conditioning

A stylist applies a moisturizing and/or strengthening hair mask and uses heat (from either a dryer or a flat iron) to increase penetration.
Time investment: 20 to 90 minutes.
Cost: $25 to $85.
Worth it?

Yes, if…
■ **You like being pampered at the salon.**
■ **You have severely damaged hair** and you want to spend the extra money for it to look its best until your next shampoo.

No, if…
■ **You just want to deep-condition your hair.** "You can get much of the same results at home with a hair mask, a plastic shower cap, and a blow-dryer," says Alan Tosler of Tosler.Davis salon in New York City. You can even wear a mask overnight under a head wrap.
■ **You expect one treatment to permanently restore your hair's health.** Brittle, frizzy, and dull hair has usually been overprocessed, says Tosler. Talk to your stylist about what to avoid (bleaching, daily heat styling, coloring, retexturizing).
Bottom line: Save time by applying a mask at home. ●

Age: The Real Tip-Offs

There are about 35 of us beauty editors at a presentation of a company's new product. I'm new, too, new to the job of beauty editor, just learning the ropes. Most of the women are lovely, sparkling, and girlish; only a few of us have seen 40 (and fewer yet, like me, are peering fondly back). A convivial young man standing at a wooden podium welcomes us. "Thank you all for coming," he says, sparkling a little himself. "I have a question for you," he says. He leans against the podium professorially: "Can anyone tell me, what are the four signs of aging?" I generally do well in classroom situations, and greenhorn though I am, I know the answer he's looking for: fine lines, sagging skin, excessive dryness, etc. But I'm reluctant to raise my hand. Because if I do, and I give him the answer I believe is true, I'm afraid I might put a blight on the magazine I love and now represent. What if the young man is offended because I'm not playing along? So I sit on my hands and regretting, regretting, bite my tongue.

Today, however—two years of experience and a lifetime of antiaging presentations later— is a different story. Ask the question again; in fact, I dare you to ask the question. Because now I am very sure there is only one right answer, and it is my happy responsibility to give it.

What are the four signs of aging?

They are Wisdom, Confidence, Character, and Strength.

Look for them not with dismay, but with hope.   —*Valerie Monroe*

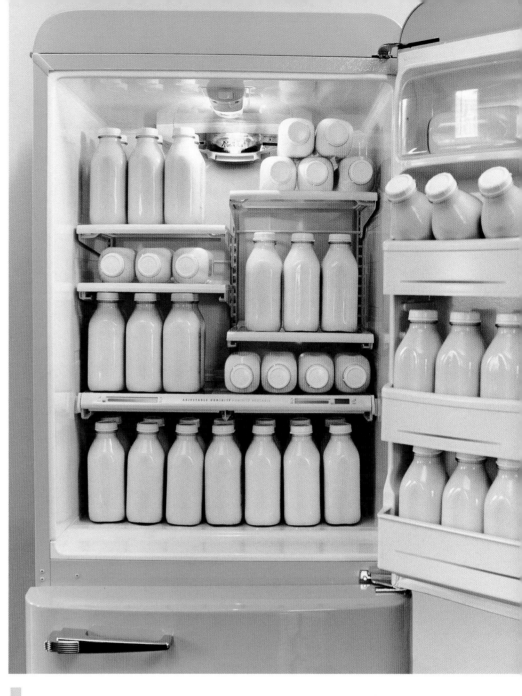

You think there's nothing you can do to prevent osteoporosis. But the truth is, no matter what your age, chances are you can stop the disease in its tracks. **BARBARA PAULSEN** reports.

Your Lovely Bones

"IF YOU'RE WEARING STOCKINGS, please remove them now to help speed the line," we're told by a white-jacketed young woman. Luckily, I'm wearing pants, but several on the queue reluctantly make a beeline for the bathroom nearby. A woman with long, curly black hair surveys the line, slips off her princess-heel shoes, and shimmies out of the pantyhose beneath her skirt in a flash. "I don't want to lose my place," she says. Geez, it's like opening day at a giant clearance sale. But this group of women—about two thirds in their 40s and younger—isn't hoping to score the latest fashions at half price. We're at a women's wellness conference at the University of

California at San Francisco, waiting to get our bone density tested.

Why would so many of us want a glimpse into our skeletal futures? Because we're worried about osteopenia, the latest diagnosis in town. It means your bones are thinner than average and you may well be headed for osteoporosis. A survey of 202 women ages 21 to 50 found that nearly one in four has it. In December 2001, the National Osteoporosis Risk Assessment (NORA) study reported that 40 percent of the 200,160 postmenopausal women they tested, ages 50 and older, did, too. Their study also found that the women they continued to follow with

Three glasses of milk per day provide most of the calcium you need.

osteopenia were almost twice as likely to break a bone in the next year—usually in the wrist, rib, hip, or forearm, or in the spine, where, with time, a series of often painless fractures caused by compression will eventually result in the classic dowager's hump. Of course, for those of us who have been counting on hormone replacement therapy to save our bones from such a fate, the news that HRT increases the risk of breast cancer, heart disease, and stroke is more than a little rattling.

And some women should be more worried than others. In my case, I'm a small-framed white female who hates milk and loves Pinot Noir—all of which puts me in a higher risk category for both osteopenia and osteoporosis. Caucasian and Asian women tend to have thinner bones than Hispanics and African-Americans. Small-framed women and those who don't get enough calcium or exercise are also more vulnerable, as are smokers. And some studies show an increased risk for women who often indulge in more than one drink a day. That would be me.

As our bone-wary procession waits to be tested, we trade tidbits about the disease known as the silent killer among the elderly. The skeletal crumbling is so debilitating that it interferes with one's ability to eat, not to mention get around, compounding other health problems and precipitating an often fatal decline. According to various statistics, between 16 and 18 percent of women over 50 have osteoporosis; half the people who break a hip will never walk again unaided; of those over 50, a quarter will die within a year.

At the very least, the thought of progressively stooping is enough to send anyone running to her doctor for a bone density scan—which I did, only to be informed that since I'm 43, my insurance won't pay, and my doctor doesn't think I need it anyway. "As long as you're still menstruating, there's no reason to think you're losing bone," she said. And she's right: Scientists know that the skeleton is constantly breaking down and building itself back up (although the building side of the equation begins to slow in your 30s). But it's only when estrogen levels take a nosedive at menopause that tiny bone destroyers called osteoclasts get aggressive and start

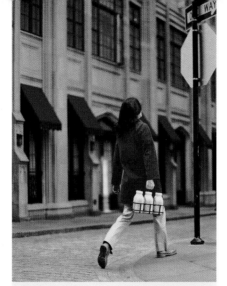

THE BARE BONES

- **OSTEOPENIA DIAGNOSIS:** It means you have thinner-than-average bones and are at higher risk for osteoporosis. If you haven't reached menopause, there's nothing to do except what you should already be doing—exercising, not smoking, and getting enough calcium. If you're postmenopausal and are diagnosed with osteopenia, you should get tested in a year and may want to consider taking drugs.
- **OSTEOPOROSIS:** Loss of bone tissue leads to bones that can break under the slightest strain. You can reduce your risk by making sure you get enough calcium and exercise.
- **CALCIUM:** Every woman under 51 should consume 1,000 milligrams a day; after menopause, 1,200 milligrams a day. If you don't get enough from your diet, take a supplement.
- **EXERCISE:** Aim for doing 30 to 60 minutes of weight-bearing exercise (walking, jogging, racket sports, dancing, etc.) four times a week, along with two resistance-training sessions per week.
- **SCREENING:** Official recommendations suggest initial bone density screenings at age 65, unless you have risk factors for osteoporosis, in which case you should be tested at menopause. But many experts advise all women to get baseline screenings at menopause. The risk factors include having a small frame, a fracture after age 50, a family history of osteoporosis, and being a smoker. If the test is normal, then screenings should be repeated at least every two years.

gnawing away at bone like a dog with a lamb chop. Once that starts, you could lose up to 20 percent of your bone mass in five to seven years.

But no one's checking our ages at this wellness conference, and besides, the bone scan is free (so-called peripheral tests like this one, which look at the heel or wrist, normally cost between $38 and $75; the more definitive dual energy X-ray absorptiometry, known as DXA or DEXA, scan measures the spine, hip, and/or limbs, and runs upwards of $200). So I take my turn in a chair and a technician swabs my heel with a gooey gel before placing my foot in an ultrasound machine that looks like it's designed to measure shoe size. The test shows I'm a 0.6. That's my T score, a measurement based on how my bone mineral density compares with the peak density of a young adult woman.

The technician says any score over zero means a woman is at low risk, and I'm instantly reassured. Still, I feel a twinge of bone envy when, on the way out, an African-American woman says she scored a 1.6. A slender white woman in her late 40s looks a bit shaken and avoids eye contact. Later she tells me she got -1.5 on her test (-2.5 indicates osteoporosis) and probably has osteopenia.

SHE NEEDN'T PANIC, AS IT turns out. "Osteopenia is a nondisease," says Steven T. Harris, MD, an endocrinologist at the University of California at San Francisco. Lots of women in their 30s and 40s will be diagnosed with osteopenia, he explains, but that doesn't mean they're destined for osteoporosis.

"The bone density test results are being misunderstood," adds Ethel Siris, MD, an endocrinologist at Columbia Presbyterian Medical Center who led the NORA study. Even though the study found that women with osteopenia were almost twice as likely to fracture a bone in the following year, these were solely postmenopausal women—and, Siris says, in any case, their absolute risk was relatively small. In younger women, unless they've stopped menstruating because of extreme exercise, anorexia, or a metabolic disorder, an osteopenia diagnosis doesn't mean they're losing bone, she explains. "Most of these women have never had high bone density, simply because they're not big people. If you're five feet two and 103 pounds, your bone density might well be lower than average."

The only real advantage of finding out you're osteopenic before menopause is in knowing that you'll need to be even more vigilant about doing what we all should be doing anyway to prevent osteoporosis: getting plenty of exercise and calcium. Most women who exercise and eat a calcium-rich diet, and then use appropriate medicines if they start losing bone after menopause, can prevent osteoporosis, says Siris. "We know we can stop bone loss."

FRACTURE-PROOF YOUR BODY: A THREE-PART PLAN

Exercise. Just as muscle grows stronger the more you use it, a bone becomes denser when you place demands on it—certainly until your early 30s. The best bone-building exercise is resistance training—lifting free weights, using the resistance machines at the gym, even Pilates and yoga. But any kind of weight-bearing exercise—where your legs support your body—helps prevent osteoporosis (jogging and dancing count; swimming and stationary bicycling are not weight bearing and therefore are less helpful). And it's never too late to start, according to several studies. In one, postmenopausal women who lifted weights for 45 minutes twice a week for a year increased their bone mass by 1 percent, while the control group, which did no resistance training, lost 2 to 2.5 percent. Experts recommend doing weight-bearing exercise at least four times per week for 30 to 60 minutes and resistance training two or three times, long enough to work each muscle group.

ANN RICHARDS BONES UP
By Sarah Wildman

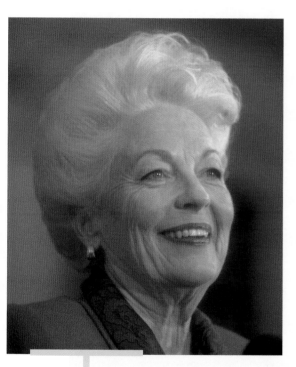

Talking to Ann Richards, the quick-witted former governor of Texas, it's easy to believe that nothing short of an act of God could slow this woman down. As she runs from her public relations job to television appearances to charity balls, you would never know that she fights every day against the disease that sucked away her mother's life and took a swipe at her own: osteoporosis. This is, after all, the woman who was catapulted to political stardom when she cheekily took on then vice president George H.W. Bush at the 1988 Democratic National Convention. ("Poor George," she sighed on national television. "He can't help it; he was born with a silver

foot in his mouth.") When Richards came into office, she promised her constituents that "opportunity knows no race or color or gender" and then appointed more minorities and women than any other governor in Texas history. "From the very beginning of her public involvement, if Ann got interested in something, she would go learn everything she could about it," says Mary Beth Rogers, her former chief of staff. "She was a woman in a man's world, and you knew you had to shine if you were going to command any attention or respect."

It was that passion that ultimately saved her life. In 1995, after she left the governor's mansion, Richards fell and broke her hand. She was 62 years old. And then, Richards says in her famous Texas drawl, "I realized I was shrinking, my collars didn't fit my neck anymore, and I'd lost probably an inch, inch and a quarter, in height." She became aware of osteoporosis when her mother was breaking bone after bone, getting more and more disabled until she died at age 86. The grip osteoporosis had on her mother galvanized her to request a bone density test. Richards was right to ask. She had osteopenia, which meant, even though she was in her 60s, she could do something to protect herself. "I started a really intense regimen of weight-bearing exercise, which helps build bone density," she says. She also changed her diet to emphasize fruit, vegetables, and

fish; and being postmenopausal, she was able to benefit from taking the bone-strengthening drug Evista.

"It's been a little more than five years now," says Richards, "and the bone density in my spine is now normal. So I know that you can build your strength to support a fragile frame." And once she knew, being Ann Richards, she started bugging her friends and acquaintances to lift weights. She also started giving speeches about her health turnaround. Women who heard her told her she had motivated them to change their habits. A publisher who happened into her audience convinced her that she could reach more women if she wrote a book: The result—her second book, *I'm Not Slowing Down: Winning My Battle with Osteoporosis*.

That Richards went, as Mary Beth Rogers puts it, "whole hog" in her battle against osteoporosis—while trying to get other women to do the same—doesn't surprise her friends at all. "She takes advantage of every experience she can to enrich her life and the lives of others. She represents a certain freedom to women," Rogers says—a freedom to both be themselves and to take charge of their lives.

"I can think of no greater gift to the people I love than my good health," Richards says. "I want to remain vital and strong, as long as I possibly can. I am 69 years old, and I don't think I've ever been in better physical health."

Calcium. Every woman under 51 should be aiming for 1,000 milligrams of calcium a day. Raise that to 1,200 after menopause. Most women are falling short. To figure out how you're doing, add up the servings of yogurt, cheese, milk, and calcium-fortified orange juice or cereal you tend to get every day. One serving is an average of 300 milligrams. Recently, there's been some controversy about whether or not dairy products are a good source of calcium. A few experts are arguing that these foods actually leach the mineral from your bones (they reason that the dairy proteins raise levels of sulfur-containing amino acids in your blood that the body then must neutralize with calcium it raids from your skeleton). But Robert Heaney, MD, of Creighton University in Omaha, one of the country's top calcium experts, says not to worry: He has analyzed scores of randomized studies showing that dairy foods help keep bones strong.

The advice about supplements can get as finicky as the mineral itself. Calcium isn't easily absorbed in large amounts, so it's best to break up your daily intake into two to three doses and to take it with meals, says Heaney. For the calcium to reach your bones, you need to make sure you're getting 200 international units (IU) of vitamin D a day if you are 50 or younger; 400 IU, ages 51 to 69; 600 IU, 70 and older. Your body probably produces enough of the vitamin if you simply step out into the sunlight every day. But you may need to take a D supplement if you're super-vigilant about sunscreen or if you're African-American, since melanin acts as a shield. You may have heard that supplements with calcium citrate are absorbed more easily than the calcium carbonate found in antacids, but Heaney says the evidence for both is equally strong. And if you can't be bothered with rules, just down your daily quotient all at once. It's better than not taking any at all.

Drugs. Calcium and exercise can only do so much. Andrea, 46, a lawyer in San Francisco who asked that her last name not be used, had a heel scan at a health fair, which indicated she was in the danger zone. When a DXA scan confirmed she was

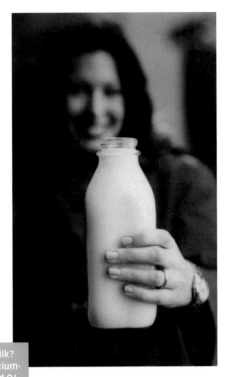

Hate milk? Try calcium-fortified OJ.

osteopenic, her doctor prescribed Fosamax, which prevents the tiny cracks caused by the osteoclasts. The drug, along with a similar drug, Actonel, has been approved to treat osteopenia—but because the osteoclasts don't get truly destructive until after menopause, the approval is only for postmenopausal women. If a woman simply has delicate bones, there's no evidence either drug will help. "I'd rather err on the side of prevention," says Andrea, who hasn't hit menopause yet. She knows several other women in their 40s whose doctors put them on the drug as well.

"That's my worst fear," says the NORA study's Siris. "A woman in her 30s or 40s finds out she has low bone density and her doctor puts her on expensive drugs she doesn't need. It's incorrect for a healthy premenopausal woman to be on Fosamax."

Evista, a third drug approved to treat osteopenia in postmenopausal women, is a selective estrogen receptor modulator, or SERM, which acts like estrogen in some parts of the body but not others. Though Evista is known to slow bone loss in postmenopausal women, it has never been studied for this purpose in younger women. And the first drug that actually stimulates bone growth, Forteo, has been approved by the Food and Drug Administration, but again only for women who've been through menopause (it involves a daily injection). None of these drugs has been studied for long-term safety.

Medication is an option for postmenopausal women with osteopenia, although even then, there's no need to rush into it. No one goes from osteopenia to osteoporosis in a year. "If your bone density is low, you might decide you want to get on one of those drugs, and that's a reasonable choice. Or you might wait and get retested in a year," says Siris. The good news is that the osteoporosis drugs have dramatically helped women who already have the disease, reducing their fracture risk by as much as half.

WHEN TO GET TESTED

Many experts think it makes sense to get tested at menopause, or even earlier so you have a baseline score to compare later scans. The peripheral heel or wrist scan has been shown to be an accurate initial screening tool; if you get a low score, you should follow up with a DXA scan. "My personal opinion is that all women at menopause should be tested," says Felicia Cosman, MD, clinical director of the National Osteoporosis Foundation. "But we can't recommend that officially because it would cost too much." So for now, the foundation advises that women first get tested at menopause only if they have certain risk factors, including: a small frame or weight of less than 127 pounds, a family history of osteoporosis, a personal history of fracture after age 50, or a smoking habit. Otherwise, you're counseled to wait until you turn 65. After that, the most recent guidelines from the U.S. Preventive Services Task Force recommend screenings at least every two years.

Whenever you do get tested, try not to panic about the results. It's normal to be worried about your bones if your mother has osteoporosis. Or if you are a slender white woman who hates milk and loves Pinot Noir. And it's right to want to take charge of your health. "But the thing to remember," says Siris, "is that if you have osteopenia, it doesn't mean your bones are going to fall apart overnight. And there's a lot you can do to keep them strong right now." •

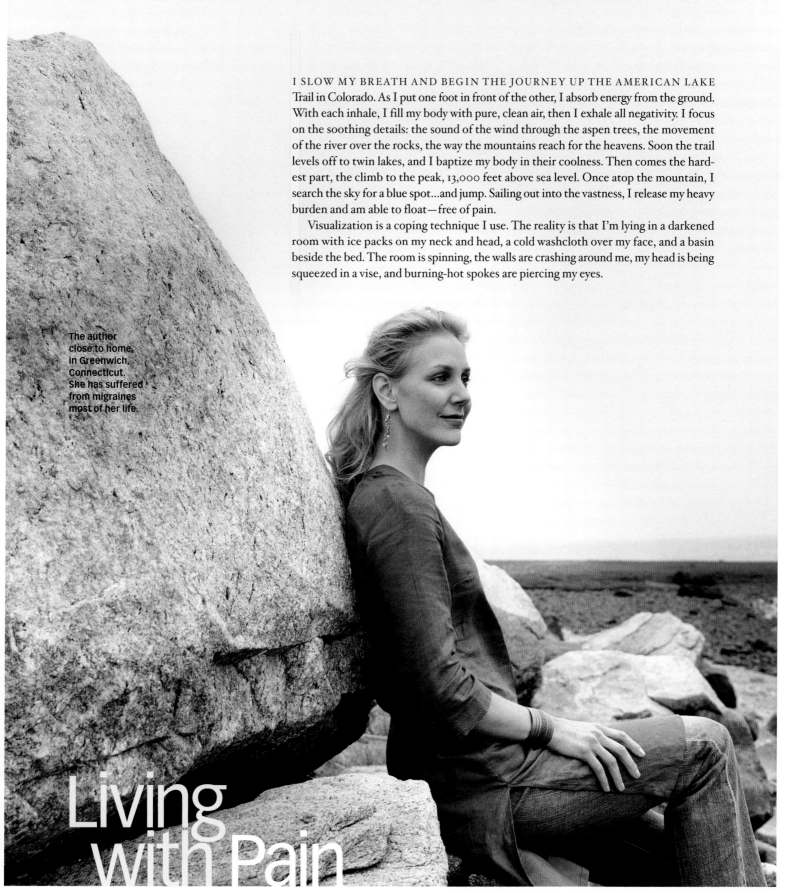

I SLOW MY BREATH AND BEGIN THE JOURNEY UP THE AMERICAN LAKE Trail in Colorado. As I put one foot in front of the other, I absorb energy from the ground. With each inhale, I fill my body with pure, clean air, then I exhale all negativity. I focus on the soothing details: the sound of the wind through the aspen trees, the movement of the river over the rocks, the way the mountains reach for the heavens. Soon the trail levels off to twin lakes, and I baptize my body in their coolness. Then comes the hardest part, the climb to the peak, 13,000 feet above sea level. Once atop the mountain, I search the sky for a blue spot...and jump. Sailing out into the vastness, I release my heavy burden and am able to float—free of pain.

Visualization is a coping technique I use. The reality is that I'm lying in a darkened room with ice packs on my neck and head, a cold washcloth over my face, and a basin beside the bed. The room is spinning, the walls are crashing around me, my head is being squeezed in a vise, and burning-hot spokes are piercing my eyes.

The author close to home, in Greenwich, Connecticut. She has suffered from migraines most of her life.

Living with Pain

Imagine: constant, mind-blowing agony every day for 24 years, no cure. **SUSANNE RUPPERT** tells how she's survived the vise in her head.

At age 8, I was diagnosed with a combination of migraine, cluster, and tension-type headaches. Many migraineurs have suicidal thoughts, and I once read that clusters can be more painful than an accidental amputation. Over the past 24 years, my migraines have become intractable—pain 24/7. New research suggests that constant headaches may cause the brain to lose its natural ability to fight pain. I fight anyway. This chronic condition isn't always visible to others. Sufferers are trapped in a different dimension, one between life and death, where invisible assailants take up permanent residency. The curse and the blessing of this existence are the same: It won't kill you.

CURRENTLY THERE'S NO cure for a migraine, but there's a loophole in the devil's plan: This brain disorder can be managed. And that's what I cling to in my search for healing. Exploring complementary treatments and conventional medicine, I'm open to all options: acupuncture, chiropractic, physical therapy, homeopathy, herbs, reiki. I've taken medications with incapacitating side effects—some that could cause bleeding in the brain, some that prevent me from driving and impair memory, speech, and thought. I've swallowed more than 50 types of pills and participated in studies with drugs that haven't yet been approved by the Food and Drug Administration. Gained weight, lost weight, lost hair. Needles have been injected into my neck and head, and nerves in my neck have been burned. *The harder the battle, the sweeter the victory,* I think. And to show my opponent it hasn't won, I hold down a full-time job, go white-water rafting down the Colorado River, trek glaciers in Norway. And I laugh—often at myself.

For the past 14 years, I've been a patient at the New England Center for Headache in Stamford, Connecticut. Last year my doctor sent me to the Michigan Head-Pain & Neurological Institute for advanced-care hospitalization—my second in-patient stay in a headache unit. The faces and actions were familiar: the wearing of sunglasses inside to brace against even the dimmest light, grown men crying, helpless parents begging for their children's release from pain. Some patients had taken too much medication and become addicted to opiates or thrown off their body's pain-control system, causing "rebound" headaches.

In this clinic, patients can be treated aggressively with daily intravenous protocols and drug cocktails. There's also instruction on relaxation techniques (biofeedback, visualization, meditation, self-hypnosis) to help move through, not against, the pain; information on food triggers; lessons in behavior modification (slow down, pace yourself, breathe, adjust your goals); psychological counseling (dealing with the depression and anxiety that often accompany pain); and physical and occupational therapy. All this offers a stronghold to someone who's climbing a cliff without a harness. Most patients, like me, leave with significantly less pain.

Going through the motions of life is my survival strategy. I don't think about the week or even the day but tackle each moment. Baby steps. Most nights I go to sleep completely drained and awake wondering if I'll be able to get out of bed. The ghosts of whys and wherefores hover above me: *Why have I been dealt this card? Why aren't I strong enough to overcome it?* There's guilt over missed days of work, canceled social plans, sacrificed goals. Maybe I'm being imprisoned for something I did in a past life. After all, pain derives from the

The curse
and the blessing of this existence are the same: It won't kill you.

TYPES OF **HEADACHES**

According to the American Council for Headache Education (ACHE), approximately 95 percent of women and 90 percent of men have had at least one headache during the past year. If you consistently have three or more headaches a week, you should notify your physician. Keep a diary of headache frequency, severity, and triggers to help your doctor identify what type you have and how to help you.

HEADACHE	DESCRIPTION	PERCENTAGE OF ADULTS AFFECTED
Tension-Type	Steady ache, usually affecting both sides of the head. Lasts anywhere from 30 minutes to several days.	Up to 90 percent
Migraine	Throbbing or pounding pain that can target one or both sides of the head or the area behind the eyes. Associated with nausea, vomiting, and sensitivity to light and sound. May be preceded by visual disturbances known as auras. Lasts anywhere from four to 72 hours.	About 12 percent (18 percent women; 6 percent men)
Cluster	Severe but brief pain (lasting one to two hours) that typically focuses around one eye. Attacks occur in groups (clusters) for weeks or months.	Less than 1 percent (about 85 percent men)
Chronic	Daily or near daily headaches for more than 15 days a month. Two of the most common types are tension-type and migraine.	About 4 percent

Latin word for punishment, *poena*. I yearn for 7000 B.C., when a hole was drilled in the back of the skull to release the evil spirits.

But I close the door on self-defeating thoughts—sometimes slowly, as if pushing against a fierce wind, other times matter-of-factly, as if locking the house before I leave. And then I take a left at the fork in the road and follow the sign marked faith. There's one thing I won't abdicate to this dominating force—my hope. Hope that though salvation may not be mine today, I'll discover it tomorrow.

Chronic pain demands a proactive mind-set. You need to help yourself at a time when all you want is for someone to save you. In attempting to prevent a more severe attack, I take a handful of medicine three times a day. I try to separate the idea of pain from that of suffering: I can't control the presence of pain, but I can control how I react to it. I move my thoughts away from what hurts and focus on breathing, relaxation tapes, the feel of wet sand between my toes. I practice biofeedback to mentally relax my muscles. And when neither these methods nor painkillers mitigate the pounding—when defeat tries to crawl under my skin, hissing, *Nothing will help, you're running out of options*—I tell myself that I'm narrowing my to-do list, getting closer to a solution.

Other ways I attempt to take control are by avoiding triggers and by following consistent sleep, eating, and exercise routines. To drown out sounds that exacerbate headaches—cars, voices, noise—I wear earplugs. I go to sleep and wake up at the same time every day, no naps. I adhere to a migraineur's diet—abstaining from alcohol, caffeine, chocolate, nitrites, and aged or pickled foods, among many other things—and try to avoid smoky, loud, or bright places. I've minimized my schedule and said goodbye—for now—to my athletic days. Walking, tai chi, and yoga have replaced running, soccer, and tennis. Twice a day I meditate, my mantra being "There is no pain"—believing that by repeating it, it will become true, that my mind will listen to my heart.

Isaac Newton said, "Truth is the offspring of silent and unbroken meditation." One day my truth will be no pain, but until then life finds ways to keep me going—

through the support of my family and friends, the sweet tartness of a lemon square, the comfort of a hiking trail beneath my feet, the touch of my husband's lips on mine. It's been 24 years of fighting for resurrection, more than two years since I've experienced a pain-free moment. I mourn for the person I could be, but this is my existence. I accept it yet refuse to be defined by it, so I'll continue searching for my lesson and for my freedom. I don't know where the chronic pain will lead me or where I'll take it. What I do know is that life is a challenge—sometimes a disappointment, sometimes a standing ovation—but always a gift. ●

THE LATEST TREATMENTS

Migraines attack approximately 28 million people. Doctors believe that they occur when various internal and external triggers—from hormones to weather changes to foods—set off nerves surrounding certain blood vessels in the brain, causing inflammation in those areas. The result can be incapacitating head pain, nausea, vomiting, and sensitivity to light and sound. According to the National Headache Foundation, 70 to 80 percent of sufferers have a family history of migraine. Here are some developments:

MEDICATIONS More than 50 drugs are used to treat migraines. Many of them are approved for other disorders, such as hypertension, epilepsy, and depression. According to Fred Sheftell, MD—cofounder of the New England Center for Headache and coauthor of *Conquering Headache*—triptans are the most effective medications once an attack occurs. They include Imitrex, Zomig, Amerge, Frova, Maxalt, and Relpax. To help reduce the frequency and intensity of attacks *before* they start, preventive drugs—such as Topamax, Depakote, Inderal, and Elavil—can be taken daily.

COMPLEMENTARY THERAPIES
Alexander Mauskop, MD, director of the New York Headache Center and coauthor of *What Your Doctor May Not Tell You About Migraines,* recommends biofeedback, acupuncture, and vitamin supplements—daily dosages of 400 milligrams of magnesium and 400 milligrams of riboflavin (B2), or 150 milligrams of Coenzyme Q10 (CoQ10). Herbs that may help migraines include feverfew and ginger. Preliminary studies suggest that some herbs or supplements might lower the efficacy of migraine medications or cause them to reach toxic levels, so consult your doctor before taking any.

NERVE CONNECTION According to Joel Saper, MD, founder and director of the Michigan Head-Pain & Neurological Institute, a migraineur's brain is more sensitive to triggers than the average person's. So the goal is to stop pain messages from reaching the brain and causing headaches. When standard treatments alone don't work, the following techniques might be considered for chronic sufferers:

■ **Botox.** This toxin, derived from the bacteria that cause botulism, is known for its ability to erase wrinkles. Studies are under way to assess its ability to prevent migraines. It was initially thought that Botox relieved headaches by relaxing tense muscles in and around the head and neck. Newer studies, however, suggest that it might inhibit nerves from sending pain signals to the brain.

■ **Trigger-point injections.** Numbing medications are injected into muscle and nerve sites for short-term relief.

■ **Facet joint and occipital nerve blocks.** Areas around the head and neck are injected with Novocaine-like drugs or steroids to reduce inflammation. If this relieves pain, nerves may be frozen or burned for a more long-term solution.

■ **Neurostimulation.** This experimental technique involves surgically implanting an electrode beneath the skin, which sends impulses to the nervous system and peripheral nerves to block pain signals.

For more information, go to achenet.org and headaches.org.

Ask for What You Want
100 Percent of the Time

Actor Evan Handler was diagnosed by the hospital staff with acute leukemia—and extreme pushiness. He believes his aggressive, persistent style saved his life. Surviving, **CYNTHIA GORNEY** discovers, isn't about being voted most popular patient.

EVAN HANDLER KNEW HE WAS going to be trouble the first time he walked into his new hospital room. He wanted to plug in his VCR.

His own VCR—not the hospital's, which was attached to a television that could be reserved in advance except that nobody ever seemed to know where it was. Handler was 24, newly diagnosed with acute myelogenous leukemia, and terrified. He was pretty sure he was going to die before long. He wanted to watch movies. He had the idea from reading he had done that watching humorous movies might help his chance at recovery, and anyway he wanted to watch them when he wanted to watch them, not when somebody in a hospital uniform thought movie-watching time had arrived. "So I brought a VCR with me, but I was told I couldn't plug it in," Handler says. "I was told the electrical outlets were needed for emergency equipment."

Handler wrote a book and performed an off-Broadway piece about his four years in cancer treatment; he's a bicoastal actor,

known for his role as the divorce lawyer Charlotte falls for and marries on *Sex and the City,* and was rather celebrated, for a time, as an Angry Patient Advocate. His 1996 memoir, *Time on Fire: My Comedy of Terrors,* is full of ferocious, unsentimental stories about what it's actually like to be a cancer patient. There's an abundance of physical pain in Handler's book ("If you can imagine what it might feel like to a bowl of chocolate pudding if you sucked some of it up through a straw, that's what it feels like to have a bone marrow aspirate"), but his real expertise turned out to be in survival, both physical and psychic, which he accomplished, in some large measure, by being—how else to put this?—pushy.

He declined, for example, to relinquish his VCR. When the nurses left his hospital room, he put the VCR discreetly under his bed, hooked it up to a tiny television friends had brought him, and stuck the plug into the outlet. "I was going to watch *Annie Hall,*" Handler says. "If they needed emergency equipment, they could unplug it."

He closed the door to his hospital room sometimes—even though the staff appeared to disapprove—and taped up a DO NOT DISTURB sign. He figured out how to arrange his IV lines so he could have sex with his girlfriend in the hospital bathroom. He announced that he would not wear hospital gowns, because they made him feel foolish and helpless, and wore his own sweatpants and T-shirts on the ward. "I was capable of more life than the hospital gown symbolized," Handler says. "I felt it was like wearing a concentration camp uniform."

Handler has been healthy for more than a decade; after a harrowing bone marrow transplant he was finally left cancer-free. And although he knows much has changed since his recovery, both in hospital practice and in the availability of medical information to patients—"The Internet would have made things so much easier, and managed care might very well have killed me," he says—he still has strong ideas about what he would say to a friend just commencing a serious round of ›

» "It's possible to be courteous without being meek. **Bring an advocate with you.** Make noise."

Who's the BOSS?

How to ensure you get A-plus medical care.

Being a vigilant health care consumer is a challenge. We want you to be well armed with strategies for getting the best possible medical attention:

1 Before a visit to the doctor, prepare a list of questions in writing and consult it during your appointment. **The Agency for Healthcare Research and Quality offers a helpful list of questions to ask before surgery, ques-**tions that can be adapted to other medical situations. (Visit www.ahrq.gov or write to AHRQ, 2101 East Jefferson Street, Suite 501, Rockville, MD 20852.)

2 Don't leave a medical appointment until you are satisfied that all your questions have been answered—**even if the doctor seems to you to be getting impatient. It's the physician's job to explain, and your job not to say you understand when you really don't.**

3 It's very easy to tune out bad news or complicated information. **If you're getting test results, bring a friend or family member with you to the appointment to take notes. Or tape the session; a good doctor shouldn't object.**

4 If you're discussing a new diagnosis or treatment, you'll probably want a second opinion; a good doctor will encourage you. Get physicians' names from your primary care doctor, your state's medical society, or your health insurance company.

5 Bring a list of all the medications you're taking, and the dosages, including herbal remedies, vitamins, and over-the-counter drugs. **If it's appropriate, bring copies of your X-rays.**

6 When you're seeing a new doctor, make sure that your old doctor has sent your records ahead. **If there's no time to mail them and you're too sick to pick them up yourself, ask a friend to do it.**

7 To spare yourself aggravation, **call the office before your appointment to see whether the doctor is running late.**

8 If a doctor calls you by your first name, feel free to use his or hers. **You'll be making it clear that you'll accord the doctor the same degree of respect that he or she offers to you.**

9 A few days before any lab test, **ask for an instruction sheet so you can properly prepare for the test.**

10 Once you've been diagnosed, talk to other people who have the same condition. **You can also do research on the Web. Medline Plus (www.nlm.nih.gov/medlineplus) is a good place to start. Smart patients become experts in their illnesses.**

11 In the hospital, treats are a great way to soften hearts, lift spirits, and make yourself real to the hospital staff. **If, for instance, someone brings you brownies, leave some in the staff room for the nurses and doctors. If your window ledge is overloaded with flowers, present a bunch to the grumpy aide on the night shift.**

12 Stay pleasantly feisty by reminding yourself that the doctors and nurses aren't doing you a favor by taking care of you; **you're paying for their services. You're entitled to good care—and a lot more. To view a copy of the patients' bill of rights, visit www.consumer. gov/qualityhealth.**

—*Judith Stone*

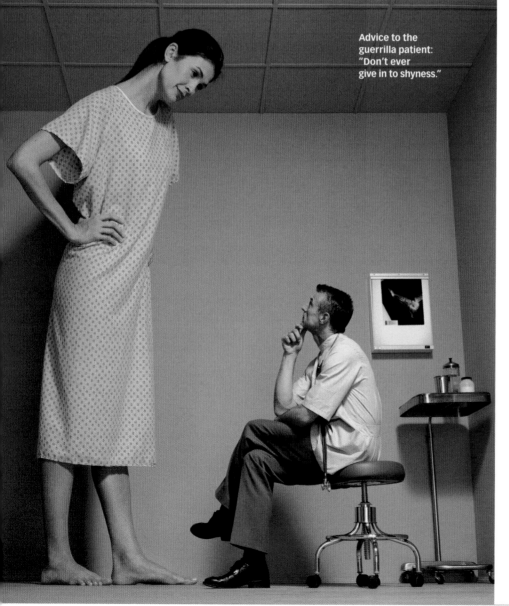

Advice to the guerrilla patient: "Don't ever give in to shyness."

medical care. There must be doctors and nurses who to this day remember Evan Handler as the eccentric oncology guerrilla, the guy who invited a psychic healer to his room, reminded nurses that he reacted badly to Benadryl even though that's what they had been told to give him, and forged the doctor's signature in order to get his blood test results from the alternate hospital lab, the one that didn't make him wait all day.

"You just have to keep constant surveillance," he says. "Information is power. The more you know, the better equipped you are." Don't be cowed into silence by uniforms or vague references to "procedure," Handler says; as a patient it's possible to be courteous without being meek. Bring an advocate with you. Make noise. Get over the fear of being regarded as demanding. "Ask for what you want, a hundred percent of the time," he says. "Be willing to hear no. Be willing to negotiate. It sounds simple, but asking for what you want is difficult to do."

Here's how difficult: A while ago, in a doctor's office waiting room, mildly feverish and feeling low, Handler found himself gazing at a receptionist who had just told him to go wait for the doctor in the examining room—because she needed to step away from the desk for a few minutes, and the doctor would want Handler to be ready for him. "Now, I know that in the waiting room there are cushioned chairs and magazines, and it's warmer," Handler says. "And I was supposed to go sit in a hard chair in the cold examining room."

To his astonishment he hesitated, Handler says, and then said he believed he would stay where he was. "I said, 'Doesn't the doctor have legs? Couldn't he walk up here and find me?' She looked at me like I was out of my mind. And I was amazed to find that it was still hard for me, as a somewhat famous patient advocate, having been through everything I'd been through—here was this little young woman...So my main piece of advice is, don't ever give into that shyness. There's no reason not to say, 'You know, that doesn't work for me.' I don't know why that's so difficult to say. But it just has to be overcome." •

The Real Health Clubs

Joining a group, any group, is a way to lift depression, boost your immune system, and maybe even help you get pregnant.
LAUREN GRAVITZ reports.

Community not only lifts the soul but may also be beneficial to your health. Although the science can be squishy, with many contradictory results, a growing number of studies are showing that different kinds of socializing, from playing bingo to participating in support groups, can do a body good.

● **The church effect.** People who attend church or other religious services at least once a week are more likely to live longer, stay healthier, and be less susceptible to depression than those who don't go as frequently, according to one of many studies by Harold G. Koenig, MD, associate professor of psychiatry and medicine at Duke University Medical Center. "It's likely that immune function is influenced by spiritual well-being," says Koenig, who notes that there's been a groundswell of research looking at how positive emotions—such as forgiveness, gratefulness, and altruism—are associated with physical and mental health.

● **Join the club.** Americans 65 and older who participate in social activities like bingo reap the same longevity benefits as those who exercise, according to a study published in the *British Medical Journal*. (But it may work only in America: Researchers found that when they compared the lifestyles of elderly Swedish men and women who were either solitary or social, physically active or inert, the only significant survival benefit was for men who engaged in active hobbies—alone.)

● **High-yield personal bonds.** Numerous studies by psychologist Janice Kiecolt-Glaser, PhD, and her husband, immunologist Ronald Glaser, PhD, both professors at the Ohio State University, indicate that the more support a person has

from friends and family, the more protective his or her immune system is. One of their earliest studies, on perpetually stressed medical school students, showed that those who were more isolated and lonely were less responsive to a series of hepatitis-B vaccines. Women with close ties to family and friends also have more energy and are physically stronger than those lacking such relationships, according to a study of 56,436 women ages 55 to 72 conducted at Harvard Medical School and Brigham and Women's Hospital.

● **A healthy dose of company.** The benefits of support groups for women with breast cancer have been documented by a host of studies. Although the talk sessions don't seem to increase survival, women who participate in them report feeling less pain than those who don't. They're also less prone to anger, anxiety, and depression, according to a study published in *The New England Journal of Medicine* in December 2001. A separate study in the journal *Cancer* indicates that online support groups confer many of the same advantages, including a reduction in depression and stress.

● **Baby, you've got friends.** Women trying to get pregnant can also benefit from weekly support groups. An infertility study headed by Alice Domar, PhD, assistant professor at Harvard Medical School, followed 184 women for one year and found that those who attended support groups for ten weeks were more than twice as successful at conceiving than those in the control group. In fact, many women chosen as controls dropped out of the study to join the group sessions because they worked so well.

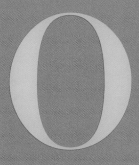

Balance

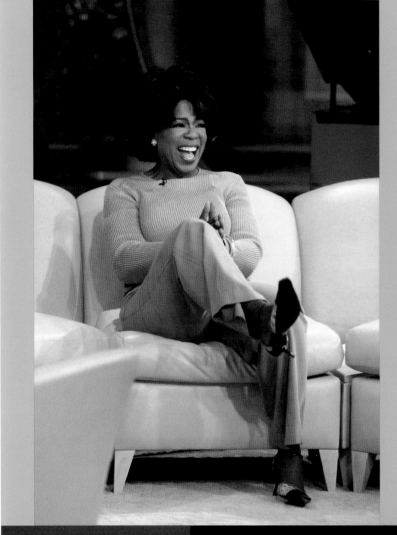

Reserve, restore, take off Sundays...
Oprah's Energy Policy

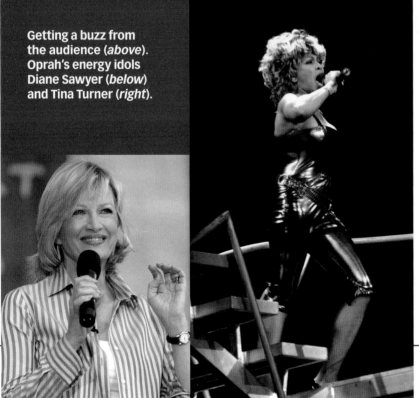

Getting a buzz from the audience (*above*). Oprah's energy idols Diane Sawyer (*below*) and Tina Turner (*right*).

I WAS IN MY 20S WHEN I FIGURED OUT HOW to regulate my energy. I'd taken a job as a reporter and was working hundred-hour weeks, trying to be a team player. It was only after I became depleted that I realized I had only a certain amount of energy—and I needed to conserve and restore it. I understood that I had to keep giving back to myself, to refill my tank.

Now when I begin to feel exhausted, I pull back. If I'm at work and people are lined up at my desk with one request after another, I literally go sit in my closet and refuel. And I always give myself Sundays as a spiritual base of renewal—a day when I do absolutely nothing. I sit in my jammies or take a walk, and I allow myself time to BE—capital B-E—with myself. When I don't, I absolutely become stressed, irritable, anxiety-prone, and not the person I want to be in the world.

The way you eat makes a difference in terms of sustainability, which is why I avoid sugar—I don't want a high followed by a fall. I don't do energy bars or caffeine. I've learned to listen to my body. I know I'll be hungry at ten o'clock every morning, about the time I finish taping my first of two shows. At four in the afternoon, I'm ravenous. "Must be ten of four," I'll announce during a meeting, "because I could eat this cushion." That's when I have my biggest meal of the day—usually a protein and some kind of fruit or vegetable.

But feeding yourself is more than food. I believe we're all connected to each other's energy fields—whenever you walk into a roomful of people, your energy is either re-stored or taken away from you. If I'm around someone who saps me, I have to put up a barrier—a nonphysical wall that keeps that person's negative vibes away. I also have a couple of energy idols—people whose energy amazes me. Diane Sawyer is one. I don't know what I would do if had to get up at three or four in the morning. And there's nobody like Tina Turner. How does she do that? And how does she do that in Manolo Blahniks?

Energy is the essence of life. Every day you decide how you're going to use it by knowing what you want and what it takes to reach that goal, and by maintaining focus. That means asking yourself, *Is what I'm doing part of my overall plan—and can I release the energy I'll need?*   **—Oprah**

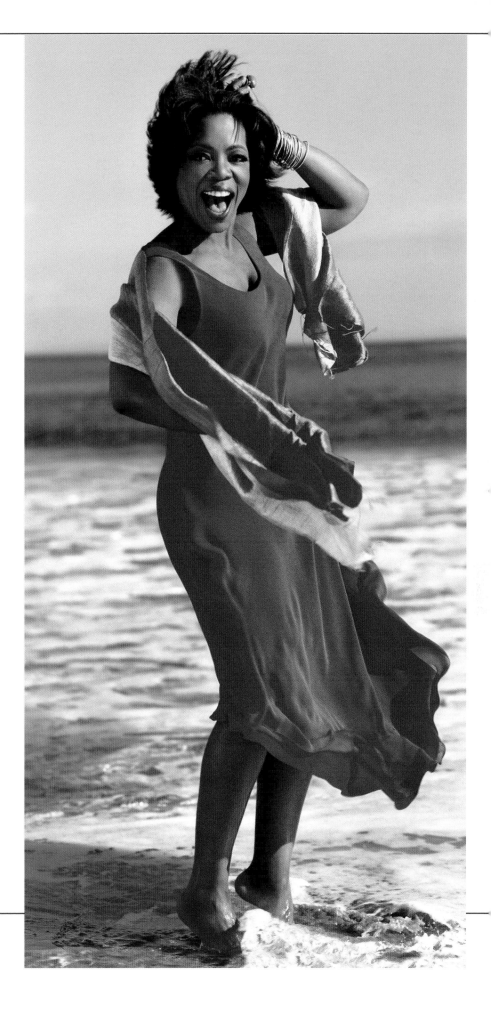

Putting Yourself First*

*Think it's selfish? Think again.
By Valerie Monroe

I learned the hard way how to put myself first.

Almost 20 years ago, my husband's identical twin brother killed himself. He was addicted to drugs. My husband—also addicted, I soon discovered—began a rapid descent along the same ruinous path, forsaking me and our 1-year-old son for grief's dark embrace. I tried to help my husband, became, in fact, almost sick with trying to help him and take care of our baby and our precarious finances. Family and concerned friends phoned me constantly to find out how my husband was doing and how I was holding up. "I can handle this," I told them. "I'll be fine." And compared with my husband, I did seem fine. But the tentacles of worry that had gripped me fitfully when I first discovered his addiction now snaked around me always, tighter and tighter, choking my appetite, my sleep, and my belief that he would ever get well. I would sit up all night waiting for a phone call—from him (I hoped) or from the police (I dreaded)—and then face another full day of chasing around an active toddler. "Keep this up and you *will* get sick," someone said, "and then who'll take care of *you*?"

There was no one to take care of me. Well, yes, there was: me. And so I did, because I had to. I got help to look after the baby and started going to a support group, and once my husband was recovering in a hospital rehab, I treated myself every visiting day to a fine steak dinner at a nearby pub. "I think I'll order a steak," I'd say to the baby as he sat in a plastic booster seat, sucking on his bottle. "Baked potato or mashed?" He'd kick his feet and slap the table with his chubby hands. "Good choice," I'd say. "Mashed it is."

Why is it hard for many of us to do things for ourselves before we do for others? Maybe we believe the "good" woman sacrifices herself for her family and, increasingly, for her work. "In terms of our relationships, women often feel they're responsible for everything—which is not a complete misperception," says nationally syndicated columnist and life coach Harriette Cole. "We are the ones who usually lead the way. But somehow we get from there to the idea that the world won't work if we don't help it along."

Taking on responsibilities that might be well or even better handled by others is one of the ways we begin to lose our balance and slide down the slippery slope from generosity to martyrdom. Because

women are likely to be the primary caretakers for husbands and children as well as for aging parents, we have ample opportunity to fall into the pattern of serving the people we love before we serve ourselves. But there are good reasons to be judicious about that. "If you always put someone else first, there's a tendency for others to depreciate you, to lose respect, because respect for another comes from an understanding that that person has her own wishes, dreams, and desires," says Ethel S. Person, MD, author of *Feeling Strong: The Achievement of Authentic Power.* Besides, why must there be only one person in first place at a time? "It's possible to have equal concerns for yourself and for loved ones," says Person. "There aren't always conflicting priorities."

In fact, being skilled at taking care of yourself may improve your capacity to care for others; if you're not fulfilled, you're only able to see other people through the filter of your own needs. And studies suggest that not taking care of ourselves is unhealthy for those who depend on us. At the Beth Israel Deaconess Medical Center in Boston, researchers found that greater levels of caregiver stress were associated with increased respiratory problems among the infants in their charge.

A friend who does a lot of pro bono work in addition to demanding full-time paying projects seemed to be in a debilitating cycle: She'd work till she collapsed, when she'd have to take a couple of weeks off to recuperate (during which time she lost both momentum and money), and then she'd fall back immediately into the same frenzied work routine. Because she is a brilliant woman, and kind, her family and friends often called on her expertise in matters professional and otherwise. Her appointment book looked like the diary of a *Survivor* contestant. Which, in a way, she was. But though she had won many hard-earned victories for other people, she herself was barely surviving. (Not incidentally, her house, quite literally, was falling down around her.) So she started to make exercise—which sometimes meant just a vigorous walk—a priority, planned her meals thoughtfully rather than eating on the run, turned off the telephone after 11 P.M. so she could get a full night's sleep, and settled in with a guy who happened to be terrific at fixing things, like leaky plumbing and loose shingles. Guess how all this affected her work: Because she is now more engaged and energetically enthusiastic, her projects are reaching (and therefore helping) more people than ever before.

I recently read about a kind of therapy advocating that when we're stressed or suffering, we put our hand over our heart or touch our cheek as we might touch the cheek of a child we love, and say simply, "I understand." In that moment, we're accomplishing one of our greatest responsibilities; without feeling loving-kindness and compassion for ourselves, we can never really know what they are.

It's the easy way to put yourself first. And it only takes a moment. ●

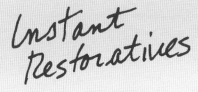

Instant Restoratives

Six things that work like magic to bring you back home to yourself.

DANCE.

THERE ONCE WAS AN UNHAPPY MARRIAGE. The woman, in her mid-60s, was feeling sad and low. One afternoon her grandson, just 4 and unaware of her problems, had an uncontrollable urge to dance, which for him meant flapping his arms and churning his legs in such a way as to appear as if he were hopping madly around on a bed of hot coals. "Dance with me, Grandma!" he said, hopping closer to her. She danced. And remembered delight.

HAVE SEX.

Three kids (grown), two demanding jobs, and one dead air-conditioner later, they lay naked and sweating in their large, connubial bed. "God," she said, "I'm hot." "That's right," he said, "you are." He raised himself on one elbow, and with his face almost touching her, he began to blow lightly, from one of her shoulders to the other. The room, already warm, heated up. Endorphins were released. "I'd forgotten," she said, finally. "Forgotten?" "I'd forgotten we were hot," she said.

FILL YOUR EYES WITH GREEN.

It's the color many jewelers use as a backdrop when they're working on a delicate piece; green is said to be the easiest color for the eye to see. It's also thought to balance emotions and bring on a feeling of calm. Have you ever been mesmerized by the dense green of a palm as it swayed in a tropical breeze?

STAND IN A STEAMING SHOWER.

And let the hot water loosen the stiff muscles in your neck. Lean over and feel the water pound your back. Stand again and breathe in the steam, which carries moisture to your airways and your skin, where it replenishes the water that has evaporated from your cells.

SWEEP.

Too tired to dance? Husband on a trip? Middle of winter? Can't sleep? Sweep. Depending on how you do it, it's either the most productive way to be mindless (sweep that dusty attic floor) or the most mindful way to be unproductive (sweep the patio of falling leaves; they keep falling, you keep sweeping, sweeping, doing only this).

BREATHE.

She used to get panic attacks. Then she learned how to "square breathe." Picture a square; choose a corner. Count to four as you slowly inhale. Count to four as you exhale. Reach the next corner on the inhale, leave it on the exhale. Four corners. Four deep breaths. Her heartbeat, which would suddenly gallop away, slowed to a comfortable trot. (Deep, slow breaths increase the amount of carbon dioxide in the body, which reduces the panic response.) —*V.M.*

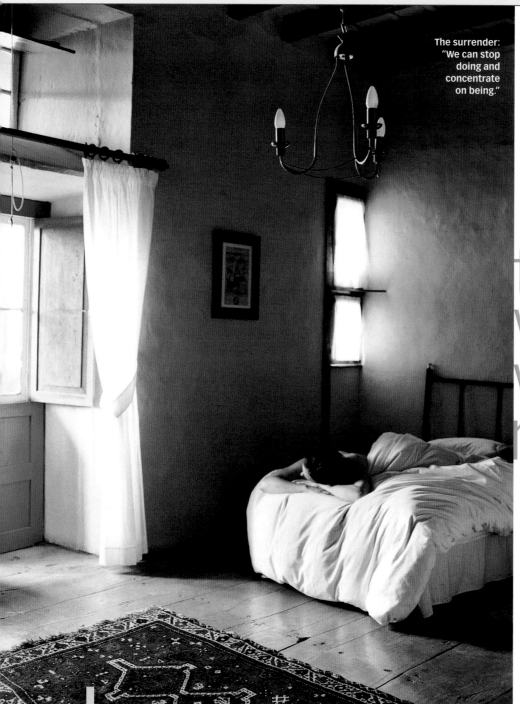

the weary woman's manifesto

Instead of scrambling for ways to keep on trucking in the face of fatigue, she committed a radical act: She rested. **Kathleen Norris** on the amazing grace of calling it a day.

I AM A HIGH-ENERGY PERSON, AND THE FIRST TIME I WENT ON A spiritual retreat I assumed I would be able to accomplish many things that were difficult to do in my everyday life. Without phone calls, other interruptions, and the responsibilities of family life, I reasoned, I could read the books I'd been longing to read, I could sit and think and write. To my dismay, I found that for the first two days I did little but sleep. I managed to stagger off to morning, noon, and evening prayers with the monks and go to meals but often napped afterward. When I tried to read in the evenings, my eyes kept closing, and by 8 p.m. I was ready for bed.

When I complained to an elderly monk about having no energy, he responded, "Oh, we hear that all the time from our guests." He added casually, "Sometimes the most spiritual thing you can do is sleep."

I was shocked. I had just been given permission to rest. It was permission I seldom granted myself. Even as a toddler, I resisted taking naps because I didn't want to miss out on anything. My poor mother, who must have longed for some free time, quickly learned that if I slept in the daytime, it was a sure sign I was ill. And here I was, in my mid-30s, being told that sleep was good for my soul.

In a way, it felt like liberation. I was free to say yes to the weariness that had seeped into my bones. Until I was in my room at the retreat house, in fact, experiencing silence and solitude for the first time in weeks, I had no idea I was so tired. I have since learned that this is a common experience among retreatants. We push ourselves so hard in our ordinary, workaday lives, and we become very good at pretending we're just fine, ready to face the next demand, take on the next task. But just a few moments spent alone in quiet reflection are enough to reveal our true condition. "My God, I'm tired," we say, as our house of cards collapses. If we're lucky, we can give in and rest without feeling guilty. We can stop doing and concentrate on being.

But it's not easy. There's so much to do, so many legitimate demands to meet. Why surrender to my lack of energy when I could reinvigorate myself any number of ways: take a brisk walk, drink a glass of orange juice or a cup of coffee. Isn't it just laziness on my part if I give in and do nothing?

Normally, I feel that it's important to keep going. In this I take after my mother, who at 86 is in the gym of her condominium every morning at 5:30 and attends a tai chi class three times a week. On the rare occasions when she has no energy, my mother complains. The last time it was because she had a head cold, and I advised her to take it easy. To my amazement, she stayed in bed most of the day. The next morning she phoned to say that although she did feel better, she still didn't have the energy to exercise. "Stay in bed," I said. "But I did that yesterday," she replied, indignant. I hope that I will have something of her outlook at the age of 86.

But sometimes I have to admit that I simply need to rest. I need to listen to my body when it tries to call a halt, and above all I need to remember that I am not so important in the scheme of things that I can't give up control (or the illusion of control) long enough to take time out. It's hard for me not to feel guilty when my energy isn't up to the tasks at hand. But I've found it is surprisingly easy to alter my plans, to reschedule a meeting, even—and here I do battle with my most basic instincts—to put off until tomorrow something I could do today. Today I would do it badly. Tomorrow, God willing, I'll be more rested and alert, and I'll be able to do it right. The trade-off is that sometimes I have to give up events I would love: a concert, a movie, a dinner with friends. If I can't reschedule, I lose out.

I have also had to set some ground rules. If I lack energy because I haven't slept well, I might change my habits in the evening so that I am more ready for sleep. If I've worn myself down with too much activity, I try to pace myself. And if I sense that my weariness is more than physical, if I find myself disconnecting from the world in an unhealthy way because of emotional exhaustion or depression, I seek help.

I now understand that the old monk's wisdom was grounded in that of the Psalms he'd recited every day for more than 60 years. The Psalms remind us that whether we are full of energy or drained of it, we are in God's presence. Several Psalms imply that it's when we are asleep, and not so full of ourselves and the noise of our lives, that we are best able to hear God speak to us. In Psalm 16 we read, "I will bless you, Lord. You give me counsel, and even at night direct my heart." When I can truly accept being drained of energy, I see it not as an opportunity, because that implies too much control on my part, but as an opening. It's as if a window has opened, or a door, inviting me to listen. It is liminal (literally, "threshold") time, the fertile ground between waking and sleeping, between doing and being. It is when I am half awake, before my list-making brain takes over and pretends it's in charge, that my best ideas come. But on my off days, when I am stripped of energy and feel too stupid even to think, all I can do is pray.

I might pray for those whose energy is sapped by serious illness or the depredations of old age. I might turn to the Book of Common Prayer and try to adopt the bravado of one of my favorite morning prayers: "This is another day, O Lord.... If I am to stand up, help me to stand bravely. If I am to sit still, help me to sit quietly. If I am to lie low, help me to do it patiently. And if I am to do nothing, let me do it gallantly." ●

I was shocked.
I had just been given permission to rest.
It was permission I seldom granted myself.

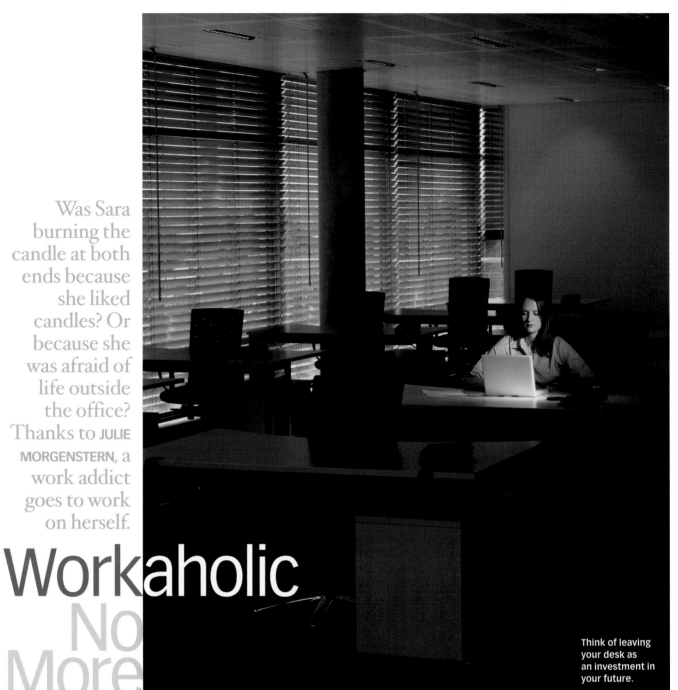

Was Sara burning the candle at both ends because she liked candles? Or because she was afraid of life outside the office? Thanks to JULIE MORGENSTERN, a work addict goes to work on herself.

Workaholic No More

Think of leaving your desk as an investment in your future.

SARA, 35 AND SINGLE, HAS NEVER led a balanced life. Every New Year's, she resolves to spend less time tied to her job at a public relations firm—but her resolution never lasts. Warm, giving, and dynamic, she's notorious among friends and family for canceling plans at the last minute because of work conflicts. En route to a brunch at her sister's one Sunday, she stopped by the office to check e-mail and never got back out the door. She joined a supper club six months ago to meet people, and has attended only one event.

The advice friends gave her was too dramatic: "Quit your job; move out of New York!" The goal of our work together was to help her make smaller, more digestible changes.

Sara's honesty was striking, a sure sign she was ready for a breakthrough. In her e-mail asking me for help, she confessed, "I give the appearance of having an incredibly demanding job, but the truth is, I often use work as an excuse for getting out of social engagements."

It's not hard to understand why work

can be a comfortable refuge. Work offers tangible results—you get the report done, land the contract, run a successful meeting. The payoffs of a personal life are harder to measure—a feeling of fulfillment, balance, energy, love.

Sara allowed that once she gets over the hump, she enjoys people's company, but getting there is a huge struggle. I asked her why. After careful thought, she said: "I get maxed out at work, taking care of my staff and clients. And many of my friends are very, very needy."

"Are all your relationships like that?" I asked. "Do you have any that give to you?"

She couldn't think of a single one. No wonder she avoided going out! Sara explained that her parents divorced when she was seven. Her mother worked constantly and her younger sister required attention, so as the oldest, Sara managed everyone's needs. She grew up with a strong work ethic, but the flip side was a deep-seated belief that it was bad to have any pleasure, relaxation, or fun.

We decided on a program of incremental, gentle changes and started by brainstorming three activities for her to try: one that would be easy, another that she felt passionately about, and a third that would be extra-challenging.

When Sara was younger, she loved taking long walks alone in nature, so her first assignment was to go on a hike. Her second was to volunteer with the elderly, a lifelong passion because her grandmother had lived with her while she was growing up.

"When I ask 'What's in it for me?' I feel selfish."

Sara's most challenging assignment was to attend the next supper club event—with a brand-new focus. Changing patterns is always easier in new relationships than in old ones. So she wouldn't jump into the role of caretaker, we came up with a rule: If someone describes a problem, *do not* offer a solution. Instead say, "I know just what you mean." And then Sara would relate a similar problem of her own.

Finally, I suggested she get a journal and record her observations, asking herself questions like *What do I enjoy? What brings me pleasure? What can people do for me?*

I checked in with Sara a week later. Although she'd made some progress, it sounded like she was pretty uncomfortable. She'd made an appointment with the volunteer coordinator of a local senior citizen center and had gone on the hike. The walk gave her moments of contentment, but it also forced her to reflect on how long she'd been hiding behind work, and she was scared. She wrote in her journal: "I don't think I have anything to offer except my help. When I look at a situation and ask 'What's in it for me?' it feels selfish and bad. If I let go of this caretaker role, is there anything else?"

Tonight was the dinner, and I could hear that Sara was terrified of being around

people without the comfort of her familiar identity, so I revised her assignment. She needn't leave the caretaker role behind completely, but she had to ask for help on a matter of her own. I gave her a question to pose to at least three people: "How do you find time for a social life?"

The dinner was a huge success. No one thought she was sucking them dry by asking advice; in fact, the entire group became captivated with the topic. Sara was stunned to discover that many people were as devoted to their personal lives as they were to their work lives. One woman explained that skipping her exercise classes was simply not an option—they make her happy, and more effective at work. Perhaps the biggest revelation of all was that these were nice, normal people—no one had horns or a tail!

Soon Sara got another lesson. Feeling the flu coming on, she took some medication and had an adverse reaction that put her in the hospital for two days. Flat on her back, unable to move, she had two shocking realizations. There were people who wanted to take care of her—but she had never let them. Despite her adamant insistence that she'd be fine, her father drove up from North Carolina, her best friend came in from D.C., and her sister came to the hospital every day. She also learned that her laissez-faire approach to making plans was hurtful to the people she loved. Sara had always thought it was easier to say yes now, to make the person feel good in the moment, and then cancel later. But her sister, her dad, and her friend confided that it made them feel unimportant every time she didn't show up. It had never dawned on Sara that her fierce independence, something she'd developed to be less of a burden, could be seen as a rejection. She ended her hospital stay determined to take her commitments more seriously.

Sara is starting her volunteer work next week, and has planned a one-week trip to Spain with her sister. She's getting together with a smaller group from the supper club on a more frequent basis. Even her coworkers have commented on how happy and productive she is. It seems, in taking care of herself, she's gotten even better at taking care of others. ●

Getting a **Life** A few steps toward balance.

- Give yourself some quiet time and ask what you're afraid of. The more honest you are, the easier it will be to address the real problem.
- Think of creating a personal life as an investment in your work. If you're refreshed and balanced, you'll be more productive.
- Measure your doses. Workaholics sometimes fear that if they take a break from work, they'll permanently lose their momentum. Start small, and slowly increase your time off as your tolerance builds.
- Keep a leisure log to track your activities—how long you spent, whether you enjoyed yourself.
- Study people whose lives are more balanced. Ask them how they do it.
- Plan something time-sensitive for immediately after work: Take a class, meet a friend for dinner, have a particular train to catch. A nonnegotiable deadline will get you out the door on time.
- Get a buddy who will leave work with you. You'll motivate each other.

I'VE ALWAYS BEEN A TYPE A, HARD-working girl, from babysitter to candy striper to part-time bank teller during my college years. My parents taught me that I could do anything and be anything I wanted to be. The good news: I believed them. The bad news: I expected to earn gold stars in everything. Moving to New York for my marriage and a career in advertising and marketing ratcheted up the pressure.

With my high-energy, can-do style, I created extra assignments and tougher deadlines—a perfect match for a fast-paced industry. I turned on the office lights many mornings and made friends with the late-night cleaning crew (kind of a class nerd turned office lunatic). After 15 years of hard work, I became CEO of a large New York ad agency with big-time, demanding clients.

My title came with a price—my life. Family vacations shrank to long weekends punctuated by frequent voice-mail checks. I was still the perfect-attendance girl, thanks in part to good health, but more because I refused to miss a day. I suppose I was guarding a mythical permanent record that couldn't withstand a single bad mark. At night I'd crash, dead asleep until I'd bolt upright at 2 a.m. to scribble ideas and leave voice messages for my associates.

Her high-stress job was eating her alive. She had no downtime at all. Then MARY LOU QUINLAN took a five-week vacation. She had no idea she was about to reinvent her life. A recovering workaholic explains it all to you.

I thought this showed how committed I was. (Looking back on it now, I imagine that "committed" was what they wanted to have done to me.)

I also harbored a secret scheme for getting some rest. I fantasized that I'd be hit by a car. Not a life-threatening accident, just a broken ankle or leg, enough to get me into a cast, off my feet, and off-limits to everybody's demands. Then one workday, a real car accident sent me to the hospital on a stretcher. Two broken ribs should have been scary enough. But far scarier was my reaction: Strapped to a gurney in the ER, I grabbed my husband's cell phone to freak out with apologies for being late for a presentation.

By 1998, midsize agencies like ours were being squeezed out, and the emotional overload took a great toll. Like many women, I was empathetic to everyone's problems but my own. Finally, a concerned friend suggested I needed some serious downtime. That obvious insight had never occurred to me, but I was so exhausted and at my wit's end that I turned a mental corner.

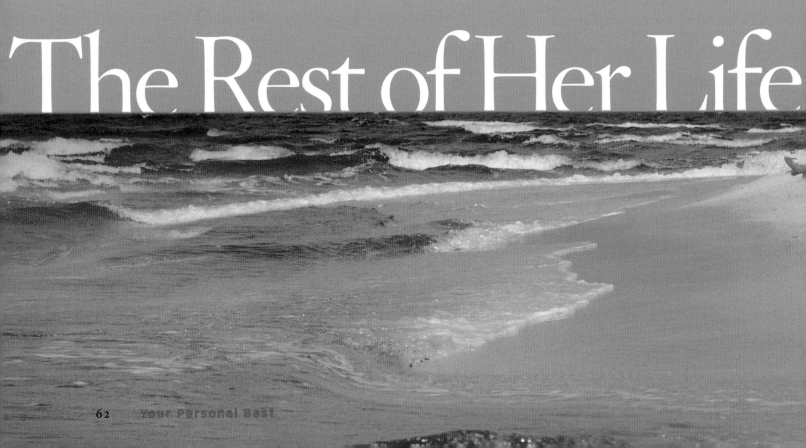

The Rest of Her Life

I decided to ask for five weeks, and I was so intent on taking them that I was prepared to quit if my boss—the head of our parent company—said no. I put together a "while I'm away" plan that, in type A fashion, included nine client events that I would still attend. "Give me your pen," my boss said. He drew a line through the entire list. "Make this the most selfish time of your life."

My 45th birthday was day one. For the next five weeks, I went cold turkey: no calls, no correspondence, no meetings, nothing. What I loved best were the pages and pages of blankness on my calendar. I was so used to seeing my days chopped into half-hour slots, each minute clogged with someone else's agenda. Instead I'd wake up and ask, "What do I want to do today?" and fill my un-agenda with fun or rest or people I love. I admit that for the first two days, I checked my office voice mail. Then I just let go.

I learned what it felt like to sip coffee while the sun shone in my apartment. I wandered around my Greenwich Village neighborhood. I watched my high school girlfriend teach poetry to her class of 8-year-olds. I dated my husband. I went to Latin dance lessons, had lunch with friends, decaf-ed myself, and took naps. I became reacquainted with the girl I once was and the woman I had become.

And I was able to think about what I wanted to do next. I'd always been fascinated by women consumers, and I started to visualize a business that would help companies understand them better.

At the end of the five weeks, I said two words I had never said in my life: I quit. It wasn't what my boss was hoping to hear, but he was intrigued enough by my concept to invite me to start up the venture within the framework of my agency's parent company, a real financial boost. Best of all, I could create the business to fit my time and my goals and still have room for a life.

That was five years ago. I didn't turn from a type A to a type zzz. Many days I work just as hard as I did at the agency. The difference is that I'm doing things I love, and I protect my rest stops. I work out regularly. I don't do the late-night shift any-more. Weekends are weekends. And my family comes first.

Many women tell me they can't take a break because they have children or money worries or feel vulnerable in their jobs. But I think the real reason is that we resist being selfish. Perhaps we unconsciously make our list of "shoulds" so long that our turn never comes; we're afraid of what the quiet hours might reveal to us.

If you're postponing your own time off, answer these questions: When did you last feel really happy about the day ahead of you? If you picture yourself six months from now living the exact same schedule, how do you feel? If you've been at this pace for ten years or more and can project working another 20 or 30, isn't there one little window that you could carve out as your own?

I believe it's time women give themselves permission to rest. Perhaps we can begin a movement together. Here's what I can tell you: From day one of my sabbatical, I felt this incredible lightness. I enjoyed the first good night's sleep I'd had in years—but not the last. It's your turn. ●

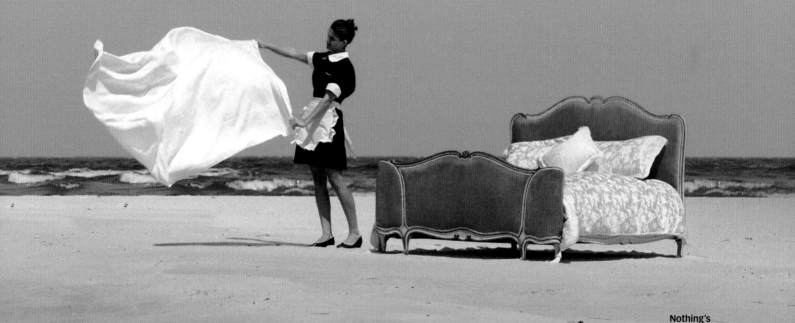

Nothing's as invigorating as mentally cleaning house.

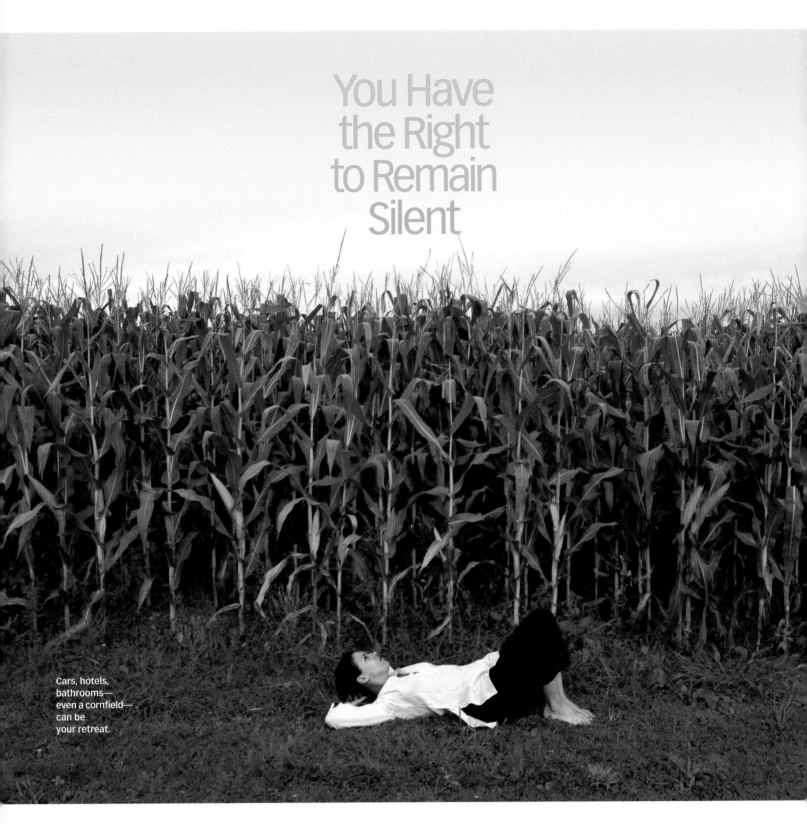

You Have the Right to Remain Silent

Cars, hotels, bathrooms—even a cornfield—can be your retreat.

Your cell phone is ringing. Your in-box is overflowing. Your friend wants to discuss her son's glue-sniffing habit. MARTHA BECK has news for you—you don't have to Be There for all people all the time. Just follow her escape routes.

THIS MONTH I SET OUT TO WRITE a thoughtful essay on the art of disconnecting. My thesis: The great English writer E.M. Forster may have valued connection above all else, but for us 21st-century folks—with our jam-packed Rolodexes, e-mail from intimates and strangers, phone messages left by friends, colleagues, passing acquaintances, and the occasional deranged stalker—disconnection is as necessary as connection for creating a healthy, happy life. When we force ourselves to connect against our heart's desires, we create false, resentful relationships; when we disconnect from the people who deplete us, we set them free to

Martha Beck's Favorite Disconnection Techniques

1. Hide.

I'm sitting in my room at a beautiful wilderness retreat where intelligent, sensitive, wonderful people come to renew their spirits. I've been running a workshop meant to stir the deepest reaches of the participants' fears and dreams. I've also been living on tap water and protein bars because the thought of going to the dining hall, where I would end up connecting for another hour with those intelligent, sensitive, wonderful people, makes me want to shoot myself.

calm my strung-out nerves—or yours. If you don't already have a cornfield, find one now.

2. Go primitive.

We all know that technological advances have made connection easier than ever before. They've also led some people to think that breaking away is a violation of the social order. Friends call to chastise each other (well, anyway, my friends call to chastise me) for being slow to return text messages or e-mail, as though the ability to communicate in half a dozen newfangled ways makes constant attention to every one of them morally imperative.

[**I've been known to hide** for days, but even a few minutes can calm my strung-out nerves—or yours. If you don't already have a "cornfield," find one now.]

find their tribes while we find ours. I planned to illustrate these thoughts with snippets of Greek philosophy, and perhaps even the poetry of Robert Frost.

But it has just occurred to me that this refined approach is not how I actually disconnect—and I need to disconnect a lot. Overconnection is my major occupational hazard.

My job is all about soulfully linking with others, and this is truly as much fun as I've ever had with my clothes on, but after doing this with many people for many hours, I often feel as if I've watched ten great movies back-to-back: dazed, frazzled, longing for silent solitude. I'm not up to gracious separation; I need quick-and-dirty ways to save my sanity, right now.

So I've listed some of my favorite disconnection strategies below, in the hope that you might find them useful. Please remember that this advice is not for the E.M. Forsters of the world but for those of us who are already connected up the wazoo.

I packed for this trip with disconnection aforethought, tossing in 20 protein bars with the express intention of hiding out. Blame my high school English teacher—I'll call her Mrs. Jensen—who married at 17, bore her first child at 19, and was a farmwife and mother of four by age 22. When she felt overwhelmed, she'd retreat into a field of tall corn near her house and hide there, listening to her children search for her, until she heard a cry of genuine pain or felt ready to reconnect, whichever came first.

"Martha," Mrs. Jensen told me, "every woman needs a cornfield. No matter what's happening in your life, find yourself a cornfield and hide there whenever you need to."

All these years later, this advice still gives me permission to sit here by myself contemplating whether I should eat the nondairy creamer from my in-room coffee setup, just for variety. I've used hundreds of other "cornfields" over the years: cars, forests, hotels, bathrooms. I've been known to hide for days, but even a few minutes can

At such times, I become downright Amish, religiously committed to avoiding all modern communication technology. I unplug phones, computers, intercoms, and fax machines, risking opprobrium because I know that if I don't lose touch with some of the people who are trying to reach me, I'll lose touch with myself. The overconnected me is a cranky, tired fussbudget. Silence is golden if it keeps me from broadcasting that fretful self into my network of treasured relationships.

3. Play favorites.

Your ability to connect is a resource much more precious than money, so manage it well. Make a list of everyone to whom you feel bonded, then consider what kind of return you're getting on your investment. Which relationships make you feel robbed or depleted? Which ones enrich you? Notice that there are many ways for "connection investments" to pay off. One person may be good at helping you solve relationship problems, while another can fix your home computer and another makes you laugh. A baby's trust may be the only return you get on a massive investment of time and energy, but it can feel like winning the lottery.

It may sound cold-blooded to say you must divest yourself of the relationships that give you consistent losses, but unless you do this, you'll soon run out of capital, and you'll have no connection energy left to invest in anybody. So please, decide now to deliberately limit the time and attention

5. Be insensitive.

A friend I'll call Zoe once went to a world-famous psychologist to discuss her recurring nightmares. After months of waiting for an appointment, she finally met the therapist, who asked why she had come.

"I'm having terrible dreams," Zoe explained.

"Yeah?" grunted the famous psychologist. "So what?"

Zoe blinked, then stammered, "Well, they keep me awake."

"Uh-huh. So?"

an airport, eager to share personal problems and ask for solutions, I may point behind them and say, "Oh, my gosh! Is that Dr. Phil?" Then, when their head snaps around, owl-like, I sprint for the nearest restroom.

I'm sure you can come up with better getaway lines than these, but do take the time to rehearse several reliable alternatives. Because when you're exhausted, a practiced excuse can keep you from wading deeper into relationships you don't need and can't handle.

> I know that if I don't lose touch with some of the people who are trying to reach me, I'll lose touch with myself.

you spend on "low yield" relationships. Above all...

4. Get rid of squid.

Squid is my word for people who seem to be missing their backbones but possess myriad sucking tentacles of emotional need. Like many invertebrates, squid appear limp and squishy—but once they get a grip on you, they're incredibly powerful. Masters at catalyzing guilt and obligation, they operate by squeezing pity from everyone they meet. They can make you feel entwined to the point of rage, desperate to escape their clutches, unable to see a means to extricate yourself.

Getting a squid out of your life is never pretty. (Excuses don't work—tell a squid you're on your way to a colonoscopy, and they'll come along to sit beside you, complaining, while your doctor performs the procedure.) Since you can't make a graceful exit, don't try. Scrape off squid any way you can. Tell them straightforwardly that you want them, yes *them,* to leave now, yes *now*. This will be unpleasant. There will be lasting hurt feelings. Don't worry. Squid love hurt feelings. They hoard them, trading them in for pity points when they find another victim—er, friend. Let them go, their coffers bulging.

"Well...," stammered Zoe, "I guess I never thought of it that way." And her nightmares went away, never to return. Once she stopped treating bad dreams like the end of the world, her mind had no reason to replay them.

I'm not suggesting that you say "So what?" every time someone turns to you for help, but I like to think that therapist was famous for a reason. I suspect he could feel the difference between something that required deep discussion and something that didn't. He was willing to be insensitive, alerting Zoe to her own hypersensitivity.

This is a very compassionate way to use your own psychological instincts. Instead of connecting with every person's problems, let yourself feel whether someone really needs your attention, or whether the best gift you can give might be a little abruptness.

6. Rehearse escape lines.

When I'm overextended, I paradoxically become worse at setting boundaries. I end up resorting to rehearsed exit lines. "Oh, there's my doorbell!" I might say to end a client call that's run 20 minutes over (this is technically true: My doorbell is, in fact, there). When someone collars me in

7. Be shallow.

Even staying in touch with a reasonably small number of high-quality people can be overwhelming if you tend toward emotional intensity. In such cases, shallowness can be a delightful alternative. So instead of discussing Schopenhauer with your beloved in meaningful, calligraphed epistles, e-mail a stupid joke. Gather your friends to watch TV shows in which strangers paint one another's rooms the color of phlegm and then feign mutual delight.

Once you know you can swim in the deep end of human connection, it's fun to splash around in the shallows.

I HOPE YOU FIND THESE DISCON-nection strategies as useful as I do. By striking a balance between the imperative to "only connect" and the need for individuation, you really will relax your psyche and your relationships, making your life as a whole more joyful, more loving.

Maybe someday we'll meet to compare notes, to share disconnection experiences as well as time, space, and perhaps a protein bar. But right now, I'm sure you'll understand when I say that I'd like to eat this one all by myself. ●

O
Happiness

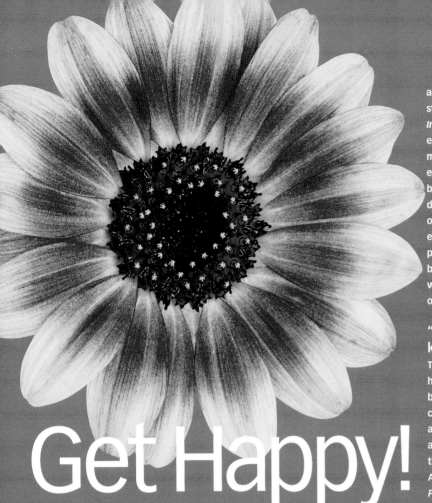

Get Happy!

We've all got little homegrown tricks for cheering ourselves up. **Lauren Gravitz** finds out why they actually work.

I've succumbed to full-blown depression just once, and the only good that came of it was learning that I never wanted to experience anything like it again. So I started collecting little mood-boosting tricks—not cure-alls for clinical depression but small, helpful ways to pull myself back from the edge. After polling friends and colleagues, I discovered that many of them had stumbled upon the same techniques, and they gave me a few new ones, too. Science is beginning to explain why they actually work, which means that these days I don't feel completely ridiculous when I'm in my car and someone catches me belting out a Beatles song.

"I rent a bunch of stand-up comedy DVDs."

THE SCIENCE A smile, even a forced one, can improve your mood. In a widely confirmed study, psychologist Fritz Strack, PhD, and his colleagues at the University of Mannheim in Germany had participants view a cartoon while gripping a pen either between their teeth (to simulate a smile) or between puckered lips. The first group found the cartoons funnier, supporting the theory of "facial feedback"—the idea that facial expressions can stimulate emotion. A Fairleigh Dickinson University study showed that laughing brightens mood even more than smiling.

"I go for a run."

THE SCIENCE Research has consistently shown that exercise can significantly impact depression and improve overall mood. A 1999 study published in the *Archives of Internal Medicine* showed that exercise could be as effective as medication. Scientists aren't exactly sure why it works so well: because it relieves stress, acts as a distraction, stimulates production of neurotransmitters (including endorphins—which have painkilling properties and can bring feelings of euphoria—as well as serotonin and dopamine), or all of the above.

"I try to commit acts of kindness."

THE SCIENCE Volunteering at a hospital or shelter, tutoring a budding reader, and even donating clothes to Goodwill facilitate a "helper's high." The benefits of altruism are most apparent when there's person-to-person contact. Allan Luks, author of *The Healing Power of Doing Good,* has found that simply recalling a charitable act brings back the same, albeit less intense, good mood.

"I listen to Madonna, sing loudly, and dance around the living room."

THE SCIENCE A number of studies suggest that listening to music stimulates the brain to release endorphins. Recent research at the University of Manchester in England showed that listening to loud music activates a part of the inner ear called the saccule, which is connected to an area of the brain responsible for drives like hunger, sex, and pleasure seeking.

"I buy bright red tulips."

THE SCIENCE A 2001 Rutgers University study on the mood-lifting effect of flowers showed that 72 percent of seniors who received one or two bouquets over a six-month period were happier than they had been. In a separate study, flowers evoked a stronger response than other gifts.

"I hang out with friends."

THE SCIENCE Numerous studies have documented the benefits of social support, while others have shown that isolation can lead to depression. According to a study at the University of Michigan, even more important than social support is a sense of belonging: Connecting with and confiding in close friends can allay despair.

"I snuggle the dog."

THE SCIENCE Two studies published in 1999 showed that both AIDS patients and senior citizens benefit from having pets; those with animals were less likely to suffer from depression than those without. An earlier study showed that pet owners were also at decreased risk of heart disease.

"I make like a cat—I find a patch of sunlight streaming through the window, curl up, and fall asleep in the warmth."

THE SCIENCE A common cause of depression is seasonal affective disorder (SAD), in which lack of sunlight increases the production of melatonin, a hormone that affects sleep patterns and mood. Some therapists believe that even people not affected by SAD can reap the rewards of sunshine— one study of depressed pregnant women showed that a daily dose of bright light for three weeks had a beneficial effect.

"I change the landscape."

THE SCIENCE Perhaps it's the calming properties of the ocean or a starry sky, or the way a new setting can take you out of yourself and provide a sense of perspective. Although scientific research is scarce, a good number of people mentioned that a change of scenery, especially one that gets you back to nature, is an instant head clearer. ●

Can New Shoes Make You Happy?

Yes, of course they can. Call us shallow, but we're buying **Valerie Monroe's** case for the therapeutic properties of pretty things.

MY ANCIENT AUNT ESTHER WAS often cranky, but when I was little I didn't notice. She allowed me to sit very close, enveloped in a cloud of her powdery lilac-water scent, close enough that I could take one and then the other of her soft, perfectly manicured hands in mine, run my small fingers over her pink, slightly opalescent nails, examine her bracelets—burnished gold bangles and links laden heavily with charms, one or two from each city she had visited around the world. Her earrings—only clip-ons—were intricate: tiny, coralline Bakelite blossoms or clusters of freshwater pearls. Aunt Esther was captivating, a museum of adornment and style. Seeing her, despite her unpredictable disposition, always made me happy.

Most of us have an intrinsic interest in pretty things. Don't you? At a work-related party the other night, I was standing around with several other beauty editors waiting somewhat impatiently for the action to begin when I suddenly noticed that the woman next to me was wearing—along with a lovely but understated skirt and sweater set—crimson pumps. "Oh, your shoes!" I said admiringly, and she smiled as she raised her foot, turning it this way and that so I could see the delicate princess heel. "They make me so happy," she said. "All I have to do is look at them, and it lifts me right up."

No surprise in that, says Valerie Steele, PhD, director of the Museum at the Fashion Institute of Technology. "Buying a new pair of shoes, or something even as small as a lipstick, resonates with the idea that we are loved, because it is a kind of gift we give to ourselves." It may also make us feel renewed, transformed. Ornament yourself with a pair of sparkling earrings or a rope of creamy pearls, a brilliant, rich lipcolor or

a quiet, delicate one, and people can see that you have made an effort, a choice to do yourself up. There is meaning in that effort, says Anne Hollander, historian and writer on art and dress; you are honoring and respecting your physical self and presenting it to the world. But it's not only your intention that lifts and engages you, she says, it's the response: Though appreciative glances may go by in a second, when we get them, they make us happy.

Adorning ourselves seems to be as profoundly human as speech, says Steele; we are the only species that does it. Even in cultures where people don't wear clothes (or much of them), they will drape themselves in jewelry (or flowers, shells, and other nature-made treasures) or ornament their hair. It's one of the ways we communicate, says Steele.

On a warm July day about ten years ago, I boarded a bus in a small city in India; I think I was the only Western passenger—I'm pretty sure I was the only Western woman. I know I felt like a foreigner in my khakis, white blouse, Keds, and a head scarf I'd never wear at home. Just as the bus lurched into traffic, I found a seat next to an Indian woman wearing a sari and sandals and lots of interesting jewelry. She politely scooched over a bit to make room for me. From the moment I sat down, we began to peek at each other from the corners of our eyes. My glance fell again and again on the

richly embroidered fabric of her sari, on her beautiful glass bangles and silver rings. She was glancing at my own silver bracelets, the pink-gold Deco pinkie ring my father had made for my mother in the 1940s. Finally, seeing that she was looking at my ring, I held my hand over for her to examine it. "Do you like it?" I asked, at which point she turned toward me and we began a very lively and intimate exchange about what each of us was wearing and where it all came from. I learned where she bought her sari fabric and how she came by her bracelets; I learned that she was a lawyer on her way to work and that she was planning one day to travel. I don't remember her name. But I do remember her resplendent carnelian ring and the happiness we both had admiring it. •

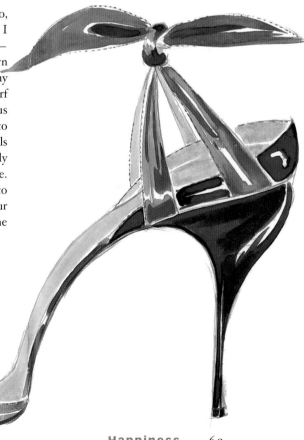

The Pursuit of Cold, Hard Happiness

No, money can't buy you happiness (you knew that). But happiness can work wonders for your bank balance. SUZE ORMAN **does the math.**

MONEY AND HAPPINESS ARE TWO of the most powerful forces in our lives, but what's so interesting to me is how we've convinced ourselves that there's a powerful connection between them: We seem to think that if we were rich, our lives would be perfect. My friends, I hope I can convince you otherwise.

The Money Myth

In my years of talking to thousands of people who've had no money, some money, and heaps of money, I've found that it doesn't create or sustain happiness. That's not to say that money isn't an important factor in our emotional state—if we can't pay our bills and support our families, we carry a great deal of stress on our shoulders and in our hearts. But it's seriously flawed logic to jump from a position of "money is important" to "money is the key to happiness." Need some proof? How about the articles we've all read about lottery winners who buy a ton of goodies after they hit the jackpot, but within a few years tell the world how out of control and miserable their lives are? I know a lottery winner who was doing just fine before she won a penny, but since her big payday she's become a financial disaster with more debt than she had in her pre-winning days.

My friend's situation is not unique. Money often compounds unhappiness because, mistakenly, we think that spending will make us feel better. It reminds me of how some of us have a screwy relationship with food. When we're unhappy, we gorge on comfort foods that we believe, either consciously or subconsciously, will make us feel better. Sure, that hot fudge sundae might give us a nice temporary lift, just like buying a great new handbag or outfit—but it's temporary. Those indulgences do nothing for our true sense of happiness. In fact, they can create unhappiness in the form of unwanted weight gain or a huge credit card bill.

Truth and Consequences

The average U.S. household has a credit card balance of about $8,000. It's hard to be happy when you carry an $8,000 balance on a credit card that charges 18 percent interest. My message to you is that happiness is not tied to how much money you have—how much you had in the past or hope to have in the future—but how you deal with what you have right now.

I want to be very clear that I fully understand that it's far more difficult to live on $20,000 a year than $200,000. I know this from personal experience; until I was 29, I was a waitress bringing home $400 a month. But I also know that we all have the capacity to take control of our lives—regardless of our bank accounts—and to commit to making the right decisions for ourselves and our family. When we do that, we're on the road to happiness. Without a sense of well-being, all the money that flows into our lives will quickly flow out. When we're strong and happy, we don't feel the need to lease a fancy car we can't afford only to impress our friends. We don't need to buy the latest fashions if it means running up a credit card balance. We don't need to spend $70 a month on lattes and then complain we have no money to invest in a retirement fund. When you're happy, you create your own financial stability by living within your means.

So how do we get to the place where we have a healthy relationship with our money and are not expecting it to change our lives? "Finances: The Spring Cleanup," below, lists some of the ways I think unhappy people deal with money. If you can tackle those roadblocks, not only will you be more financially stable but your fears about money will vanish. I've also included practical advice to get you moving toward a happier you, but your biggest challenge is to first clear out the obstacles in your head and heart that keep you from making smarter financial moves. Money won't determine your emotional state of being, but your emotional state of being certainly will affect how you deal with money. With the right approach, you can be happy no matter the specifics of your financial situation.

Power Moves

In my experience, most people are unhappy because they aren't being honest with themselves. Being truthful with yourself plugs you into your inner power.

> When you're happy, you create your own financial **stability** by living within your means.

Whether it's your relationship with money or with a partner, you aren't going to be content or successful until you are connected to your heart and operating with all your energy. And that requires a commitment to a life based on honesty in every aspect. If you can pull that off, it's virtually impossible not to be happy. When friends invite you to dinner at a fancy-pants place

that will break your budget, you'll be honest and tell them you would love to get together, but because you're watching your finances, could they meet at your place for potluck instead? You won't run up a big credit card balance, and you'll find a way to start paying more than the required monthly minimum so you can get rid of your debt. By getting your hair cut every seven weeks rather than every five, you could save $30 to $60 a month. Going to the movies twice a month rather than three times could save close to $40, when you consider the cost of two tickets plus popcorn and soda. Quite simply, by making the right choices from a position of strength rather than weakness, you are bound to be happy. In part you'll feel better because your finances are in good shape, and also because you took the initiative to create a life based on honesty. In my book, that's the priceless route to ultimate happiness. ●

Finances: The Spring Cleanup

It's always a good time of year to do some spring-cleaning in our financial lives.

You know you need to reach for the mop if:
- You don't pay off your credit card balance every month.
- Your credit card balance exceeds your monthly paycheck.
- You pay your bills late, incurring costly fees.
- You spend $10 a day on coffee, snacks, and cabs, yet you don't invest in a retirement fund.
- You eat at expensive restaurants that are so out of your price range that you lose your appetite.
- You have clothes that have never been worn and still have their tags.
- Your closets are jammed with impulse purchases—grills, dehumidifiers, toys for the kids—that have never been used.
- You buy things you can't afford.

If you recognize yourself in this list, what you can do now is:
- Make bill paying a monthly ritual—with your partner, if you live with someone. Put on some good music; open a bottle of wine. Do whatever it takes to commit to this.

- Always pay your bills on time and never go over your credit limit, which can save you $25 a month or more. By paying on time and paying in full, you'll save yourself a lot of money and stress.

- Find an extra $50 or $100 a month so you can pay more than the monthly minimum on your credit card balance. Come on, give up one trip to the movies and one dinner out a month and you'll save about $50. Do you realize how much more money you'll have if you stop paying the credit card company 18 percent interest?

- Once your balance is paid off, keep making those extra payments—to yourself. That's your retirement fund, the money to pay off your student loan, or the down payment on your first home.

- Clear your closets of every unused and unwanted item, and donate it all to charity. The tax deduction is a great financial move.

- If you haven't been balancing your checkbook, it's time to start over. Open a new checking account. Pay off your outstanding bills from your old account and close it. From now on, do all your banking from this new account. Balance it every month and track those ATM transactions. By closely following your spending, you will never live beyond your means.

Please take these steps to living a life that's truthful. Once your finances are in shape, you're bound to be happy.

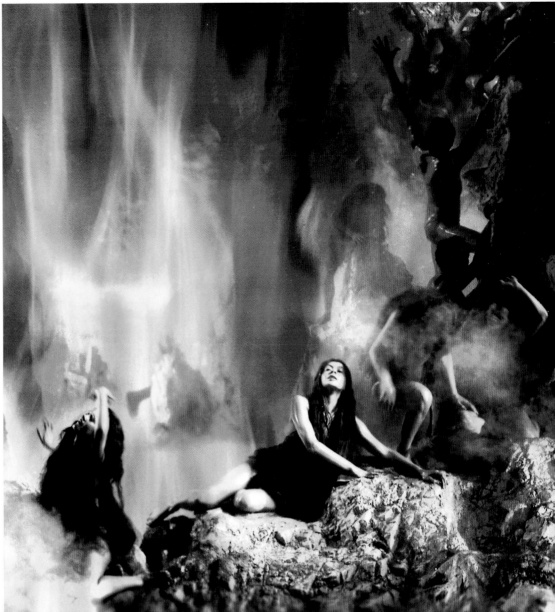

Is it hell being you? Good news: You may have just taken the first step toward finding peace of mind. **DAWN RAFFEL** sits down with an inspired pair of psychotherapists.

The Divine Therapy

IF YOU'RE SEEKING PEACE OF MIND, emotional fulfillment, and a sense of your place in the world, try looking in hell. We're not talking about your Sunday-school teacher's fire-and-brimstone inferno but the one you've built for yourself in the privacy of your own mind. According to husband-and-wife psychotherapists Bonney and Richard Schaub, the road to enduring solace begins,

Break out of the inferno of your self-created torments.

inevitably, with a tour of your home-honed torture chambers.

The Schaubs' personal journey, which led to their book, *Dante's Path* (Gotham), began 30 years ago. Frustrated that traditional therapy failed to address spiritual needs—and that so many apparently successful people they met seemed to feel lost in their lives—they stumbled on the work of an Italian analyst named Roberto Assagioli. A student of Freud, Assagioli had rejected the master to develop something called psychosynthesis, which rests on the belief that we're each capable of reaching beyond our personalities, that we can grasp transcendent wisdom—but only if we first take a long, hard look at how we contribute to our suffering.

Born in a Jewish ghetto in 1888, Assagioli was no stranger to the kind of hardships we can't control. He was imprisoned by the Fascists (for being a pacifist), then freed, only to be forced into hiding during the Nazi occupation. Shortly after the war, his only child died. He deeply understood the pain that life can visit on us, yet insisted that a profound, healing wisdom is always

accolades—anything to fill the emptiness inside); jealousy; intentional cruelty; betrayal; and addiction. We're in "purgatory" when we become aware of our self-created torments and consciously work to release ourselves, and rise to "paradise" when we tap into our higher wisdom, our universal connection with others.

Combining traditional therapeutic techniques with meditation, visualization, and even contemplation of art, the Schaubs have helped cancer, cardiac, and AIDS patients gain relief from depression and rage. They've also led clients with marital strife, career anxiety, and garden-variety angst to recognize their role in their problems as a first step in getting unstuck.

The Schaubs' view of addiction is particularly eye-opening: "It isn't just about drugs and alcohol," Bonney says. "Some

I'll do that, and if X happens, I'll do Y—so she probably won't end up on the street. Then she feels temporarily relieved, as though she had a drink. But it's destroying her stomach," Richard says. "To liberate your consciousness, you have to recognize these patterns and actively help free yourself."

Looking in your dark corners takes guts—but the eventual payoff might be extraordinary. "So many people feel a nagging sense that they're not getting something, some promise hasn't been fulfilled," Richard says. "Our understanding is that we have potentials we don't have a name for and we don't know how to make them active. That's part of the spiritual journey, to discover those capacities."

"When Dante started to write *The Divine Comedy,* he had lost everything," Bonney says. "He needed to face his losses

> "We all use a limited amount of **consciousness.** If it's absorbed
> in hell patterns—fear-based instincts and the reactions
> we develop around them—that means we're unable to
> discover other parts of ourselves."

available. He found his internal Mapquest not in modern science but in Dante's 14th-century masterpiece, *The Divine Comedy*. Written while Dante was in exile, this epic poem depicts the progress of "the Pilgrim" on a guided tour of hell and purgatory, and finally into an illuminated paradise. While Dante's frame of reference was Catholicism, Assagioli read his work metaphorically, as an exploration of our inner realms, a model of personal transformation.

"The idea," Richard Schaub says, sitting in the Manhattan office where he and Bonney use psychosynthesis to treat clients with 21st-century problems, "is that we all use a limited amount of consciousness. If it's absorbed in hell patterns—fear-based instincts and the reactions we develop around them—that means we're unable to discover other parts of ourselves." We create our own hell, the Schaubs believe, through indifference (attempting to protect ourselves by assuming an air of not caring); greed (insatiably craving money, stuff,

people say, 'I'm a shopaholic,' or that kind of thing. But the next step is to understand how habitual *thoughts* stop us. For example, someone I work with has a hard time taking in all the things she has accomplished. There's a part of her that's tremendously envious of other people." She can now watch that misery-making process start in her thinking, Bonney says: "She goes into a social situation and compares herself—that person looks better than she does, that woman's younger, that person makes more money. It becomes completely self-defeating. It takes over the way a drug does. But it goes back to her survival instincts from childhood. This was her way of taking care of herself—having to always be the best and the smartest and the prettiest to get the attention she needed."

Worry, Richard says, can also be addictive. "I know a highly successful woman with tons of money in the bank, but she obsessively thinks about every horrible thing that could happen—*If this goes wrong,*

and then find a way to still feel hope and connection." Dante spent the last years of his life reaching for higher states of consciousness, and he taught that love—an ego-transcending unity—is the source of all joy. "I see people today who are so identified with a job and then the job isn't there, and the first response is, *Oh my God, this is unimaginable*. But once they get past the shock, a lot of people start to reconnect with what's really important to them. And they're grateful. They wouldn't have chosen to be thrown into this position, but it got them to reevaluate what they want to do with their lives, what they want to put their energy into." And their vulnerability can bring them closer to other people, "to a sense of union as opposed to separateness," Bonney says. "Having listened to so many people's stories, I can read what Dante wrote and recognize it as true and feel tremendously encouraged by the fact that literature and art can touch human truth at such a deep level." •

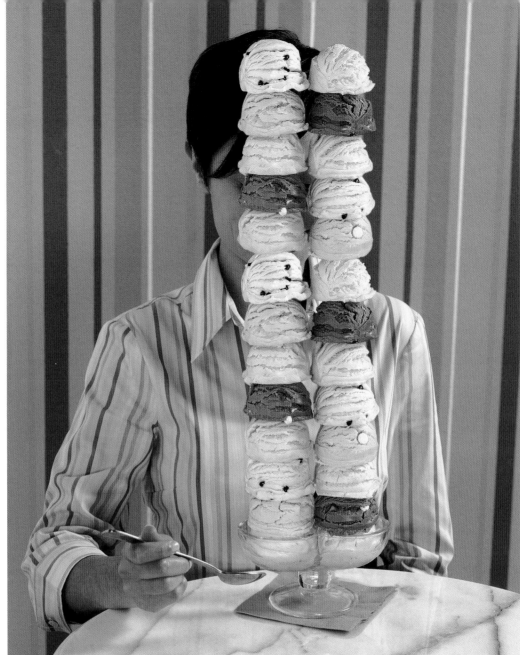

The Joy Diet

In her delightful book, **MARTHA BECK** concocts a recipe for a fuller, happier, all-around zingier life. If that sounds appetizing, may we suggest menu item no. 10?

I HAD JUST TRAVELED HOME FROM SINGAPORE TO ATTEND my sister's wedding. Now, a week later, I was back in Asia. My circadian rhythm was bewildered by two massive time-zone changes, so I was pleased to stumble across a magazine article about overcoming jet lag. The key, it said, was scheduling food intake. Travelers are supposed to eat at certain times and strictly abstain from food the remainder of the day. The article listed "feast/fast" schedules for several travel itineraries. I eagerly looked up mine. The chart said something like "feast, fast, feast, fast, fast, feast," as if the author were sending a message in some kind of dietetic Morse code. But in my bleary-eyed

Sundaes are good, but the Joy Diet has feasts for all the senses.

incoherence, I misread the words. I thought the prescription said "feast, feast, feast, feast, feast, feast."

I felt a spontaneous smile ripple through my whole body. I was authorized for constant feasting! As an American female, I was accustomed to thinking that the occasional ounce of chopped celery was a righteous and appropriate diet. The word *feast* brought back memories of childhood Thanksgivings, when I was too young to be diet conscious; the lovely chaos of sounds, sights, and aromas that swirled around me as my enormous family sat down at a heavily laden

HOW TO THROW A FEAST

The most common definition of the word *feast,* of course, is a large meal. Most Joy Diet feasts, however, don't involve food, and a big bunch o' food won't always qualify as a Joy Diet feast. A compulsive eating binge, for example, is the opposite of feasting. It is isolating and tasteless and sickening; it robs delight from both the senses and the soul. On the other hand, hearing a symphony or touching the curve of your lover's elbow could definitely count as a feast, provided that you pay the right kind of attention.

not. For example, you may follow the same pattern of actions every night before you go to sleep, when you drink a cup of coffee, or when you exercise. In the spaces below, write down anything you do that typically involves a set pattern of action.

**Celebratory Rituals
I Already Observe**

1._____
2._____
3._____

Don't hide love. If you feel it, express it—not to demand that others love you back, but simply to live outwardly the best of what you feel inwardly.

table. Those feasts had been loud and obstreperous and wonderful, and I had given them up for lost.

Within a few seconds, I realized that I'd misread the jet lag article. No, I did not have permission to indulge myself in nonstop feasts. I remember sighing with disappointment, but even so, something had changed. For the first time in years, I'd allowed myself to picture life full of feasts, and that glimpse was so seductive that it never completely faded. It took another decade or so, but I finally decided that I not only could but should "feast, feast, feast, feast, feast, feast."

Now I live that way all the time. I don't mean that I never stop eating. I mean that every day I remind myself to return to the spirit of feasting. This is part of a program I call the Joy Diet, a regimen designed not for the body but for the inner self (the word *diet* originally didn't mean an eating program; it was a way of living). To go on the Joy Diet, you add certain simple behaviors to your daily routine, practices that will improve your life whether you're feeling just a bit dreary or utterly confined to the pits. Feasting (Joy Diet–style) means adding an element of attention and structure to events that otherwise might slip by as too ordinary for comment. Doing this can turn the most ordinary situations into celebrations.

It helps to perform some kind of ritual that will direct your attention to the symbolic significance of your actions. A ritual, however simple, creates a border around an activity the way a frame does around a picture. It sets this activity apart from regular life in a way that emphasizes beauty and uniqueness, ensuring that those who participate in it become more aware of its meaning.

I've watched my own children, who grew up with very little ritual, develop their own ways of formalizing celebration, as though the need to do this came precoded in their brains.

One year, while learning the distinction between Christmas, Hanukkah, and Kwanza, the kids asked me about their own ethnic heritage. I explained that their ancestors were Celtic and Scandinavian, so we should probably observe the winter solstice, maybe by—I dunno—wearing Viking helmets, painting our faces blue, and eating venison. I was joking, but my children were so entranced by this idea that we actually started doing it (though we substitute steaks for wild game). This is now one of our family's cherished yearly rituals, one that strengthens our bonds to one another by reinforcing other people's belief that we are insane.

You probably perform dozens of small rituals already, whether you realize it or

If the most meaningful rituals you already observe involve preparing the washer for the addition of fabric softener, you might want to add some with a bit more psychological oomph. Here are some suggestions for ritualizing, and thereby feast-ifying, some ordinary events that can and should be extraordinary.

FEASTING ON FOOD

Though the Joy Diet isn't a typical food regimen, it does have two strict rules about eating. They are:

1. You must eat only what you really enjoy.

2. You must really enjoy everything you eat.

This means that if you want a fudge sundae and you substitute raw broccoli, you're totally blowing your diet. On the other hand, if you're happily inhaling your sundae and you start to feel uncomfortably full, the Joy Diet requires that you stop eating immediately.

I settled on these two rules to normalize my own eating, which, believe me, was no easy task. Having danced a few youthful numbers with an eating disorder, I've done plenty of fasting, as well as my share

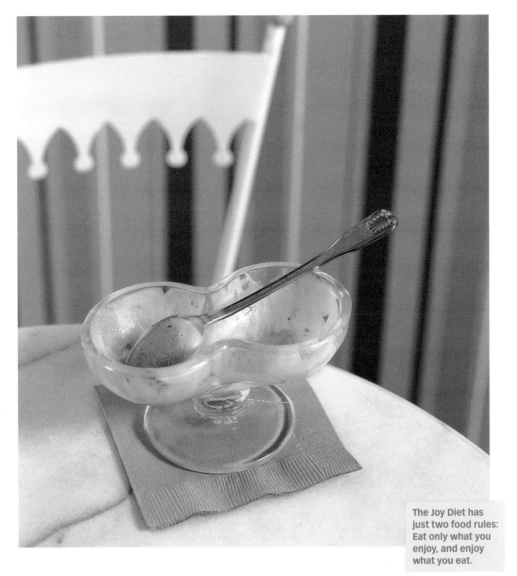

issues, eating what you enjoy and enjoying what you eat can turn the simplest meal into a festive event. At each meal, feed your body what it requests, without judgment or stinginess. Spend an extra buck on a really satisfying snack, rather than a cheaper but less tasty substitute. Get the original-recipe treat instead of the gritty, boring, low-fat foodlike product sitting next to it. Keep asking your body—it will tell you exactly what it prefers.

FEASTING ON BEAUTY

Food-feasts are particularly gratifying to the senses of taste and smell. However, the Joy Diet encourages you to indulge in feasts for the other senses as well. We usually apply the term *beautiful* to things that appeal either to our eyes or our ears. Seeking these kinds of delights is what I call a beauty-feast.

I had a beauty-feast right after my first book tour, a grueling affair that involved discussing the book I'd written until I hated to talk about it. By the tour's end, the thought of saying another word made me want to hurl myself into a volcano. I retreated home with just one thought in my head: orange. I don't mean the fruit, or even the word *orange.* I was obsessed with the color. I was entranced by sunsets and poppies, but also by traffic cones and bags of Chee-tos. I bought a canvas and spent several days painting it with orange of every tone and hue, parking myself in the visual right side of my brain while my verbal left side recharged its batteries. It was one long, delicious feast for my eyes, and a much-needed rest for what little was left of my mind.

A visual beauty-feast can be even more enthralling if you add auditory pleasures, such as music, the thunder of waves, or crickets' song. In the spaces below, jot down three things that appeal to your eyes, then to your ears.

Ideas for Beauty-Feasts
1. I love the sight of:

(a)_____

(b)_____

(c)_____

of uncontrollable bingeing. When I first considered obeying my natural appetite, it sounded like leaving the fox in charge of the henhouse. I expected to stuff myself so unstintingly that I'd end up the size of a municipal library. But after years of apprehensive experimentation, I realized that my body just wanted to establish its ideal weight and eating patterns.

True, for a while I ate enough chocolate to cause a price spike in the world cocoa market, but this was not so much my body's wish as a psychological reaction to denying myself yummy things for years. I believe that our psychology—and also our body chemistry—wants us to hoard whatever pleasures seem to be in short supply. Starve yourself, and your body will want to

binge. Then it will store every calorie as fat, bracing itself for the next period of famine. On the other hand, if you give yourself permission to eat whatever truly makes you feel good, you may be surprised by how dietetically correct your body wants to be. Pediatricians tell us that left to their own devices, children will choose a balanced, healthy diet. Adults will do the same—unless they are eating for reasons other than physical hunger.

If you are using food to soothe feelings other than hunger, you won't be able to tell what your body really wants, or to really enjoy what you eat. The rest of the Joy Diet will help you address the psychological issues that may result in this kind of emotional eating. Once you've resolved those

2. I love the sound of:

(a)_____

(b)_____

(c)_____

It's amazing how long we may go without feasting on things we find beautiful. We may own dozens of CDs and a great sound system but virtually never listen to our favorite music. We hate the mustard color of the bathroom but never get around to painting it our favorite shade of periwinkle. I often force clients—not at gunpoint, but almost—to revisit and reclaim the things they find most beautiful. When they seek out beauty for their daily feast requirement, the world abruptly becomes more vivid, often breath-snatchingly lovely.

FEASTING ON FEELING

So far we've covered four senses: taste, smell, sight, and hearing. The remaining sense, touch, can provide the most amazing feasts yet. Leading the list of tactile feasts is good sex—need I say more? A

ing, skipping, dancing—anything that moves your body in a pleasurable way can be a feast.

Another entry I'd put in this feasting category is that sublime nourishment, sleep. Our economy loses billions every year because of problems caused by widespread, chronic sleep deprivation. I myself slept for approximately 15 minutes between 1986 (when I started graduate school and had my first baby) and 1993 (when I finished my degree and sent my youngest child to preschool). Since then I've slept pretty much continuously. If your lifestyle doesn't permit you to sleep until you feel rested, commit to changing it. If you have insomnia, see a doctor. Reclaim naps not as the refuge of the lazy but as the birthright of every creature able to snooze. There may still be times when you won't be able to have as many sleep-feasts as you want, but these should be rare.

FEASTING ON LOVE

In the end, there is one sort of feast that eclipses all the other kinds put together,

toward what we think will be a love-feast, offer our hearts, and meet rejection. It's true that this hurts. But you'll find that love-feasts are so incredibly nourishing to your soul that it's worth the risk of heartbreak to attend even the smallest or most crowded one around.

Here are some ways to make sure you never miss a love-feast you could have attended. (1) In Benjamin Franklin's words, "If you would be loved, love and be lovable." Love-feasts are always potlucks: Each person must bring the ability to love, somehow, some way. If you're waiting for someone else to supply 100 percent of the love you need, find a therapist who's willing to accept reciprocation in the form of cash. (2) Don't hide love. If you feel it, express it—not to demand that others love you back, but simply to live outwardly the best of what you feel inwardly. The worst that can happen to your heart is not rejection by another person but failure to act on the love you feel. (3) If you have a choice between a feast of love and any other option, go with love.

Compared to other activities, love-feasts will mess up your life, complicate your

I often force clients—not at gunpoint, but almost—to revisit and reclaim the things they find most beautiful.

luxurious massage can be added to or substituted for this kind of pleasure, depending on your state of mind and social calendar. Then there are other spa-type activities: facials, manicures, elaborate baths. Just making sure you have appealing textures next to your skin can make the day feel festive. Flannel pajamas are a feast for a tired hide. So are fuzzy slippers or your favorite old T-shirt.

There's a sort of feeling called proprioception, the sensitivity that tells you how your body is positioned and how it's moving. Just lying down and relaxing can be a feast for the body, especially if you can get away with doing it for a few minutes in the middle of the day. Stretching, scratch-

and that is a feast of love. If you don't know what I'm talking about, keep searching until you do. There are as many different love-feasts as there are moments when one person reaches out to another, and all of them are wonderful.

To me a feast of love is any instant (or hour or lifetime) when human beings exchange affection. I see my 14-year-old son and his friends giving each other gentle punches on the arm; that's a love-feast. A client tells me that I actually helped, and I tell him it was his doing, not mine; that's a love-feast, too. A crowd shows up to cheer for the runners in a marathon, and the runners wave back. Massive love-feast. It's true that sometimes we head hopefully

career, wear you out, make you crazy. But I guarantee that when you look back over the time you've spent on earth, the feasts of love will be the events you'll remember most joyfully, the experiences that will make you glad you have lived.

Consciously choosing to have at least three square feasts a day may simply cause you to notice the sacred and wonderful ceremonies that already fill your life. Or it may remind you to discover and enjoy things you would otherwise never experience. Either way, it will ensure that you have a more joyful, balanced life, a life lived in the conscious pursuit of your dearest longings and grandest hopes. Now, that's what I call a healthy diet. ●

Health, **Happiness,** and the Well-Lived Life: A Doctor's Prescription

What is well-being? Can it be found in a doctor's office or a bottle of pills? Or is it something more headlong, passionate, risky? **RACHEL NAOMI REMEN, MD,** speaks her mind.

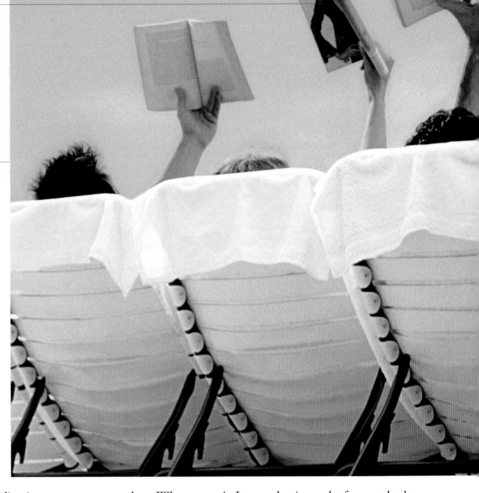

LAST WEEK AT A BREAKFAST MEETING with three healthy women friends who are each more than 20 years younger than I am, I was stunned to watch one of them take a box out of her purse and swallow 10 or 12 capsules and pills of various sizes and colors. Seeing my surprise, the others laughed and told me that they, too, take a handful of pills with their breakfast coffee, among them ginseng, ginkgo, CoQ10, soy concentrate, multivitamins, megaminerals, hormones, and the diet supplement Metabolife. "Health is everything," one of them told me.

But perhaps not. I have a chronic disease as a lifetime companion. I have survived eight major surgeries and several minor ones, and somewhere there is a stack of medical charts with my name on them that is by now taller than I am. Yet everyone at that breakfast table takes more pills every morning than I do.

I wonder how we have become so worried about our health and so dependent on medication to support ourselves. When did life become a disease that we need to prevent?

I WAS ACTUALLY RAISED TO BE fearful about life. When I was small, my Russian mother tied red ribbons to my crib and my carriage. As I grew older she would often hide little pieces of red ribbon in the pockets of my clothes or in my shoes. They were meant to protect me from the evil eye.

As I remember it, much of my mother's communication was about saving me from danger, about Button up! Watch your step! Hold your purse! Don't talk to strangers! In my family, where doctors are almost as common as people, it was assumed that medical knowledge was all that was needed to be safe and live well. Yet all of these warnings made me uncertain.

Many women have told me that they, too, feel watchful and uncertain about

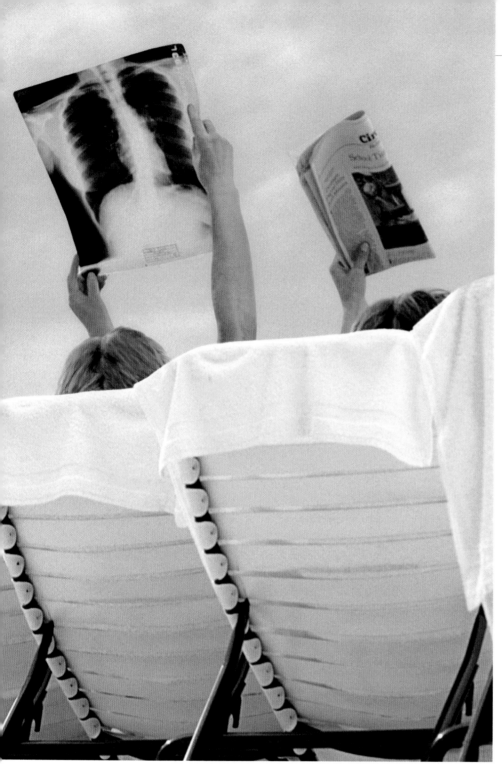

their health. Perhaps such fearfulness is just an inside-out way of saying that life is valuable and important, too important to lose or misplace. If so, it might make sense to put more of our energy into celebrating life rather than defending it.

This is especially true in times when uncertainty surrounds us. I now know that medications I once confidently took to achieve an ideal weight or protect myself from osteoporosis can actually hurt me far more than having thinner bones or carrying 20 extra pounds. The very things that science told us to do a few years ago may cause us irreparable harm. The long-range effects of taking daily megadoses of vitamins and minerals, of using powerful hormones to increase muscle tone or ease the discomfort of menopause are just not known.

But we may not need the answers to these questions in order to live well. Per-

haps what we really need to know is not "How do I choose among the many medical options that science can offer?" but "How do I choose life?"

Maybe we do not need to relentlessly pursue our physical health in order to live a good life. Maybe we are not broken. I stopped looking for the right combination of medicines and supplements when I finally realized that no pills would make me happy. Happiness is about living with passion, coherence, meaning, and integrity—becoming satisfied not with my health but with my life.

MY MENTORS IN LIVING WELL have been the many women with cancer I have cared for in 30 years as a physician. Being with them has made me less frightened and far more alive. They have shown me that health is only a means to an end and not an end in itself.

Life-threatening illness can shuffle our values and priorities as if they were a deck of cards. One of my patients, a successful businesswoman, tells me that before her illness she would become depressed unless things went her way. Happiness was "having the cookie." Unfortunately, the cookie kept changing. Some of the time it was money, sometimes power, sometimes beauty, sometimes fitness and perfect health. At other times, it was the new furniture, the biggest contract, and the most prestigious address. Two years after her cancer diagnosis, she sits shaking her head ruefully. "It's like somewhere along the way I forgot how to live. When I give my son a cookie, he is happy. If I take the cookie away or it breaks, he is unhappy. But he is 2½ and I am 43. It's taken me this long to understand that the cookie will never make me happy for long. The minute you have the cookie, it starts to crumble or you start to worry about it crumbling or about someone trying to take it away from you. You have to give up a lot of things to take care of the cookie. You may not even get a chance to eat it because you are so busy just trying not to lose it."

My patient laughs and says her illness has changed her. For the first time she is happy. No matter if her business is doing well or not, no matter if she wins or loses at tennis. "Two years ago, cancer asked me, 'Okay, what is really important?' Well, life is important. Life any way you can have it. Happiness does not have anything to do with the cookie; it has to do with being really alive. Before, who made the time?" She pauses and begins to laugh. "Damn, I guess life is the cookie," she tells me.

MOST OF US LIVE HOMELESS, IN the neighborhood of our true selves. A few years ago, I asked a group of women to prioritize a list of goals according to what was most important to them in their professional lives. The list included such things as approval, love, power, fame, comfort, adventure, friendship, security, respect, influence, kindness, wisdom, meaning, and money. Then I asked these women to prioritize the list of goals according to what was most important to them personally.

Of the 300 women who did this, only 10 came up with the same list. Most were stunned to discover that they believed one way and lived in quite another. Their work actually violated their personal values. While we may not know the long-term effects of many of our medical choices, we can all choose to live closer to our true selves than we do. The stress of living divided like this has a far greater impact on our lives and even on our health than not taking the right pill.

Our health is important but not as a major focus of our lives. We may just need to care for our physical well-being in some simple and commonsense ways:

■ Don't be the first on the block to take a new medication. Wait and see.
■ Eat a good and balanced diet as a source of the vitamins and minerals you really need. The vitamins in food may be far more useful to your body than those you presently buy in bottles.

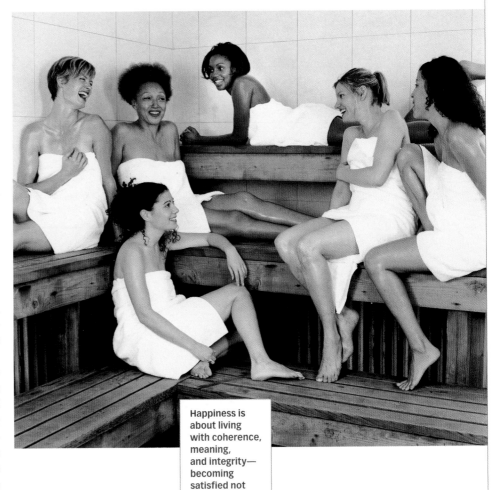

Happiness is about living with coherence, meaning, and integrity—becoming satisfied not only with your health but with your life.

■ Read before you eat. Avoid foods that have chemicals in them or on them.
■ Pay more attention to your environment, to what you put on your lawn and paint on your walls.
■ Listen to yourself more closely and to the life experiences of other women. Respect the wisdom that has helped others to live well.

THERE ARE MANY THINGS WE CAN control that make us less vulnerable to illness. None of them comes in a pill. We can learn to understand ourselves better, to know what will fulfill us and to pursue that in large and small ways no matter what others think. We can reach within to find a place of personal truth and live from there. And no matter if we are sick or well, we can learn to live passionately.

After 50 years of Crohn's disease, I can now say that perfect health is not the sine qua non of a good life. The wisdom to live well is not about holding on to everything you have at all costs. Living a full and rich life may require us to focus beyond our physical health and learn the direction in which our wholeness lies—to take risks and let go of what we have outgrown, over and over again, until all we are following is our own dream of ourselves. ●

» There are many things we can control that make us less vulnerable to illness. None of them comes in a pill.

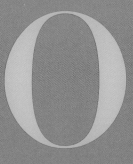

Confidence

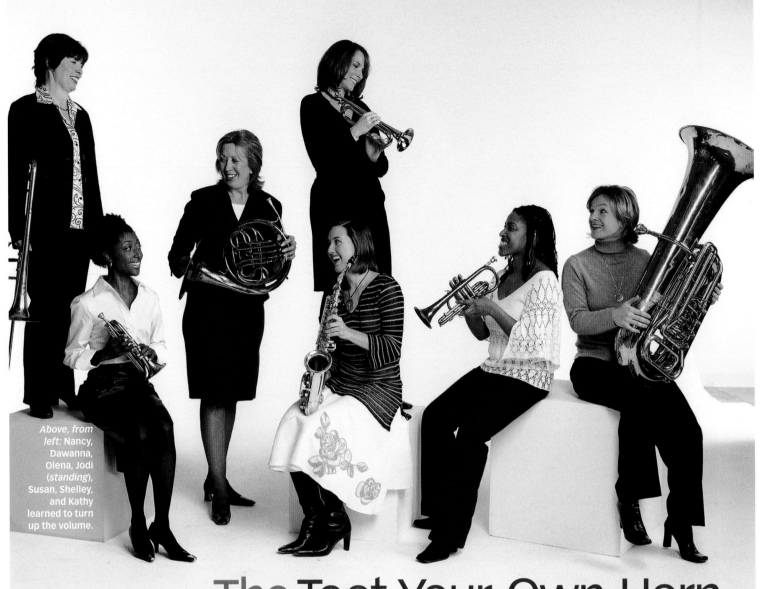

Above, from left: Nancy, Dawanna, Olena, Jodi (*standing*), Susan, Shelley, and Kathy learned to turn up the volume.

The Toot-Your-Own-Horn Workshop

Most women don't know how to sell themselves. **RONNA LICHTENBERG** shows you why modesty isn't always the best policy.

AS MUCH AS WE WISH OTHER PEOple would notice our talents and shower us with recognition, more often than not, just like in New York traffic, it takes horn tooting to get someone's attention. The problem, as I've learned in my experience as a management consultant, is that even women who are great at selling something or someone else have a tough time doing it for themselves. That's why I leapt at *O* magazine's invitation to conduct a seminar to help women break through their mental blocks and trumpet their strengths.

Our eight participants had varying backgrounds. Some were starting new ventures, like Dawanna, 34, who'd just gone out on her own in real estate development, and Shelley, 32, a freelance researcher at *O*, who'd recorded a CD and wanted to expand her singing career and record label. A few women worked for major corporations. Among them were Kathy, 33, a project manager at a medical device firm, who needed to sell her ideas internally, and Olena, 47, a vice president of finance at a Fortune 500 company, who feared her division would be disbanded and she'd need to make a fresh start.

To give these women a broad range of expertise, I invited executive coach

Aven Kerr, a human resources veteran who now runs her own business, and Valrine Daley, a senior executive in organizational development for Salomon Smith Barney, to help run the workshop.

We started with everyone sitting around a table, brainstorming about why it's important to toot your own horn. We came up with a long list of reasons—everything from "recognition, money, and influence!" to "It's going to be a long wait if you're expecting someone else to do it for you. You're waiting to be anointed—and even if you do find a champion, she could leave." Jodi, 35, a senior marketing manager, put her finger on the problem: "It's tough to find the balance between tooting your own horn and showing off."

This seemed like a good time to begin the first exercise. I asked each woman to introduce herself using only four sentences, which meant she had to set priorities about what she'd reveal. Rather than focus solely on accomplishments, the women mentioned family and hobbies, and even made little jokes. Then I handed out neckties and asked everyone to try again—this time as if she were a man. Not a single woman introduced herself the same way. Instead, they went straight to their successes, backed up by data. Acting as a guy, Kathy, the project manager, cheerfully admitted to some exaggeration and embellishment.

Over the years, I've seen that women try to show a rounded picture of themselves, including their personal lives, to create intimacy, whereas men immediately try to gain respect. The point is to be aware of the choices you're making; in some situations where you have a limited amount of time to make a pitch, the typically male "bragging" approach can be more effective.

With the exercise fresh in our minds, Aven introduced the concept of "discounting behavior"—ways women often unwittingly undercut ourselves. For instance, we preface our message with "You probably don't remember me..." or "I haven't really thought this out, but..." We deflect praise by saying, "Well, the idea needs a lot of work." We protect ourselves by saying, "Oh, I've never been very good at..." or "I'll try and see if I can do it." When Aven noted that six of the eight women had included some kind of dis-

THE PANIC ROOM

Sometimes you know you're going to be called upon to toot your own horn, and sometimes you don't. Knowing it's coming can be harder because you have time to get anxious. That's why it's good to be able to create a safe place within your own head where you can go when you start to panic.

Take a minute by yourself, away from distractions. Bring up an image of a place where you feel secure and at peace. It may be a beautiful beach. It may be your home. Your body should feel warm and relaxed while you're "seeing" it. Practice visualizing your refuge as clearly and vividly as possible, so that when you need a safe place to gather energy, you'll be ready.

counting comment in her original introduction, Shelley gasped in recognition: "I said I had a very *small* music business."

Aven explained that we discount to avoid looking overconfident and to minimize the risk of someone's not liking our ideas. But discounting is not a great strategy. Other people might take your words

at face value—or find your self-deprecation annoyingly disingenuous.

So one goal we agreed on was trying not to discount, without getting so hung up on it that it's one more thing we put ourselves down for. ("I can't believe I discount all the time. It's awful!") Aven suggested we consider "premium pricing" instead—adding value by presenting ourselves and our ideas in the best possible light. People pay more for something that looks good. You should not only dress well but dress your ideas well, by being fastidious about written correspondence and making sure the prototype of any product you want to promote is high quality. People also pay more for ideas and products that fit their needs precisely, so do your homework by learning about the bosses or buyers you're approaching and what they stand to gain from you. Be prepared to state your strengths succinctly, and be ready, if someone asks about your weaknesses, to share the least threatening one.

Although you can't expect to get top dollar or highest priority every time out, thinking you deserve the best—at least

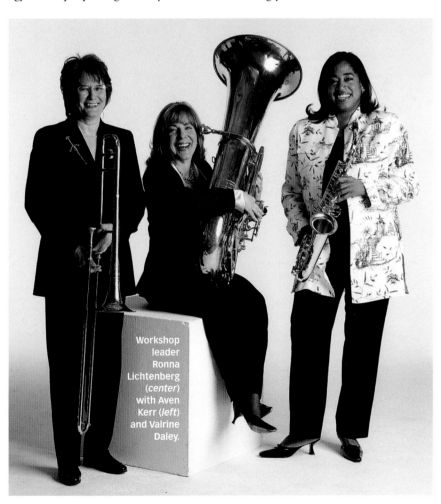

Workshop leader Ronna Lichtenberg (*center*) with Aven Kerr (*left*) and Valrine Daley.

sometimes—helps you strengthen your presentations and build your self-confidence. I warned the group that premium pricing might not feel authentic at first, or like the "real you." But showing other people the most flattering view of yourself is every bit as legitimate as leading with your flaws.

Next we decided to try some "toots." The first one was simple. I'd brought in a box of stuff from my office, ranging from a Slinky toy to a purple tape dispenser to a bud vase. We broke into pairs, and each pair chose an item from the box. One person had to sell the product to her partner. Kathy, it turned out, was particularly emphatic about the appeal of the bud vase, demonstrating what a great gift it would be and how easy life would be if you had a half dozen of them on hand. Olena, her partner, was so convinced that if you were a friend of hers and had a birthday coming up, I can almost guarantee you'd get one as a present.

Then we raised the stakes: The partner who'd played buyer had to sell herself as a potential CEO of the company that made the item. After the exercise, everyone admitted she wasn't as good at singing her own praises. And while it was easy to talk about the price of the product, no one was comfortable discussing her salary.

In the next exercise—"Miss Wonderful"—we raised the stakes even higher. Each woman had to stand in front of the group and make her single biggest business claim. I asked everyone to drive that claim home with three points that proved the case, ideally with data. By now, we were all trying to avoid discounting. Nancy, 47, a design director who was looking for a full-time job, stated, "I created a logo for my own business [TomatoDesign.net] that was so powerful that the state of New Jersey used it." Yet even with a new level of awareness about diminishing ourselves, two people said they got an opportunity "by default" and someone said of her most shining career moment, "It happened to be a success." We resolved to practice telling our stories in a more compelling way.

Before we went home, Valrine offered practical strategies for selling a pet project within an organization, whether it's a Fortune 500 or a local nonprofit where you volunteer. "You have to start by gathering a constituency—don't even try to make a big group presentation unless you've made sure that at least 51 percent of the group wants to hear what you have to say. Then lead with a strong, specific statement of the benefit," she said. "Too often we communicate by stating why we care instead of why they should." Among the biggest mis-

takes: expecting unrealistically speedy results from an overworked group that has to weigh your idea, and failing to rehearse your pitch.

Knowing how hard it can be to stick your neck out, my last piece of advice was that everyone reward herself for the effort, regardless of the outcome. We talked about what constituted a treat: "a glass of wine on my porch," "handbags!" and "20 minutes to actually drink my wine instead of carrying it around the house." The point is that you have to replenish your energy to be able to expend it again. With that, we gave everyone Tootsie Rolls as a reminder that horn tooting can be sweet.

A few weeks later, I called each woman to see how she was doing. Olena had indeed been downsized but was enthusiastic about trying something new. Buoyed by the workshop, she'd already pitched a proposal to a university for a tailor-made advanced degree. Jodi reported feeling more confident about selling a new business approach at work. And Shelley had decided to use her stage name in her day job, realizing that consistency is a necessary tool when promoting yourself.

Underneath these changes, I saw a shift in thinking from "What will they think of me?" to "What do I think will be good for them to know about me?" Each woman seemed better equipped to create freedom where there had been fear. Freedom to say, "Here I am, and here is my contribution. I may not get every note right, but I'm going to use every instrument I have." ●

TOOTING 101

1 Practice horn tooting for something you believe in. Nonprofit groups need help more than ever. Saying something good about their mission helps you learn what makes for a compelling pitch and makes you feel good about doing it.

2 Toot a coworker's horn. It's great to point out someone else's accomplishments. Just make sure you don't use it as an excuse to put yourself down.

3 Don't bad-mouth other women for promoting themselves. It's easy to ask, "Who does she think she is?" But every time we do, we're sending a message to others, and to ourselves, that it's wrong for women to say good things about themselves. Change the world—and yourself—by mentally saying "Hurrah!" when another woman goes for it.

4 Data is your friend. Particularly in the business world, numbers are an effective way to tell the story of how wonderful you are. Practice saying something great about yourself and proving it with statistics. If you can't back up your claims, think about asking for opportunities that would give you the bragging rights you need.

5 Preparing to toot your own horn goes beyond deciding what you're going to say. Make sure you know what you need to feel supported while you make your pitch and how to take care of yourself afterward, no matter how it goes.

6 Give yourself permission to experiment. Many of the workshop participants found freedom in the "male" style and plan to incorporate it into their lives.

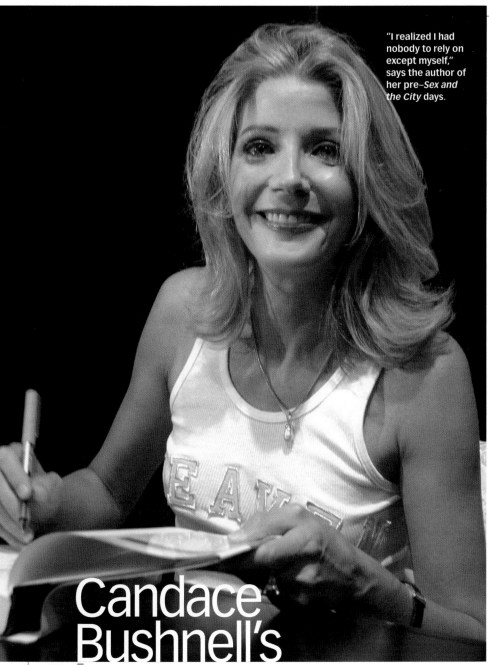

"I realized I had nobody to rely on except myself," says the author of her pre-*Sex and the City* days.

Candace Bushnell's
Aha! Moment

She was broke, afraid, and losing hope. Then she stumbled on the secret of a lasting success.

WHEN I WAS IN MY EARLY 30S, I WAS writing all the time, but for some reason none of my stuff was selling. There are periods in the life of an artist when you go through growing phases, and in order to do that, you need to be able to fail. You have to sit back, regroup, and rethink. I didn't know it then, but I was going through one of those phases.

Unfortunately, it was accompanied by being broke. I'd go to the supermarket with two dollars and cry in the aisles, *I don't even have enough money for dinner.* I ate a lot of soup. I was living in an apartment that cost $300 a month, and I got kicked out because I couldn't afford it. I was constantly worrying, *Oh my God. What am I going to do with my life?* It was frightening, and I was alone. I didn't have a husband. I didn't have a boyfriend. I had nobody to rely on, I realized, except for myself. I knew I was going to have to pull myself out of it.

So I got a freelance job writing profiles for *The New York Observer.* I worked so hard on those stories, but I was beginning to think that my big break might never happen. A few months later, though, the editor offered me my own column, "Sex and the City." I felt on top of the world; I finally had an opportunity. I remember it was a gorgeous, sunny afternoon in October. I walked up Park Avenue, which is such a beautiful street. All the doormen were smiling and saying, "Hello, Miss. How are you?" It was a changing point in my life—I experienced such a feeling of triumph. I think that's what everybody always hopes for; the chance to show off what you can do and become what you're meant to become.

One of the things I learned through writing the column is that so much of what society tells us—about women and men, what our roles are, and what they're supposed to be—just isn't true. We still tell women, *Relationships are really important— you have to find a man.* But there are certain things a relationship cannot give you. It can't give you self-esteem and won't necessarily bring you happiness. It might give you some sense of accomplishment temporarily, but not in the long term. We don't tell women enough that one of the most important things to strive for in life is some kind of personal and professional achievement. Not as a man or a woman—but as a person. Sometimes it's important to be a person first and a gender second.

When you experience some sort of *I just kicked the field goal that won the game* moment, you can go into relationships without being needy or looking for self-esteem. We, as women, need to get those things for ourselves. •

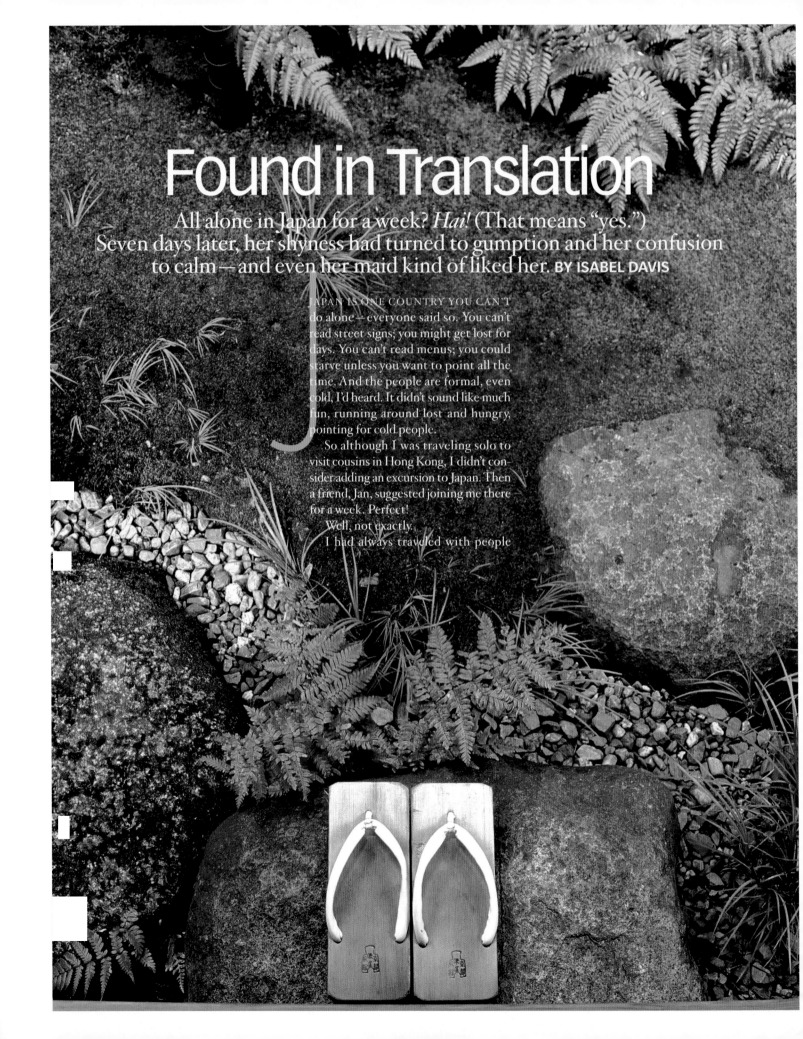

Found in Translation

All alone in Japan for a week? *Hai!* (That means "yes.")
Seven days later, her shyness had turned to gumption and her confusion
to calm—and even her maid kind of liked her. BY ISABEL DAVIS

JAPAN IS ONE COUNTRY YOU CAN'T
do alone—everyone said so. You can't
read street signs; you might get lost for
days. You can't read menus; you could
starve unless you want to point all the
time. And the people are formal, even
cold, I'd heard. It didn't sound like much
fun, running around lost and hungry,
pointing for cold people.

So although I was traveling solo to
visit cousins in Hong Kong, I didn't consider adding an excursion to Japan. Then
a friend, Jan, suggested joining me there
for a week. Perfect!

Well, not exactly.

I had always traveled with people

I knew well (mostly husbands, whom I was out of at the moment). Although Jan and I went way back, we hadn't lived in the same city in more than 20 years. Within days of arriving in Japan, we discovered our differences on just about everything. Our friendship exploded, and Jan announced she was going home. "Fine," I said tersely.

Two hours later, I was by myself in Kyoto, terrified. I sat in the hotel room trying not to panic. I thought about leaving, but—get all the way to Japan and not see it? I knew I had to conquer my acute shyness, which a shrink had told me years ago was "a luxury I could no longer afford." I'd worried that I wouldn't be able to think of anything to say to strangers. Here, all I could say was *arigatou* ("thank you") and *hai* (which means "yes," and a lot of other things I never quite figured out). How wrong could I go?

My first adventure was visiting a *ryokan,* a traditional inn. When I arrived, a lovely woman in a kimono bowed to me, letting me know she was my maid. My maid. "Your stay at a ryokan will be determined by how well you get along with your maid," the guidebook informed me.

SHE LED ME TO AN ENCHANTING room: shoji screens, a single purple blossom in a turquoise vase, a low wooden table. She gestured that I was to sit down on the floor as she served tea and sweets. She also brought a menu (in English!) for the next morning's breakfast: orange juice, bacon, and eggs. At a *ryokan?* I consulted my phrase book: *Wafuu*—"Japanese style." "Japanese morning?" she asked, astonished. "*Hai,*" I answered. She seemed pleased. I was succeeding with the maid. She showed me where my kimono was, pointed to a large wooden tub in the bathroom, and left.

I had expected from my reading to be guided through the bath, which was supposed to be communal, but apparently this *ryokan* worked on a privacy principle. Well, at least I wouldn't have to smile at naked people I couldn't talk to. I decided to do as the book instructed: I took a cold shower (to purify) and then soaked in the large cypress tub filled with scalding water ("to make the cares of the day melt away into a stupor"). Later the maid came back with an exquisite dinner. There were ten dishes

of various shapes and sizes, not counting dipping sauces. The food was sensual as a still life. I recognized only a few things: One dish, I swear, contained mashed potatoes, but these were mashed potatoes for the gods. As I ate, I began to feel my fear melt away.

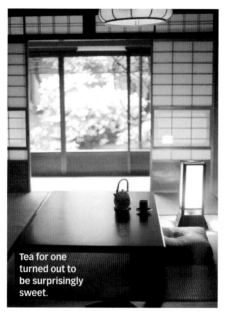

Tea for one turned out to be surprisingly sweet.

The bath wasn't communal—
so at least I wouldn't have to smile at naked people I couldn't talk to.

Next morning, I was trying to connect street signs to my map when a man stopped and asked in excellent English if he could help. "I'm trying to find Murin-an Gardens," I said. He said, "Murin-an—I've never been there. May I accompany you?" I felt awkward as we strolled along. Was he just being polite? Was he picking me up?

Turned out he wanted to practice his English and hear about America. When we left Murin-an, he said, "I admire the way you're traveling by yourself. Very interesting woman."

Energized, I divided the rest of my time in Kyoto between visiting gardens and getting lost (not without its own rewards). People were amazingly kind. As I stood baffled in front of train schedules I couldn't read, someone would always turn me in the right direction and show me how much change to put in the turnstile. Once, while a cop on a bicycle was giving me directions, it started to pour. Five minutes later, he caught up with me and handed me a plastic raincoat. So much for the cold Japanese.

Tokyo was a bigger challenge: It makes the New York subways at rush hour seem empty. Crowds push past you, smoking furiously, talking rapidly in—my God—Japanese. Ikebukero, the subway station nearest the hotel I was heading for, was so huge that it took me a full hour just to find my way out of it. After I got to my room, I carefully planned the last two days of my trip. The idea was: Stay close by. Get lost small.

Anonymity gave me freedom. When a headwaiter whom I'd asked for a table looked askance at my clothes, I realized that the New York principle of "black will take you anywhere" doesn't apply to a T-shirt and Reeboks. "This is a French restaurant, Madame," he said in English, implying that someone like me would be looking for something cheaper. "*Bien sûr,*" I replied haughtily. I'd traveled from America to Tokyo—I could afford their damn lunch. Why didn't he assume I was rich and eccentric? I ordered a fine meal with excellent wine and began to feel rich and eccentric. I was seated by a window wall, through which I could see a waterfall and golden carp swimming.

With my new attitude, I decided I would take a few photographs (maybe they'd think I was a photojournalist), and after a while, one of the waiters asked if I'd like him to take my picture. How about that? Total triumph.

Heading home, I realized that something had changed dramatically for me. I felt calmer and more confident. When I'm confronted with mundane terrors now, a little voice inside whispers: "What do you mean you're afraid? You spent a week alone in Japan." Who knows where I might go next? ●

how to talk to (nicely) yourself

How do you silence the jeering voice in your head that tells you everything you're saying is wrong and stupid and dumb and unfounded and…*stop!* Cathleen Medwick attempts to shush her inner critic.

YOU KNOW THE ROUTINE. YOU'RE in a room with your boss. Or the man you secretly love. Or the girl who tormented you in high school. Though you plan on being silent and serene, you open your mouth to answer a simple question, and out of it come words so ghoulishly inane that you immediately turn purple. You try to cover, but the more you talk the stupider you get. You can barely hear what the other person is saying, because the voice in your head is screaming, *Oh, my God, I sound like an idiot! What's the matter with me?* After you've slithered out of the room, the inner harangue continues as your eyes well up. You can't stop replaying the conversation in your head. Days later you're still rehearsing the things you should have said.

I have spent most of my life listening to the voice in my head that tells me what's wrong with me, what I can't do even if I try hard, and why things will never be any different. I'm in awe of people who seem to be full of confidence, taking every setback in stride, never losing their composure. What's their secret?

I decide to ask an expert, Martin E.P. Seligman, PhD, the University of Pennsylvania psychology professor noted for his theories on "learned optimism." Seligman wrote a book called *Authentic Happiness: Using the New Positive Psychology to Realize Your Potential for Lasting Fulfillment* (Free Press). As I read about his techniques for combating negative thoughts, I think I recognize a kindred spirit. "I am a dyed-in-the-wool pessimist," Seligman writes, "and the techniques that I wrote about in *Learned Optimism* I use every day." His theories evolved from his continuing efforts to transform himself into a more positive person, even after "I had spent 50 years enduring mostly wet weather in my soul and the last ten years as a walking nimbus cloud in a household radiant with sunshine." If this man can't help me disperse my own dark clouds, nobody can.

I dial Seligman's number, and he answers. His voice is deep, distant, and a little scary. Well, more than a little. He sounds like the Grim Reaper. I hear my own voice beginning to waffle, the way it does when I'm speaking to someone whose judgment I fear. I try to explain that I'm calling him to find out how to talk myself down, to quiet the fearful, self-critical voice in my head—but I can't find the words. I am not just vague; I am unintelligible. When I finish my baroque explanation, I ask Seligman, "Does that make any sense?"

"Not to me," he answers.

Oh, that's great, the voice in my head begins chattering, *you've managed to confuse him with the first question—typical. It's all downhill from here.* I try to be a little clearer, telling him about irrational anxieties that I've developed since 9/11 (like my fear of being in the tunnel beneath Grand Central Terminal when a bomb goes off) and how they increase my feelings of helplessness. Seligman hears me out, and then he says, "I see what you mean."

You do? Unfortunately, I'm so insecure by this time that I keep right on explaining. "Another example," I burble, "would be if you ask for more money in your job and you're told no. Your immediate thought is, *Of course not. How could I even have asked?*"

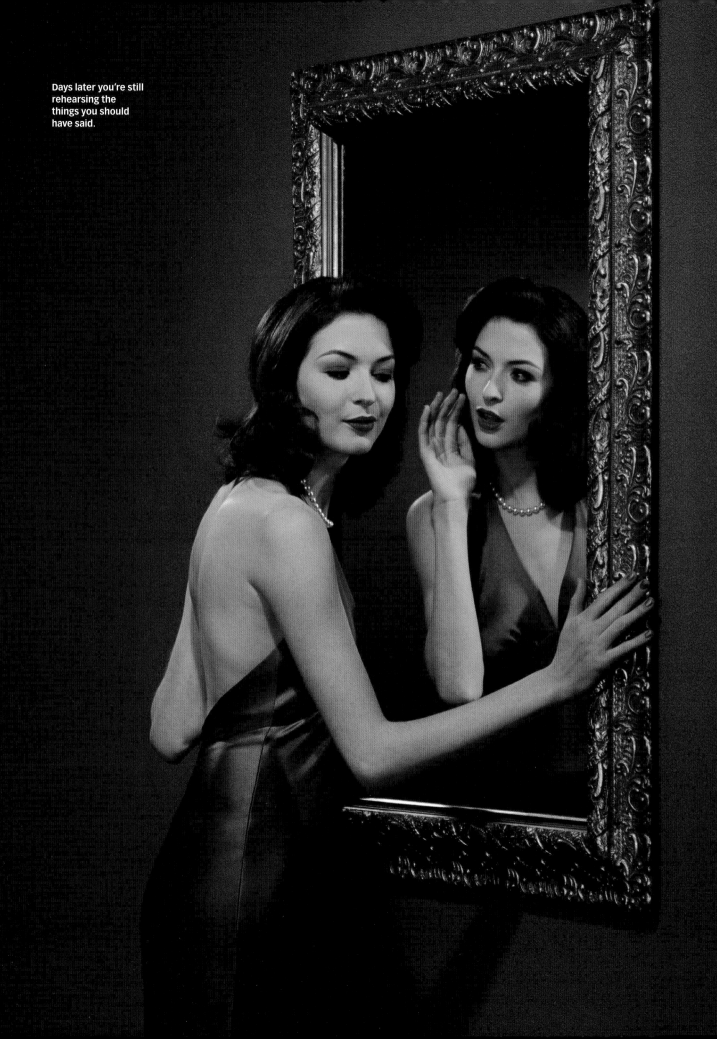

Days later you're still rehearsing the things you should have said.

That, Seligman explains, is another "catastrophic thought," and he has a three-step technique to counteract it. "First you recognize that the thought is there," he tells me. "Then you learn to treat that thought as if it were said by some third person whose job in life was to make your life miserable. And then you learn to dispute it, to marshal evidence against it."

I'm starting to rally. Maybe this interview isn't a disaster after all.

"Let's say we're doing this interview," Seligman continues, "and you say to yourself, *Gee, this interview is going really badly, I'm just not getting anywhere with this interviewee. Maybe I've lost my touch.*"

He knows I've lost it! The voice in my head is ratcheting up to a shriek.

"And so what you do in a situation like that," he says as steadily as a general mapping out a battle plan, "is first, you treat that as if it was said by a rival for your job, someone who wanted to demoralize you and accuse you of things that were unfounded. And then you start to marshal evidence, like, 'Well, what I said in the first question to my interviewee drew a blank, but then when I fleshed it out, he started to come out of himself. And consider my last interview, in which I did this, that, and the other thing.' So you've basically marshaled evidence against the catastrophic thought."

I hear only the first part of that, because I'm too distracted with worry to understand that he's meeting me halfway. I'm like a fish that continues to thrash even though the fisherman has withdrawn the hook. I'm so busy accusing myself of flubbing the interview, I don't hear that it's actually going fine.

"If somebody were saying bad things about me or trying to get my job," I find myself arguing, "I don't know that I would confront the person, because I'd assume it wasn't going to work."

"How about if they're accusing you of something grossly false?" Seligman counters. "Then you'd probably stand up for yourself. Most people do. That's a skill," he adds, "that can be learned and built."

But, I persist, suppose you have an involuntary physical reaction—like blushing,

or getting nauseous when you have to speak in front of people? Even if you "dispute" the voice that's filling you with fear and embarrassment, your body will give you away.

"Well, if you're describing a deathly fear of speaking," Seligman answers slowly, "then you're probably dealing with someone who needs face-to-face behavior or cognitive therapy for speech anxiety."

He thinks I'm crazy! I imagine myself in a Marx Brothers movie, with Groucho as the Viennese psychoanalyst: Me: "Doc, I'm so scared I'm afraid I'm going to throw up." Groucho: "What are you, some kind of nut?"

I summon up my calmest, most professional manner. Inwardly, of course, I'm 6 years old. "Sometimes I can successfully

> I'm so busy accusing myself of flubbing the interview with Seligman, I don't hear that it's actually going fine.

talk to myself," I assure the doctor, "and make myself feel better after some anxiety-provoking event. But then the bad thoughts will rush back in."

Yes, Seligman agrees, that's what tends to happen. "You're not going to still the provoking thoughts…"

I knew it!

"…you're just going to get better and better at neutralizing them."

"Well," I venture as his words finally begin to make sense to me, "that would be good enough."

"Better if you could eliminate them," Seligman says darkly. I can almost see the pessimist in him scratching to get out. "I don't think anyone's found a way of eliminating thoughts of danger and loss," he says. "It's rather that, when they're unrealistic, you become an acrobat at marshaling evidence against them."

THE INTERVIEW IS OVER. As soon as I hang up the phone, the full frontal assault begins. First, the accusation (*I made an ass of myself*). Next, the kicker (*serves me right for assuming I knew what I was doing*). Then the dread (*I'm going to have to listen to the tape!*) and the despair (*I'll never get a story out of this*). And then, as I clench my teeth and turn on the transcription machine, a revelation: This is not the conversation I remember!

Seligman wasn't going after me. He was listening very, very closely and working with what he heard—that's what psychologists do, after all. The interview wasn't going badly, and most of the time I sounded reasonable and assured. But I wasn't hearing everything he said. I was responding automatically; the voice in my head kept drowning him out. I was on the defensive, so I kept coming up with ways to challenge him, when what I really wanted to do was duck for cover. "Pessimists have a particularly pernicious way of construing their setbacks and frustrations," Seligman writes. While optimists expect their problems to be temporary, and would never dream of blaming themselves, "[pessimists] automatically think that the cause is permanent, pervasive, and personal: 'It's going to last forever, it's going to undermine everything, and it's my fault.'"

My sentiments exactly. So how do I plan on getting over my pessimism? I'll try Seligman's technique, with a slight twist suggested by a Buddhist friend who practices "loving-kindness," a way of relating more humanely to yourself and others: Instead of pretending my inner voice is an enemy, I might start thinking of her as a dear but deluded friend. Maybe I'll be able to listen to what she tells me without taking it so much to heart. Maybe, after getting a little distance, I'll begin to be able to laugh at her a little, and gently dispute what she says. I might even try throwing in a word or two of self-approval. But that's another conversation. ●

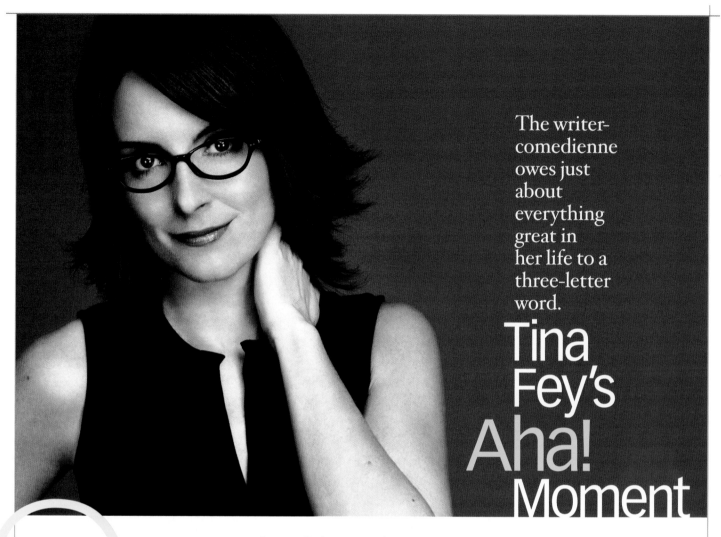

The writer-comedienne owes just about everything great in her life to a three-letter word.

Tina Fey's Aha! Moment

SIX YEARS AGO, I MOVED FROM Chicago to New York to work at *Saturday Night Live.* I packed up and was going through my things to see what I would take with me and what I'd leave behind. I found an orange folder—a regular school folder—in a bookshelf. As soon as I saw it, I knew what it was. There were quotes written all over the front of it. Some of them were: "Greet everything with 'Yes, and…'" "Make statements instead of putting the burden on others with questions." "Stay in the present, as opposed to focusing on the past or future." "The fun is always on the other side of a yes."

Years before, I was a student at Second City, an improvisational acting school in Chicago, and took a class with artistic director Martin de Maat. These quotes were some of the rules of improv he gave us. When I found the folder, I realized that taking that class had completely changed my life. It certainly sent me down a career path that I never would have ended up on

otherwise. It also sent me down a personal path—my friends were all part of the improv community. My husband was a piano player at the ImprovOlympic, and we met there. All those rules and exercises defined us and our outlook on the world.

The things I learned in that class became part of the way I live my life. A couple of times I've been called on to do things—jobs or whatever—where I've felt, *Maybe I'm not quite ready. Maybe it's a little early for this to happen to me.* But the rules are so ingrained. "Say yes, and you'll figure it out afterward" has helped me to be more adventurous. It has definitely helped me be less afraid.

"We're offering you a job here at *Saturday Night Live*—can you move here within a week?"

"Ummm, yes I can."

"You know, you haven't been here that long, but do you want to move up and try to be one of the head writers?"

Feeling completely terrified

inside, but saying, "Uhhh, yes, okay, yes, for sure."

"Do you wanna do 'Weekend Update' with Jimmy?"

Petrified. "Yes, thank you, of course!"

There are limits of reason to this idea of saying yes to everything, but when I meet someone whose first instinct is "No, how can we do that? That doesn't seem possible," I'm always kind of taken aback. Almost anyone would say, "It's Friday at two in the morning. We don't have an opening political sketch. We can't do it." Yeah, of course you can. There's no choice. And even if you abandon one idea for another one, saying yes allows you to move forward.

Sitting on the floor of my Chicago apartment, I realized that the words on the folder had a broader use than just for improvising comedy. Life is improvisation. All of those classes were like church to me. The training had seeped into me and changed who I am. •

Above: Tina Fey, coanchor of *Saturday Night Live*'s "Weekend Update."

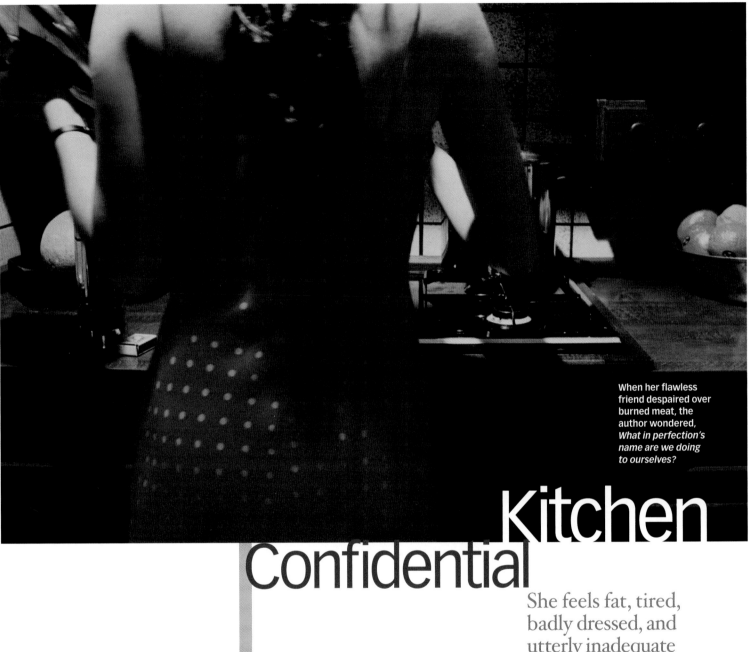

When her flawless friend despaired over burned meat, the author wondered, *What in perfection's name are we doing to ourselves?*

Kitchen
Confidential

She feels fat, tired, badly dressed, and utterly inadequate in the presence of a perfect hostess. But wait, there's a twist. **LISA WOLFE** finds out why the roast is always juicier at someone else's dinner party.

I AM STANDING IN FRONT OF MY CLOSET, searching for something that fits. So far, I have tried on a pair of black pants, which I couldn't zip up, a blue tent dress, which made me look like a tent, and an old purple skirt, which felt promising until I tried to sit down and discovered my thighs oozing out the sides and down the chair like in one of those paintings by Dalí. I have worn nothing but sweatpants and my husband's old shirts in the year since our second son was born. But tonight that won't do. Tonight we're going to a dinner party.

I used to like dinner parties. I used to like them for the reasons I am dreading the one tonight: the chance to dress up (at 5'3", with legs proportioned like a dachshund's, it's not that I ever felt beautiful, but at least I didn't feel like the beast), the chance to get to know other people (as a journalist, chatting was easy), the chance for them to get to know me (I was an associate producer at *60 Minutes,* which prompted people to say something flattering like "Wow!" when they heard this). But that was a very long time ago.

N THE PAST THREE YEARS, I'VE had two kids, quit my job, and moved into a house. Which I know is wonderful and lucky. I feel enormously blessed. And that going to this dinner party might make me cry.

But that's ridiculous. Of course I'm not going to cry. I'm going to find something to wear. This is London, where my husband and I moved for our jobs a few years ago, and dressing my sweats up with dangly earrings won't cut it. I scrounge up a plum dress I bought when I was three months pregnant with my first son and busting out of all that I owned. I put it on. I feel relieved. I head downstairs to kiss the boys goodbye.

They're sitting on the sofa with the babysitter, watching Barney. I bend down to kiss Nico, my older son, and Aidan, my younger. Nature seems to understand that Aidan, who has a form of reflux that causes him to throw up three times a day and again in the middle of the night, had better be especially sweet to me. He leaps into my arms and brushes his cheek against mine. Then he throws up all over my dress.

I head back up the stairs, angry. Not at my son, who didn't ask for his reflux, but at myself, for failing to get out of this dinner as I have managed to get out of every other we've been invited to in the past year. I have an arsenal of very good excuses, from Aidan is sick (often true) to Joe is out of town (also often true: the new job my husband took to support my hausfraudom has him away as often as at home). I tried them all again this time. But the woman inviting us—Nancy, an American I know from the playground who had her third kid when I

had my second—was persistent. And Aidan had thrown up twice in the middle of the previous night, so I was too tired to put up resistance.

I take off my dress and wipe myself with a washcloth, determined not to feel discouraged. But it's hard. I can understand not fitting into my clothes six months after having a baby, or nine, but this is 13. I am tired. I miss my job. And I feel guilty for missing my job. So who cares if I look like a tent? I put on the blue tent dress, which makes me look like I could sleep four.

"Are you ready?" asks Joe, walking into the room.

I'm about to say yes, when it occurs to me I might still smell of vomit.

I have been feeling intimidated by a woman who is in fact intimidated by me.

"Do I still smell of vomit?" I ask him.

"No," Joe answers from so far across the room he wouldn't know even if I did.

Acting on the one piece of advice my mother dared offer when I got married—if something is important to you, don't assume he knows, tell him—I don't assume Joe knows that not smelling like vomit is very important to me, I tell him. "Joe," I say, "my question may have sounded silly to you, but it's not silly to me. It's really important to me not to be one of those women who walk around smelling of their kid's vomit without even realizing it. I washed off with a washcloth, but do you think I need to take a whole shower?"

"You don't smell of vomit," Joe says, not paying any closer attention than he did the first time around. I resolve the matter by spraying myself with too much perfume.

Leaving home, alas, doesn't turn out to be half as bad as arriving at Nancy's party. Joe rings the doorbell. A tall, handsome guest opens the door and leads us to the living room, where nine or ten people have already gathered. The place looks amazing.

Though our home very much reflects the fact that we have little kids—smudges on walls, indentations in sofas from where the boys like to jump, toys if not blanketing the floor then at least overflowing from the boxes, bins, and baskets into which they've been hastily shoved—Nancy's looks more like a spread in a magazine. The living room walls are a funky shade of pumpkin, the chandelier is burning real candles, and the sofas are such a daring but dazzling crimson that I want to hide under one.

In the center of the perfect room stands perfect Nancy, looking resplendent in gray pants and a long maroon jacket, which she can wear because she's got the height, as well as her figure back, even after having had more children than I. I suck in my stomach and walk over to say hello.

"Hi!" I say, standing on tiptoe to kiss her. "You look great!"

"No, I don't."

"Yes, you do. And your house looks beautiful, too."

Nancy extends before us a platter of flaky triangular pastries. "Try one," she says. "They're stuffed with spinach. I made them myself."

She made them herself? Of course she made them herself! And why shouldn't she have? Just because I can't boil noodles these days without getting them all gunked up at the bottom of the pot doesn't mean Nancy shouldn't be able to make professional-looking pastries like it's no big deal at all. I bet they're even delicious.

I'm right. They're delicious. So delicious I remember that I might cry. "Joe," I say, swallowing hard, "you should try one. They're delicious."

Joe tries one. His eyes light up. He is one of those people who really cares about food. "You're right," he says. "They're delicious."

I duck out from under the tray and run into a happy, burly man who smiles and offers his hand. I shake it. He tells me his name, where he's from, what he does, but I don't pay much attention until he asks what I do.

"I used to be a journalist, but now I'm taking care of my kids."

"Oh," he says.

I smile lamely. The man smiles lamely.

Nancy mercifully calls us to the table. I pray this isn't a sit-your-spouse-at-the-opposite-end-of-the-room-from-you affair, but it is. I watch Joe walk to the opposite end of the room, feeling like a kid being dropped off at nursery. I will have to be a big girl now and make conversation all by myself.

The man to my right turns out to be an English barrister, who is thankfully pretty boring himself. The man to my left is more problematic. He's a German currency trader who is bright, worldly, and even, unfortunately, cute. I want to hang a sign on me that says I used to be cuter myself. I interview the guy about his work.

Nancy starts passing around red ceramic bowls filled with cold cucumber soup. I am in awe. Cold cucumber soup! Don't you have to puree for that sort of thing?

It's delicious. Everyone says how delicious it is.

Nancy stands up to start clearing bowls. I get up to help her. "Please don't," she says. "Just sit down."

But she doesn't understand. I'm not doing her any favors. Getting up would relieve the pressure of my pantyhose, which are cutting into my waist like a knife, and it would reassure me I am not an absolute loser, that at least I have good manners. "Honestly, I would love to get up," I say.

Nancy and I gather the bowls and carry them into the kitchen. As I load them into the dishwasher, Nancy whips up a fluffy white sauce and pours it over the green beans.

"How's Aidan feeling?" she asks, for not only is she beautiful and a great cook but she is revoltingly kind.

"Fine, thanks," I say, figuring I'll spare her tonight's details now that I'm standing here over her food. "How are your kids?"

"Fine, thanks," she says, opening the oven door and pulling out a roast.

A roast? Did it really have to be a roast? Would it have been such a crime to have made something less ambitious, like chicken?

"Wow!" I cry. "That's beautiful!"

"No, it's not."

"Of course it is!"

"No," Nancy insists, poking the meat, prodding it, and lifting it up to examine underneath. "This is not beautiful. It's overcooked. I wanted the center rare. I'm sure Joe would want it rare, too. People who care about their meat like it rare. But I screwed it all up."

> In the kitchen, where I have come to escape how bad I've been feeling, I find myself mopping her ego off her (stunning slate) floor.

I can't stand her being this hard on herself. "Nancy, please. Trust me, everything has been delicious."

Nancy isn't listening. She is standing at the roast and shaking her head like it was the family pet that just died.

I must do something. Something radical to make her feel better. I know! I will tell the truth. "Nancy," I say, "everything about this evening has been so beautiful—the way you look, the way your home looks, the way your food tastes—that it's intimidating to watch you."

"Right. You're one to feel intimidated." What?

I search Nancy's face for the smirk, the smile, the laugh to show me that she is, of course, kidding. But Nancy looks serious, even a little sad. Her gaze has been fixed on the roast, but now it's fixed on me. "You're so smart," she says. "You had such an interesting career."

"*Had* is the operative word. I don't have it anymore."

"You know what I mean. You are something. You're a journalist. You happen to be taking time off to take care of your kids,

but still you have that professional skill. I don't have any professional skills. I was 24 when I quit my job to come here, and all I've done since is have kids. The only thing I know how to do is cook, but look, I can't even do that! This roast is a disaster. Can you help me get it on the plate?"

I lift my end of the meat, trying to get this all straight: I have been feeling intimidated by a woman who is in fact intimidated by me. In the kitchen, where I have come to escape how bad I've been feeling, I find myself mopping her ego off her (stunning slate) floor. How can this be right? What in perfection's name are we doing to ourselves?

Nancy takes another pan out of the oven, this one with roasted potatoes. I help her arrange them on a plate. "Does Joe like his meat rare?" she asks. "Because I'm afraid no part of this thing will be rare."

"Joe," I assure her, "is happy to be eating at all."

NANCY AND I ENTER THE dining room carrying the roast, potatoes, and green beans, whose white sauce has still not lost its fluff. She does not announce to the table that the meat is overcooked and that she is an idiot for overcooking it. I admire that. I make a mental note to please try to follow her example.

The roast is, of course, delicious. Everyone says how delicious it is.

"Marvelous, Nancy," the cute German man coos.

"Ooooh…" moans Joe, in ecstasy. "This is so good. Please can I have some more?"

Nancy looks at me. I look at her. We burst out laughing. It's a big, raucous laugh, completely out of keeping with how well-mannered we've been the rest of the night. It's a laugh that will resonate in my ears for years to come, reminding me of a very important thing: I am not the only one failing to live up to my ludicrous expectations of myself; we all are. So maybe we all should relax. And instead of feeling bad that the roast tastes so good, I decide to simply enjoy it. ●

O
Dreaming Big

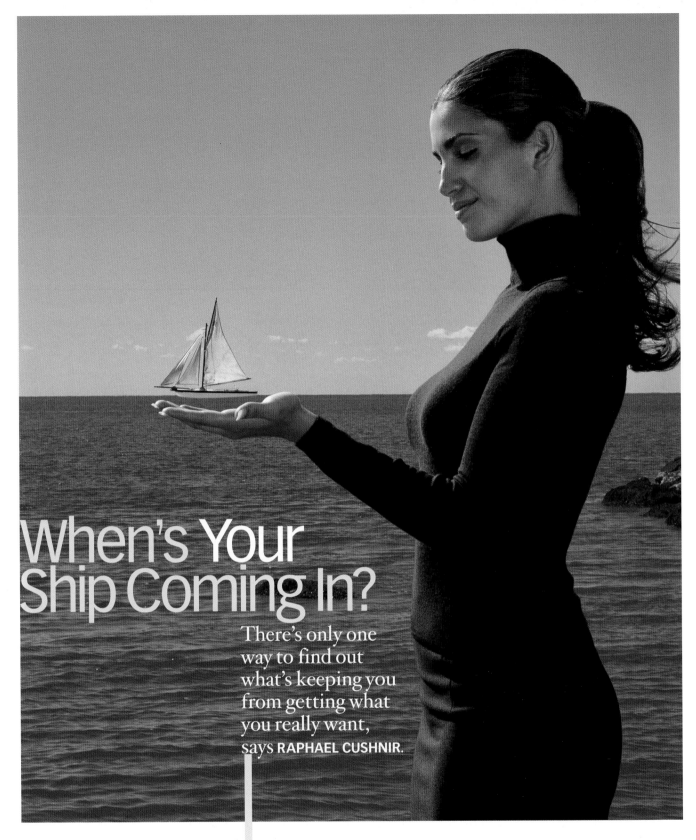

When's Your Ship Coming In?

There's only one way to find out what's keeping you from getting what you really want, says **RAPHAEL CUSHNIR**.

IT'S NEW YEAR'S EVE 1988. I'M traveling alone off the coast of Belize. After spending the day snorkeling, I've come down with a terrible infection. Racked with chills, barely coherent, I stumble across town to rouse the lone nurse from her holiday dinner. Grudgingly, she gives me some antibiotics, and I take to bed.

That night was perhaps the most important of my life. Twisted up in the sheets, raging with fever, I thought I was going to die. In those supposed last moments, I considered my life with deathbed candor. Having failed to make it as a Hollywood screen-writer after almost a decade of trying, I'd privately become convinced that my lack of success was well deserved. I believed that, deep inside, there was something wrong with me—a fatal flaw, an indefinable shortcoming.

Whenever that belief had arisen before, I'd fought it with all the resistance I could summon. Now, instead, I dove straight into wave after wave of enveloping hopeless-ness. It was excruciating, but there was also great relief in giving up the struggle. Maybe it was the semidelirium that finally melted my defenses—I'll never know. But when dawn broke and I was still breathing, the darkness inside me was lighter, too.

In the months that followed, I enjoyed my first hot streak with the studios. Within a couple of years, I had written, produced, and directed an award-winning film. It wasn't newfound discipline that had led to my turnaround. Nor was it a burst of creativity or a stroke of luck. What changed everything was my will-ingness to feel how hopeless I'd been. When I was finally ready to reclaim the part of me that was so hurting and broken-down, healing began. Out of that healing came ease, a new and natural sense of flow. And from that flow, in short order, came the realization of my dream.

ONE DECADE AND SOME major transitions later, I be-gan teaching workshops and counseling clients about how to live more joyfully. I quickly found that most people have a vision for themselves that they are not pursuing, or are approaching halfheartedly, or are chasing with all their might yet somehow falling short. The goal can be modest or grand. It might involve breaking free of a destructive habit, finding a healthy rela-tionship, or leaping into a new career. But in almost every case, there's a similarity to my own story: Whenever people aren't liv-ing their dreams, it's because of emotions they're not yet willing to feel. Once they're willing, the dream comes true—in one form or another.

Annette, for example, was an office manager. When she called me for coun-seling, her voice was small and clipped. What she'd always wanted, she told me, was to start a flower-arranging business for weddings. For almost two years, she'd had the information she needed to begin but hadn't done a single thing with it. By the time we spoke, she was avoiding her home office entirely.

When I was finally ready to reclaim the part of me that was so hurting and broken-down, healing began.

I asked Annette to imagine herself in the office doorway, about to get to work. Immediately, she reported feeling "scared to death."

"Scared of?" I said.

She paused. "Hmm. You know, I thought it would be fear of failure, but what's coming up is different." Annette went on to describe an emotional legacy from her childhood, when she learned to be seen and not heard. If she put herself forward without being asked, she was met with such fury that she quickly trained herself never to do it. So starting a new business felt like trying to get away with something.

After her fear subsided a bit, I asked Annette to tell me the worst thing that could happen if she went ahead with her project anyway.

"Well, I'm not sure," she said. "I've never thought that far ahead."

I suggested she imagine that her busi-ness was up and running, and that she delivered a floral arrangement to a client who was angry and disappointed, shouting, "Who do you think you are? You don't deserve to be a florist!"

Annette seemed to shrink and re-ported that her chest and shoulders felt wrapped up like a mummy. I encouraged her to keep her attention on that tight-ness, to regard it with as much tenderness as possible.

"It's starting to release," she told me after a few moments, "but now I feel humiliated, as though I'm being punished for the whole world to see."

"Keep feeling that, too," I said, knowing she'd struck gold. It was Annette's unwillingness to come face-to-face with this humiliation that had led to her professional paralysis. All she needed to do was stay present to the feeling, without fighting it or trying to figure it out. In about two or three min-utes, the emotion subsided. This left her a little stunned.

"Wow, that wasn't as bad as I thought," she said. It almost never is, I told her. Then I asked her, from this place of relaxation and acceptance, how she would respond to the angry client.

"I guess…" She paused. "I guess I could just apologize and see if there's a way to fix the problem."

This simple recognition, that there was life after her worst-case scenario, marked the beginning of Annette's transformation. She started going to trade shows and mak-ing cold calls. Today, while she still needs her day job, she arranges flowers for about two weddings a month. What's even more important is that she feels like a success, which provides her with the energy and motivation to persist.

You can jump-start just about any dream using these four steps:

1. Find the flinch.

Identify an important action you haven't taken. This could involve doing research, making a call, or just setting foot in your home office. It's possible that you've taken this action from time to time, but not consistently. Or you've taken it over and over with no success. What's crucial is that you recognize the moment when you ordinarily check out, not only from your dream but from your ongoing emotional flow. This is the point when you might reach for a distraction, go numb, or sink into a "What's the use?" depression.

2. Go for the jugular.

If there weren't something very challenging for you to feel, you'd have no need to check out. To find that challenging emotion, ask yourself, *What's the worst thing that could happen if I went forward in this moment?* Rather than jump to conclusions, let the answer come on its own. Once you've discovered your worst-case scenario, ask, *If this happened, what's the most awful feeling I'd have to endure?* Again, let the answer arrive naturally, without rushing to uncover it. It may be fear, failure, loss, guilt, rejection, rage, hurt, or something uniquely yours. You know you're on the right track when your original flinch deepens, when you want to run for the hills.

3. Weather the storm.

It's now time to feel what you've been resisting, perhaps for most of your life. This takes real courage, but the only alternative is an unfulfilled dream. So go ahead, imagine that the worst has come to pass, and give yourself over completely to that torment. Whether you feel it in one particular spot or all over, stay connected to its physical manifestation. Whenever you lose your focus, patiently bring it back. Let your awareness remain soft and steady,

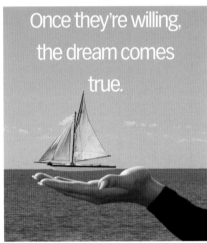

When people aren't living their dreams, it's because of emotions they're not yet willing to feel. Once they're willing, the dream comes true.

without attempting to *do* anything. Freed up in this way, your emotions will shift and change, just like the weather.

4. Repeat as necessary.

Now you know the most liberating truth: The emotion you thought was intolerable actually isn't. You have the capacity to accept it, survive it, and feel cleansed with its passing. And that means it can no longer deter your dream. You'll be able to stop procrastinating, work longer and harder, uplifted by an exhilarating flow. You will,

however, need to repeat these four steps whenever you find yourself yearning to escape. But each time, the process will be easier and quicker.

One of my clients, Noelle, was freed to have a peaceful relationship with her teenage daughter by accepting that she felt like a bad parent. That didn't mean believing she really was a bad parent, but rather ceasing to deny the feeling and therefore having to blow up every time her daughter triggered it.

Another client, Evelyn, loved to sing and wanted to create a cabaret act—but she couldn't accept that her voice wasn't great. When she surrendered to feeling "painfully mediocre," she soon found songs that played to her vocal strengths.

Perhaps the most telling example is Christine, who yearned to turn her enthusiasm and caring nature into a career as a personal coach. She'd printed up business cards and gone to a few networking events, but that was years ago. She called herself the Queen of Procrastination, and a lost cause. "It's like there's a mile between me and my dream," she told everyone at a workshop, "but I can't take the first step."

It turned out that the feeling Christine most resisted was being overwhelmed. A few moments of staring at a to-do list usually sent her straight for a bowl of Häagen-Dazs. But when she sat still and said yes to the feeling, she found she wasn't so overwhelmed after all. Instead, she felt sadness. She realized that all her role models had been even bigger procrastinators and that no one had taught her to follow through.

Christine's sadness gave way to relief, and she was able to give herself a break. She came to understand that her first job was to coach herself. In the process, she developed greater patience, an ability to ask for help, and the kind of authenticity that only meeting challenges can bring. Six months later, her coaching practice is already half-full. And what inspires her clients the most, she reports, is hearing about her own path to emotional freedom. ●

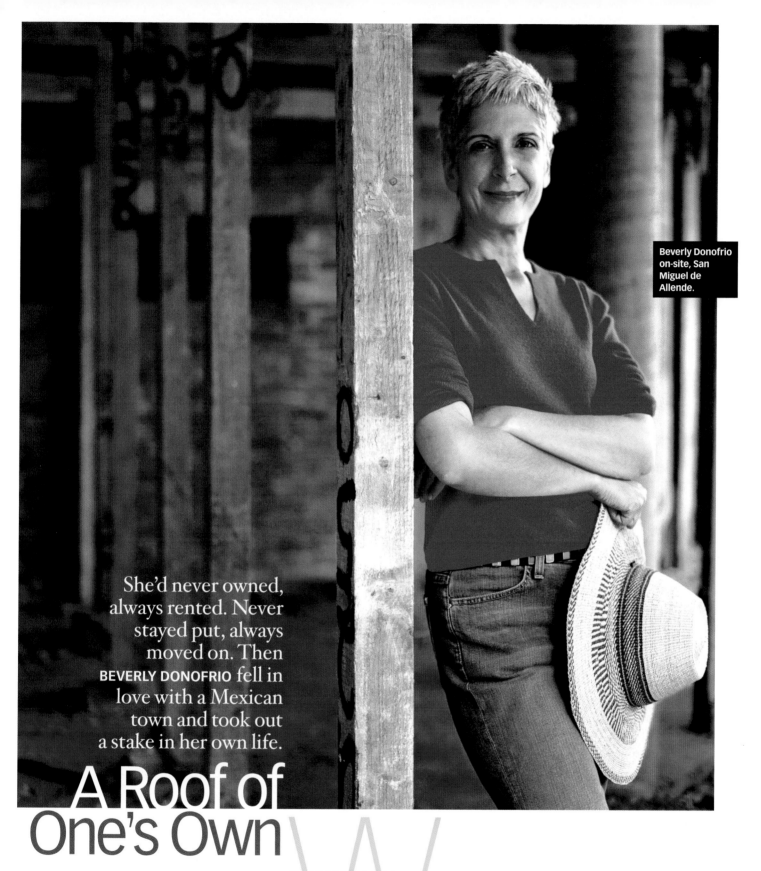

She'd never owned, always rented. Never stayed put, always moved on. Then **BEVERLY DONOFRIO** fell in love with a Mexican town and took out a stake in her own life.

A Roof of One's Own

WHEN I WAS A KID, I BELIEVED I'D BECOME A PRINCESS AND LIVE IN a castle, but then I got realistic and figured that I'd just move out of the public housing project one day and own my own home. By the time I was 51, I'd lived in another country, four states, nine towns, and 22 different rentals. Although each packing up had been a nightmare, moving had become rejuvenation, adventure, therapy, a way to take regular inventory and shed unnecessary stuff.

I still did, however, periodically fantasize about a home of my own, where I'd plant a tree and watch it grow, make improvements every year, survey my property, take stock of it and me, observe how we evolved together.

Ten years ago there was even an opportunity. In a seaside village on Long Island, I looked at a sweet little house with an office over the garage and a pristine view of the bay, selling for $120,000. I'm a writer with no guaranteed income and hardly a

I could see that by not allowing myself a home of my own, I was holding on to the feeling of being deprived.

credit history. But I did have option money coming in for a book I'd sold to the movies, and if I'd bothered to go talk to a bank, I might have found they were willing to take a risk on me. Instead I assumed they wouldn't. I told myself that it would be silly to give up my inexpensive rented house for a smaller house, huge debt...and let's not forget all the responsibility for fixing things like the plumbing, which, knowing my luck, would break down.

Through the years, as my friends and siblings proceeded to take the plunge, I was the only holdout—occasionally remembering with a prick of discomfort the little house I'd passed up and how it had increased in value to $300,000, occasionally wondering why I was not solid enough to be a homeowner. At 17 I'd become a mother, moved into another rental in the same housing project I grew up in, and by 19 I was on welfare. But eventually, I did go to college. I got a master's degree, published a few books, traveled. My parents had done none of these things. And yet in some deep way, I still felt I wasn't supposed to go beyond them or the house I grew up in. How could I claim the right?

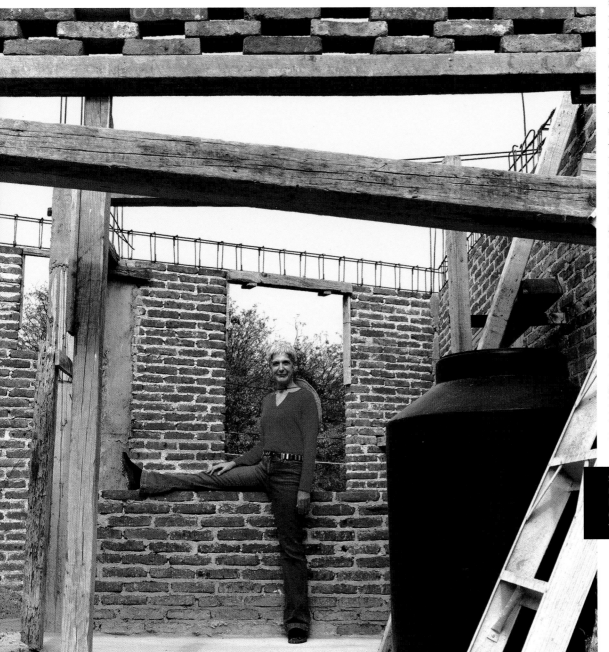

Settling for more: "I fell in love with the culture and the place."

Then in 1999, in a mountain town in Mexico where I'd come to write a book about the Virgin Mary, I fell in love with the culture and the place, and I stayed. Four rentals later, I found a jewel of a house, set in the middle of a luscious garden, with one drawback: I must relinquish the house to its owners for a month every summer. I moved in anyway, fantasizing that the owners would miraculously decide to sell it to me and, just as miraculously, I'd find the money to buy it. I painted every room, installed the plumbing for a washer, planted lemon, lime, and pomegranate trees, and converted an outdoor room into a salon, neatly overlooking the fact—as I'd always done—that every attempt to make the house my own would be thwarted by the reality that it wasn't. Only this time I'd be given an intolerable reminder every year when I had to abandon my house to its owners. To hammer that awful truth home, the second year's lease had a new clause. Either party (read: the owners) could cancel the lease with 30 days' notice. And the final blow: The owners would return to occupy my/their house from December 20 till January 2, leaving me homeless for Christmas and New Year's.

I had no choice but to experience this as a prod from the universe, which likes to send up smoke signals and when you don't read the signs starts a fire.

I began waking in the middle of the night, wanting to commit myself to buying a house but afraid I couldn't find a way. I could see that by not allowing myself a home of my own, I was holding on to the feeling of being deprived. Each time I lived in a beautiful house, I felt at once lucky to live there and deprived because it didn't belong to me. To allow myself to buy a house, I'd have to see myself as worthy of it: a stable and substantial person who deserved to be the woman of the manor even if I wasn't to the manor born. To buy a house, I'd have to be willing to shed my old self-image as the poor kid and the underprivileged adult. To stop moving from house to house would require putting down roots, becoming a woman who could shoulder responsibility, make a commitment, stop fleeing.

I was terrified. I saw no chunk of disposable income heading my way in the near future. I didn't think a Mexican bank would be willing to lend me money, and no American bank I knew of would risk money on a private house there. So how could I swing it?

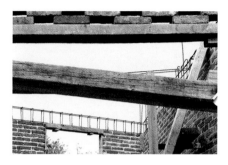

You take one risk,
do one great thing for yourself, and the universe showers you with rewards.

A few months earlier, my friends and neighbors Caren and Dave had mentioned that over the years they'd helped family and friends buy houses, and Caren had said, "If you ever…" I prided myself on being independent, considered myself self-reliant. How could I swallow my pride and find the courage to ask friends for a loan?

Then I remembered another opportunity I'd passed up. When I graduated from college, a friend's father, then the programming director at PBS, had urged me to apply for a job in the news research department. I was a working-class girl, sure I'd never be hired, and even if I were, I'd be fired. Besides, I'd missed the lesson in third grade on how to use the dictionary and hadn't mastered researching in college. I never went for the position and was stuck in menial jobs for years.

I couldn't pass up this chance. I had to make the leap and become the substantial person I wanted to be. I called up Dave and asked if we could talk. He picked me up on his motorcycle, and we rode up the mountain and sat on a rock by the lake. A lump formed in my throat. Fighting back tears, I pushed through it. "Dave," I choked out, "could you loan me money to buy a house?"

"Sure," he said. "We've been waiting for you to ask." The 6 percent interest they'd charge would be a good investment for them. When we rode back to Dave and Caren's and told her the news, she offered to help me find a place.

YOU TAKE ONE RISK, DO one great thing for yourself, and the universe showers you with rewards. On my way home from Caren and Dave's, I departed from my usual route and spotted a FOR SALE sign on the wall of an unfamiliar street. Behind it was a piece of land with a palm tree and mature magueys overlooking a canyon on one side and the ancient mosaic and gold-leafed domes of the town on the other. I began negotiations immediately, and the next week at a restaurant I was introduced to an architect renowned for designing houses flooded with light. He's retired, works out of love, and he offered to draw up the plans and oversee the building of my house for $2,000.

Three weeks later, I signed on the dotted line and was handed the keys to the gate of the property wall. I had my land. During those heady three weeks, I was invited to receive the Distinguished Alumna Award from Wesleyan University, to judge a prestigious competition for nonfiction writers, and to become president of our local chapter of the writers' organization PEN. These days I have to go a long way to imagine myself as an underprivileged adult. In fact, I am filled with awe that I've attained what I'd believed was impossible. And I'm reminded of something I already knew but seem constantly in need of relearning: If you say yes to yourself, if you let your imagination fly, if you open one stuck, fear-warped door, other doors you never even noticed fly open, pushed by a spirit strong as a hurricane. ●

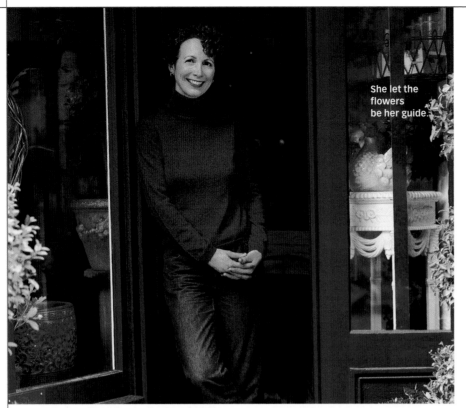

She let the flowers be her guide.

A Budding Genius

What, you ask, was she doing? Quitting her job,
going to work at a florist, risking everything.
WENDY KING FREDELL finds the perfect arrangement.

FISK & COMPANY LOOKS LIKE A shop you might find on the Left Bank in Paris. The windows display two large champagne bottles spewing tiny yellow foam balls of fizz that recycle through a hidden trough. Silk flowers in black-lacquered urns share the space with hand-painted pottery from Tuscany. As the owner, Gregg, proclaims in his ads, the shop is "a feast for the eyes!"

I stared curiously at the world on the other side of the windows. The past week had been rough for me at work. My boss, Martha, was difficult—cruel and unpleasant—and I seemed to be her main obsession. I longed for something new. Something sane.

I stepped into the store, slipping past the grapevines that looped along the walls, the giant silk hydrangeas and wicker baskets massed with roses. Gregg was standing at the counter with a big smile, as if he were expecting me. Suddenly I thought,

Why don't I work here? Impulsively I said, "If you ever need an assistant, let me know!" He took my name and number, and I left.

Three months later, I got an urgent call from him: "Can you manage my shop for me while I run my garden tour of Italy?"

"Yes, of course." (*What am I doing? I thought.*)

"You *have* designed flowers professionally, haven't you?" Gregg asked.

"Yes," I lied. (*I've lost my mind!*)

I'd never had a lesson in flower arranging. When I "fix" flowers, something other than me seems to take over. I let the flowers and my intuition guide me. I hoped that would get me through the ten days Gregg would be away.

"Can you do French provincial or the English country look?" Gregg asked.

"Oh, I lived in Europe for ten years, and I spent a lot of time poring over French and English flower design." (As I strolled by

florists, I'd study the arrangements in the windows.)

"Great. Come in this week," Gregg said. "I'll show you how to manage the shop."

With dread I tried to imagine myself running his high-end shop. *You're in way over your head,* my inner voice chided.

But I quit my job that day. Goodbye, Martha!

After a sleepless night, acid reflux, and what-in-the-hell-am-I-doing thoughts, I met Gregg for my first job-training session. It lasted only one hour and consisted of Gregg's barking instructions as he whirled around the shop: "Make sure you reboot the computer every day and see that the Dove Network is on so you can receive flower orders."

After four more days of the same training technique, I nervously asked, "Don't you think I need some hands-on training?"

"Oh, yes!" Gregg replied, as if this were a novel idea. "Why don't you man the phone and the cash register and handle the customers for a while? I need to finish these wedding arrangements." Then, inspired, he said, "On second thought, why don't you do the main arrangement for the reception?" He grabbed four massive flower-filled buckets from the cooler and set up a workspace for me in back, leaving me alone to contemplate the buckets. Sweating with anxiety, I stared at the empty silver container and wondered how I would ever pull this off. *Face the fear and do it anyway* ran through my head as my shaking hands pushed flower stems into a wet oasis. *Flowers, speak to me,* I muttered to myself. *Show me who you want to stand next to.* One hour later, it was done. Gregg returned. In silence he looked at my design.

"You are good," he said with relief. "Very talented. I feel really confident leaving you in charge!" He beamed.

Mercifully, there was no funeral the week my new boss was away. And Gregg—who found his shop still standing when he got back—turned out to be all that Martha was not. In a matter of weeks, I had learned the difference between French provincial and English country—let's just say it involves artichokes—and I'd also discovered the exhilaration of taking a leap of faith and landing in a bed of roses. •

O
Spirituality

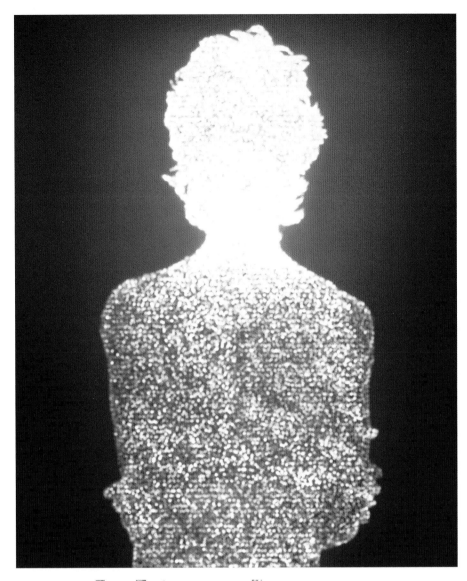

spiritual energy

Have you ever been in the presence of something so lively, engaged, selfless, and utterly radiant, it's left you speechless? **Mark Matousek** taps into the world's greatest renewable power source.

A FEW MONTHS BEFORE HE DIED, 83-year-old Spyros Sathi, widely regarded as the greatest Christian mystic of modern times, agreed to sit down and talk with me in his first American interview. Known simply as the Daskalos ("teacher"), this powerful Cypriot healer had, I'd heard, once frightened a group of hard-nosed reporters by rocking a lame child in his arms and setting him down a few minutes later on legs that were suddenly functional. The night before our interview, I'd studied the Daskalos from a distance, holding forth on a New York stage strewn with flowers; now, stepping into his hotel room with a photographer, I had no idea what to expect.

The moment he rose—six feet five in a cardigan sweater—and took my hand, all my apprehension disappeared. Something about this towering man—a glowing kindness, a welcoming ease—put me at ease, too, and for the next hour I questioned him about how it felt to have his powers. I barely understood his responses (you try interviewing a mystic), but when I stood up to say goodbye, I was so light-headed—so light all over—that I had to sit down to steady myself. The Daskalos smiled and watched me intently; then without any forethought, I asked him about a painful situation in my life. My host leaned forward, took my wrist between his fingers, and said, "You are good." Three simple words—just that—bearing no conscious link to my question; yet hearing them I wanted to weep, as if Spyros Sathi had somehow heard, underneath the surface question, a deeper confusion, a covert hunger, a secret longing to be blessed. The photographer happened to capture this moment, the Daskalos gently touching my arm, grinning at me as I beamed back at him with the same sort of lit-up expression. In the photograph, which I treasure, my face looks like a hundred-watt bulb.

I'VE NEVER BEEN A PERSON OF FAITH. In matters of spirit, I'm from Missouri—fascinated but skeptical. Were it not for meeting the Daskalos and a handful of other exceptional teachers in my travels as a writer and seeker, I would surely doubt that such a thing as spiritual energy existed—not as a miraculous fluke but a natural gift accessible to all of us. Like harmony, symmetry, and even genius, this invisible force is a mystery whose uplifting power must be encountered to be believed. Once that happens, revealing a glimpse of our awesome potential, it can never again be denied.

Daniel Goleman first became aware of spiritual energy three decades ago in Asia. The author of the best-selling *Emotional Intelligence,* Goleman was a Harvard graduate studying meditation in India when he noticed that most seasoned practitioners exuded what he calls "a special quality, magnetic in a quiet sense." Contrary to stereotype, these spiritual types did not seem otherworldly at all. "They were lively and engaged," he says, "extremely present, involved in the moment, often funny, yet profoundly at peace—equanimous in disturbing situations." What's more, it seemed to him that this quality was communicable: "You always felt better than before you'd spent time with them, and this feeling lasted."

Goleman discovered that the components of spiritual energy are as carefully quantified in ancient traditions as waves and particles are in physics. "One of the words used to describe this magnetic state is *sukha*," he says, a Pali expression denoting a sense of "repleteness, contentment, delight—a calm, abiding joy regardless of external circumstances." *Sukha* is selfless in nature and connected to a greater purpose—which is why it increases through service to others.

Traditional cultures recognize that spending time with individuals who radiate this quality is nourishing in itself. In the Hindu custom known as *darshan* ("presence"), people "tune in to someone who is already in that magnificent internal space," Goleman says, "catching it, so to speak, and carrying it out to others."

Such transmission is more palpable than a skeptic might expect, as I found with the Daskalos, and as San Francisco psychologist Paul Ekman saw after spending a week in Dharmsala with the Dalai Lama. "At the airport afterward, my wife looked at me and said, 'You're not the man I married!'" Ekman says with a laugh. "I was acting like somebody who's in love." The foremost authority on the physiology of emotion, Ekman—who is not a Buddhist—had been invited to engage in a cross-cultural dialogue between Western scientists and His Holiness, along with several monks. Ekman left the meeting deeply moved. "These monks were unlike any human beings I had encountered before," he says. "They were joyous in a way I had never seen, except, perhaps, in my daughter at two or three years old."

Ekman detected four characteristics common to people with this energy: a "palpable goodness," first of all, that went far beyond some "warm and fuzzy aura" and seemed to arise from genuine integrity. Next, an impression of selflessness—a lack of concern with status, fame, and ego—a "transparency between their personal and public lives that set them apart from those with charisma, who are often one thing on the outside, another when you look under the surface." Third, Ekman noticed that this expansive, compassionate energy nurtured others. Finally, he was struck by the "amazing powers of attentiveness" dis-played by these individuals, and the feeling he had of being seen in the round, wholly acknowledged, and embraced by someone with open eyes.

If these qualities were unique to masters, they wouldn't be half as compelling. What inspired Ekman-the-scientist was witnessing that transformation is possible for the rest of us. "It wasn't luck or culture or genes that created this qualitative difference," he insists. "These people have re-sculpted their brains through practice." Contrary to the old hardwiring theory that posited the human brain as fixed from birth, the emerging theory of neuroplasticity has revealed that our minds are reshaped through repeated experience.

In his book, *Destructive Emotions,* Goleman cites a recent study involving a monk being monitored in a laboratory while he meditates on compassion. Among other findings, scientists saw a dramatic increase

Focusing on gratitude enhances the feeling of connection.

in gamma energy (sparked in the part of the brain associated with positive emotions), proving that through concern for others we can create measurably greater well-being in ourselves.

This ability requires practice. According to Maxine Gaudio, a biofeedback pioneer and master of the energy work known as reiki, "everybody can draw, but not everybody's a Picasso." As beginners trying to kick-start our gamma, we find ourselves in an ongoing struggle with our own anger, greed, and fear. We lose sight of the fact that we're all interrelated, and that connection is central to tapping into a spiritual wellspring.

"It's our daily dilemma," says David Steindl-Rast, a 77-year-old Benedictine monk who lives as a hermit in upstate New York. "A spiritual energy flows through the universe, a superaliveness—an active *yes.* Yet even though our greatest happiness comes from feeling this eternal connection, there's a tendency in all of us to close off from it. Those who counteract the ten-dency through practice deepen their sense of belonging and free this latent energy."

Focusing on gratitude enhances the feeling of connection. "When we say 'Count your blessings,' this is a very profound teaching," Brother David assures me. "A stream of energy—of blessing—is flowing from the universal source as blood pulsates from the heart. Knowing this, I'm energized and pass the blessing along to my brother so it flows again to its source. We create a network of grateful living."

Gratitude can also arise through meditation. Tara Brach, a psychologist and instructor of mindfulness practice, counsels students to harness an active yes through something she calls radical acceptance—the title of her book. "Our basic nature is loving awareness, but we forget," Brach says. "We disconnect; we perceive separation, and along with that illusion comes most of our suffering."

An excellent means of plugging back in, Brach maintains, is to begin with self-acceptance, opening with kindness to what is. "This compassionate quality wakes us up. We have more choices, we're more connected. Spiritual practice is about remembering who we are," Brach says. "Others' awareness helps us to remember—they become our mirrors. Resting together in this energy, we're not driven to create more violence in the world, nor to violate ourselves."

Hearing these words, I can't help thinking how closely the process of connection resembles love. When I mention my observation to David Steindl-Rast, he insists, "It *is* love." Not personal or romantic love but the love described in the various gospels—the love "which passeth all understanding"—the unconditional warmth that arises naturally from our humanity. It was this that I felt with the Daskalos: enormous, embracing, unstoppable love drawing me toward its own radiance. This force could save the world, I think, melt away borders, give us hope. Another great Christian, Pierre Teilhard de Chardin, articulated this for all time. "Someday after we have mastered the winds, the waves, the tides, and gravity, we shall harness...the energies of love," he wrote. "Then for the second time in the history of the world, man will have discovered fire." •

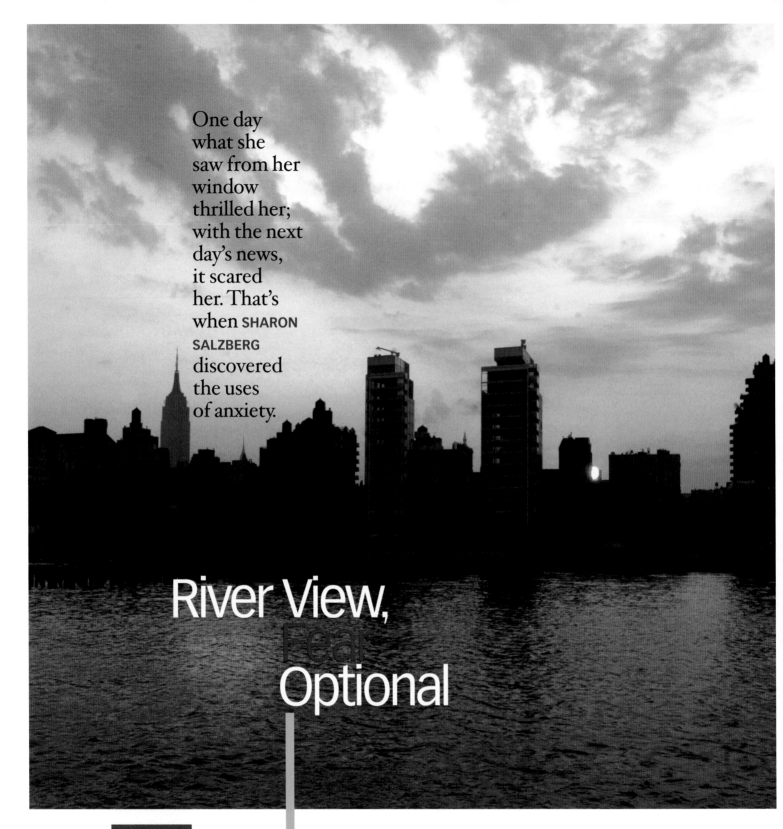

One day what she saw from her window thrilled her; with the next day's news, it scared her. That's when **SHARON SALZBERG** discovered the uses of anxiety.

River View, Fear Optional

Safety becomes a psychological destination rather than a physical one.

LAST YEAR I MANAGED TO PROCURE that most rare and precious commodity: a sublet in New York City that was both magnificent and affordable. This beautiful loft was owned by Fred, a friend who had gone off to England for an extended meditation retreat. Located on the west side of town, the loft's living room windows opened onto a panoramic sweep of the Hudson River. I was captivated by the view. To be able to look out at the river last thing at night and first thing in the morning, I slept on the living room couch. I wrote my landlord's meditation instructor, a colleague of mine, to suggest half-jokingly that Fred might derive benefit from an even longer stay in England. Keep him there, I suggested, and I'll just stay on here. Watching that river flow by, I sensed mystery, voyage, delight. I was so happy.

Then one day a friend sent me an e-mail asking if I'd heard the new warning about possible terror attacks on subways and trains. Thinking I really needed to keep up more, I turned on the television, located on the same wall as my wonderful river view. Right away I heard the newscaster's voice say, "Warnings have been issued about possible scuba-diving terrorists." I froze. Scuba-diving terrorists! Scuba-diving terrorists would need a body of water, wouldn't they? I looked from the television screen to the river view, back to the television screen, back to the river view, and I sensed devastation, horror, menace. *How can I manage to get Fred back here quickly?* was my desperate thought.

Some people claim that all danger exists simply in one's own mind, or contend that terror threats are merely the strategic tool of a political machine bent on distracting its populace. But life is made up of uncertainty. Each time we breathe out, we don't know if we'll breathe in again. Each time we risk stepping forward, we don't know what we'll encounter, but we can't just idle where we are. Despite all our efforts to picture the unfolding of events as managed, orderly, fixed, we don't know what will happen next.

B UT IT MAKES NO SENSE TO let our actions be determined by fear's blind rush, its choking certainty that everything is bad and will only get worse. The space fear carves out for us to reside in is very small. Last year I could have let my blast of worry about the river overwhelm everything else and moved inland. Living in New York City right after September 11, I was startled by the degree of strategizing that went on to try to manage a world revealed to be spinning well outside our control: "If I don't cross that bridge at that time, I'll be okay." "As long as it's not rush hour when I take the subway, things will be fine." Yet when what we fear can come

in any form at any time, safety becomes a psychological or spiritual destination rather than a physical one. Finding our inner strength, our love for one another, our aspiration to make this a better world is the only sure way to survive with our hearts intact.

I've recently learned a new term from friends who work in federal agencies in Washington, D.C.—*shelter in place.* Shelter in place is the opposite of evacuation, and it's used in the event of a chemical, nuclear, or biological attack, when it's not safe to go outside. When a shelter-in-place drill is ordered, people go to some designated windowless space, with their supplies of water and food and clothing, and stay there until they are told it's safe to leave. Before I knew what the term meant,

> Now I remind
> **myself,**
> while feeling afraid,
> to love life anyway.

I found the sound of it inspiring, even uplifting—like *Make your home wherever you are. Let your deepest understanding be your sanctuary, even in bad circumstances. Safety is not where you are, it's what you do about where you are.* That deeper sense of shelter in place is what I'd always longed for spiritually and had aimed for steadily.

I know that regardless of whatever outward measures any of us takes, we are likely to still be afraid. We live in times of immense turmoil and anxiety. Whether the threat is scuba-diving terrorists, new diseases, biological attacks, personal heartache, or what *The Wall Street Journal* suggests we should be most afraid of in terms of daily-life casualties—stairs—our lives are full of real, potential, and imagined hazards. Because of this omnipresent truth, I believe that what we need to do right here and now is work to retain our faith. We can do this no matter what our religious orientation, or lack of one, by

remembering that everything is changing all the time. This is the positive face of uncertainty. Daily reflection or meditation will remind us that if we look closely at any painful emotion or difficult situation, it is bound to change—it's not as solid and inert as it might have seemed. The fear we feel in the morning may not be present in the afternoon. Hopelessness may be replaced by calm, or even a little bit less hopelessness. Even while a challenging situation is unfolding, it is shifting, varied, alive. Once we see the inherent change in our experience, we see that we're not trapped, that we have options. Then, even if we are afraid, faith can arise.

Faith is the quality that allows us to find a way to go on, to feel empowered, to—no matter what—keep on trying. This is not a sentimental faith that everything will be just fine, according to our wishes or our timetable. Rather, it is an awakened faith that gives us the courage to go into the unknown, the remembrance that nothing is fixed, and the understanding that as long as we are alive, possibility is alive. It is the power of faith that inspires us to step forward into the center of our lives—to participate, to link up, to reach out to others and let others reach out to us, to work for a better world. And it is the vitality of faith that tells us, however easy it is to forget or be overcome by fear, that the place for communicating, for loving, for sheltering, for trying, is right where we are.

Now I remind myself, while feeling afraid, to love life anyway, to retain the certain knowledge that I will die someday and use that to open to the preciousness of what I see and touch and feel right in front of me. Now I might feel afraid but am determined to have that fear serve as a counterpoint to my tendency to procrastinate—if I have to apologize, tell someone "I love you," try to make a difference, I need to do it without delay. Now I want fear to liberate me instead of victimize me—to have it free me to go beyond embarrassment and habitual social stricture and hollow expectations to fully live my life, nothing held back. To venture to love. To enjoy every river and all friendships and each drop of air. •

What They Did for BLiSS

Once they were lawyers, investment bankers, artists.
One was a movie star. One was Jewish.
Today these 40 highly accomplished women
have given up everything to live in a unique monastery
in Bethlehem, Connecticut. They've taken vows of
chastity, poverty, and obedience, and claim that they've
never been happier. SARA DAVIDSON
goes behind the abbey walls.

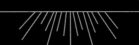

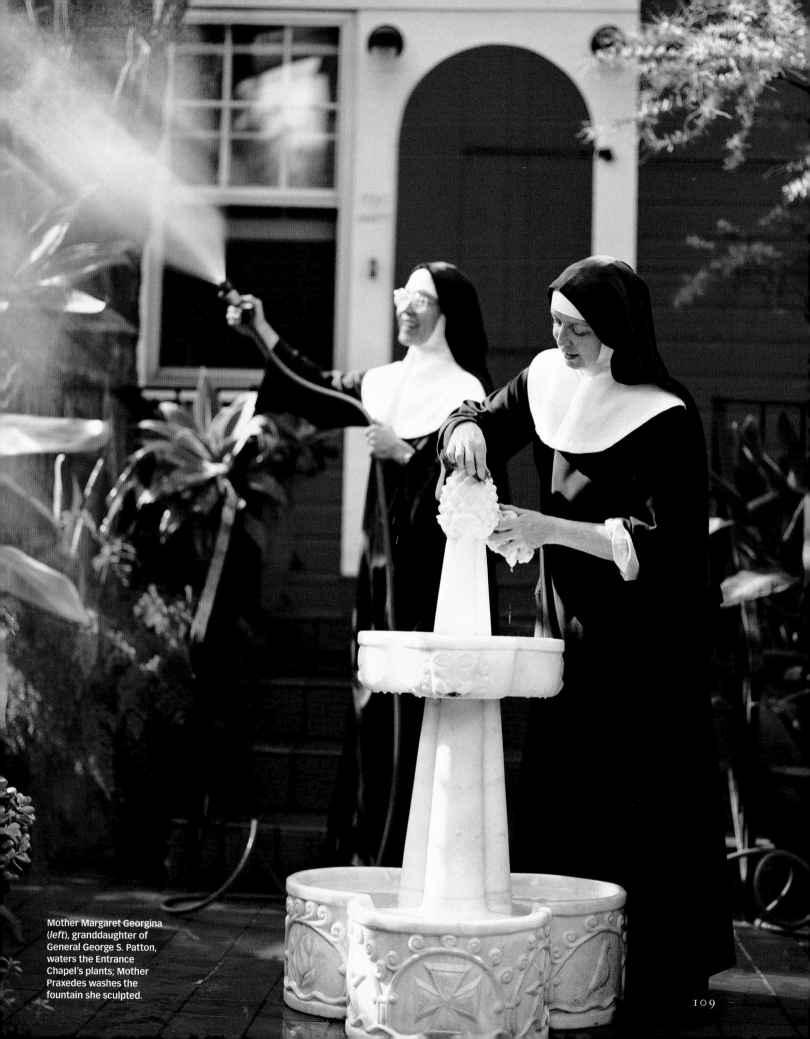

Mother Margaret Georgina (*left*), granddaughter of General George S. Patton, waters the Entrance Chapel's plants; Mother Praxedes washes the fountain she sculpted.

At a brunch near the University of Colorado last year, I met a film professor, Jim Palmer, who told me his 34-year-old daughter, Sydney, was becoming a nun. She was about to have her "clothing ceremony," when she would receive a new name and have her long strawberry blonde hair cut off to go "under the veil." Palmer was struggling to come to terms with his daughter's choice. She had been raised Episcopalian, was stylish and sophisticated, and had studied comparative literature at Smith College. "This was not the trajectory we envisioned for her," he said. Yet Palmer spoke with admiration of the women in the monastery his daughter was joining, the Abbey of

Regina Laudis in Bethlehem, Connecticut. The community is unique: 40 exceptionally bright and gifted women, many of whom attained success in the world before becoming nuns.

The founder, Lady Abbess Benedict Duss, set a standard of excellence. She decided that every woman who entered must have some gift, talent, or profession and must strive to be "equal to or superior to others in her field." From its start in 1947, the abbey has attracted strong women, including a movie star, Dolores Hart, who made two films with Elvis Presley; a member of the Connecticut legislature; a Shakespearean scholar from Yale; several lawyers; a Wall Street executive; and a sculptor whom the abbey sent to Rome to learn marble carving from the top artists in Italy.

This pattern, set decades ago at the abbey, now appears to be a national trend. Women are entering religious orders when they are older, have had careers, and long for something beyond what they've accomplished in the world.

At Regina Laudis, the nuns live on 450 acres of land where they grow their own food and make an acclaimed cheese from raw milk given by their black-and-white belted cows. Some nuns have been married and had children. Yet they live behind an enclosure, according to the rules established by Saint Benedict in the sixth century, pray in Latin, sing Gregorian chant eight times a day, and take vows of chastity and obedience.

Curious to learn what brought these women to the abbey and why they've stayed, I drove into green Connecticut last May, when it rained almost daily and lightning cracked across the sky.

WHAT STRIKES ME FIRST IS THE harmonious beauty of the gardens and buildings, which reflect a spirit that's feminine but not soft. Everything is designed on a massive scale. The Entrance Chapel is a soaring two-story greenhouse filled with tropical plants and a thrusting marble fountain carved by the sculptor, Mother Praxedes. Above the door is another work of hers, a giant stained-glass window of Mary that looks like an image

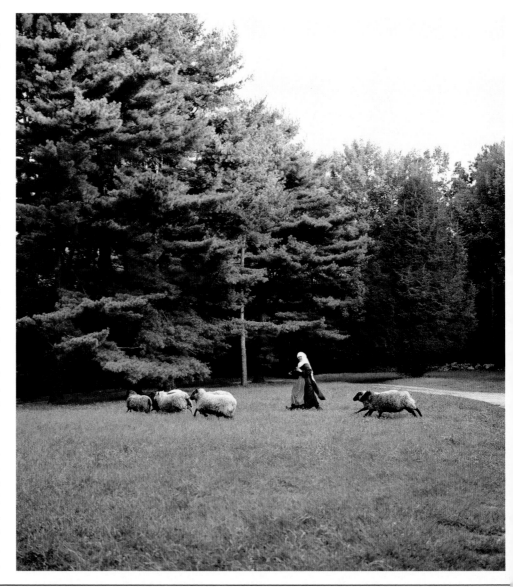

from a tarot card: Mary is emerging from the trunk of a tree, holding the sun and moon in her hands, with the infant Jesus in her flower-petaled womb.

I step inside to ring the bell, and a nun appears behind the wooden grille—Sister Angèle, who will be my guide. She drives me to the women's guesthouse and shows me my room. The stairs creak with every step, and the place has the musty smell of old New England houses in the rain. It's furnished with homey antiques, quilts, and religious paintings, and in the kitchen the nuns have left me supper in a basket: lettuce that's just been picked, three slices of the abbey cheese, freshly baked bread, and tomato soup loaded with chunks of tomatoes from the garden.

Sister Angèle, who was raised Jewish and became a nun at 50 after a career managing opera singers, tells me the abbey schedule is a paradox of "serenity and chaos." Unlike monks who sit in meditation for extended periods, the nuns are constantly rushing, working, jumping into a car to drive to Mass because they don't have ten minutes to walk up the hill.

To have an interview or conversation with a nun, one requests a "parlor," from the French *parler,* "to talk." Both men and women visitors can stay at the abbey, but they eat separately from the nuns and never enter their private quarters. For my first interview, I walk through a door into a small room that's divided in two by a wooden latticework grille. On the other side of the grille, through a different door, Mother Lucia walks in and sits down with a rustling of robes.

She takes hold of the grille and rattles it. "I was mystified by this when I first came here," she says. She and her college boyfriend had hitchhiked to the abbey in 1970 while exploring alternative forms of spirituality. "We were coming from the youth protest culture: Tear down the walls,

take off your clothes, break all the barriers," she recalls. But they were impressed by how happy the nuns seemed, at a time when the protest movement was turning bitter and fragmented.

For eight years, Mother Lucia and a group of friends of both sexes came to the abbey for the month of August to study and work. Four of her friends entered the abbey as nuns. "I was the last," she says. She had completed a PhD in literature at Yale, writing her dissertation on the breakdown of masculine and feminine relationships in Shakespeare's plays. And then, she says, "a light fell on my inmost soul." Although she had seriously considered marriage, she realized, "I was drawn to something else. What I felt at the abbey was the most intense experience of love I'd known."

Friends and family responded with alarm. "Are you crazy," they said, "throwing away your PhD after all the years you worked for it?" But Mother Lucia says that in addition to being the abbey's librarian, "I feel I'm living my dissertation now. I wrote about gender, and every day, I'm still working with that issue."

Some feminists assert that the Catholic Church has oppressed women and should now ordain women priests. Mother Lucia says, "As a community we don't feel oppressed or excluded, and we don't believe women should be priests. We have a complementary role; I think we do something different." She says that men see themselves as following Christ, "but women can see themselves as entering into union with Christ." This is why the abbey observes the Consecration to a Life of Virginity, a rite that dates from the fourth century, when women declared they would not take a husband because they considered themselves married to Christ and would spend their days apart "in prayer and good works."

In 1998 the abbey held a consecration of virginity ceremony for Mother Lucia

and eight other nuns who'd taken their final vows. The women carried candles and wore crowns of flowers. "It's on the same level as the ordination of a priest," Mother Lucia says. "You place your hands in the hands of the bishop, he slips a gold ring on your wedding finger and acknowledges your marriage with Christ." She reflects: "You feel awe: How can I live up to this?"

Mother Lucia believes women exert a power that's unique. "I don't mean to say this is all worked out, but it's the direction we've chosen to go—deeper into the truth of each gender rather than press for an equality with men that quickly becomes a power struggle." A smile of whimsy flickers in her eyes. "A gendered world is more exciting than a uniform world. What's the world without sex?"

WE'RE UP TO OUR ELBOWS IN THE warm, sweet liquid called whey. I'm in the dairy with Mother Margaret Georgina learning how to make cheese. Tall and slender, she wears round glasses and a black headband dotted with white stars over her black veil. She is the granddaughter of General George S. Patton, but when she first visited the abbey in the seventies as a flower child, embarrassed by her military family, she did not know that her grandfather had inspired the founding of Regina Laudis. Mother Benedict Duss, an American nun, was living in a French monastery in a town occupied by the Nazis during World War II. She was hiding from the Gestapo when she saw General Patton's troops march in to liberate the town, and vowed that she would found a monastery in America out of gratitude.

In the dairy, as we reach down through the whey and press the curds with our hands, they change from the consistency of custard to that of a dense sponge. The round mass feels alive, like bread dough.

Sister Angèle, who was raised Jewish and used to manage opera singers, says the abbey schedule is a paradox of "serenity and chaos."

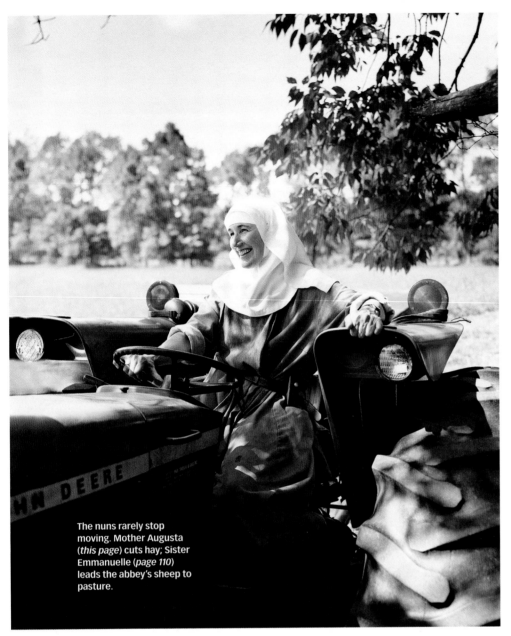

The nuns rarely stop moving. Mother Augusta (*this page*) cuts hay; Sister Emmanuelle (*page 110*) leads the abbey's sheep to pasture.

"If a piece breaks off and starts to rise," Mother Margaret Georgina says, "guide it back down gently. Use persuasion—not force." She smiles and quotes the French poet Charles Péguy: "All life comes from tenderness."

The cheese, if created with love and tenderness, "will speak," she says. "Everything we make that goes out of here speaks. That's one way contemplatives speak to the world."

She takes a wooden tool that one of the nuns brought back from France and slices the curd so it looks like a tic-tac-toe grid. We lift the square pieces and fit them, like a puzzle, into round molds and press the pieces together. My cheese is wild and ungainly, spilling over the wooden mold like soapsuds, but hers is compact and neat. We trim off the cheese I can't "persuade" into the mold and taste it. Unripened, velvety, warm from the cow, it tastes—excuse the expression—heavenly.

ON MY SECOND NIGHT AT THE ABBEY, I fall asleep in an unaccustomed state of calm and awaken with quiet pleasure. I walk to Mass through lush rhododendron, and during the service, the nuns and congregants kiss one another on the cheek—the "kiss of peace."

I ask the nuns how members are accepted. "We're always looking for new blood," one says, "but our process is slow and careful." Usually a woman will first come to visit and if she feels a connection may become an intern, living and working with the nuns but not inside the enclosure. If she "asks to enter"—a mutual decision made by the individual and the community—she becomes a postulant, wears a simple black dress and veil, and starts to follow the abbey schedule, studying Latin and learning to chant the psalms. This is a time for her to question whether the path is right for her while the community sets out to learn what the woman's gift is and how to nourish it. Mother Telchilde, the mistress of postulants, says, "If you're coming because you hate your job or don't like your life, this won't work. To be happy at the abbey, you need to have a lot going for you and a profession you love."

The next step is becoming a novice, at which time you're given the habit and a name. Jim Palmer showed me photographs of his daughter's clothing ceremony. First she appears in her street clothes, dressed up for the final time with necklaces, bracelets, and rings. She has chosen her sister, who is pregnant and has flown in from Seattle, to carry in the habit she will wear and have it blessed. Then she kneels before the abbess, removing each piece of jewelry. Jim remembers the silence, which exaggerated the sound of the bracelets dropping—*clink! clink!*—into a dish. Sydney holds up her hands, unadorned. A nun cuts her long gold hair until it's only a few inches, then fits a white veil around her face. She receives her name: Sister Chava, which is Hebrew for "Eve," the name of her grandmother, who died recently. Jim says the veiling was a moment of intense power and, for the parents, loss: Their daughter will not come home again.

After the ceremony, the novice begins her canonical year, a time of introspection when she does not receive phone calls or visits from family or friends. After that year of retreat, she progresses at her own pace and, when she feels ready—usually in another two years—takes her first vows, which are not permanent.

The last step is taking final vows, which are binding. All ownership of property must be relinquished however she sees fit. "Up to now," one sister says, "you keep your bank accounts." The nun's title changes from Sister to Mother, and she wears a black veil. The three vows are:

stability—you promise to stay in the cloister; conversion—you promise to change your life and recenter yourself in God through the community; and obedience.

Mother Deborah Joseph, a former New York debutante who ran her own interior design firm and worked as an investment manager on Wall Street before entering, says her willingness to obey was quickly tested. When the nun who'd been the beekeeper left for Italy, the abbess told Mother Deborah Joseph she would be the new one. "I was shocked. I lost my voice," she recalls. "I thought I was going to work on the abbey's finances. I went back to the abbess and said, 'I know nothing about bees!' and she said, 'Precisely. It's time for you to learn something new.'"

BELLS RING FOR THE FIRST PRAYER service at 1:50 A.M. Some of the nuns don't attend this service, because it means interrupted sleep, which was "a classical penance." Mother Margaret Georgina says, "We believe there's plenty of penance in life without cooking it up."

At all the prayer services, including Mass, the nuns sing Gregorian chant. In 1997 they produced a CD, *Women in Chant,* which became a best-seller. They have also released *A Gregorian Chant Master Class,* to make singing this music accessible.

At the end of Mass, a nun recites what they're going to pray for. She runs down a list that includes peace in the Middle East, the names of people who are sick, and finally, "for Sara and her work, we pray to the Lord." I feel a rush of embarrassment, and then, to my surprise, a sense of comfort.

SISTER ELIZABETH, 43, A FEISTY AND intellectually gifted woman, is the only African-American nun at the abbey. "It's not unfamiliar for me to be the only one," she says, sitting down across the grille from me. She earned a law degree at Stanford and worked as a corporate lawyer on Wall Street. "Hated it," she says, "so I went back to San Francisco and became a professor of law at Santa Clara University. I had everything I thought I wanted: I'd bought a house, I was publishing, I had a romantic relationship." But some piece was missing—something buzzing like an irritant in the back of her mind.

She had visited the abbey at age 19. She'd grown up in New York City with musical parents who were constantly playing Ella Fitzgerald and Duke Ellington, classical music, and Gregorian chant sung by a men's choir in France. Sister Elizabeth loved the chant and tried to find it in America. When she heard about the abbey, she took a bus there, walked into the chapel, heard the nuns singing, and thought, *This is what I've been looking for.* She recalls, "It felt like coming home."

But ten years passed while she was studying law and starting her career. In 1991 she received an invitation to the consecration of virginity ceremony of a nun who was a potter, and on the invitation was a picture of a kiln—"the red-hot, enclosed fire of a kiln." Sister Elizabeth flew to the abbey and again had the shock of feeling she was home. "I thought, *This is*

> "I had to come to a Benedictine abbey with all these white women to find a way to be black."

the piece that's missing—the fire that's burning so intensely because it's enclosed in a kiln," she says. "That intense fire is monastic life, and nothing on the outside can come close to it."

She says two events in the world also compelled her to join the abbey: the acquittal of the police officers accused of beating Rodney King, and the appointment of Clarence Thomas to the Supreme Court despite the testimony of Anita Hill. In both cases, she felt "there was a severe breach of justice." As a lawyer, she thought, there was little she could do except write an essay for a legal journal. But as a contemplative nun, she could work on a higher level.

I ask how becoming a nun could help restore justice. She says her two major forms of prayer at the abbey are music and cheesemaking. She describes how she was making Cheddar cheese and wanted it to look the way she thought Cheddar should

look—"neon orange like supermarket cheese. So I put vegetable color in the cheese. I thought, *If it's not the right color, nobody will recognize it as Cheddar.*" She laughs, and says she began to see the analogy between wanting the cheese to look orange and the pressure she'd felt to make herself look like a middle-aged white man in a Brooks Brothers suit when she walked into a courtroom.

"If I could allow the cheese to be itself, to take on its own color, that's a form of prayer. That's my prayer for Anita Hill. By allowing the cheese to be itself, I'm allowing all those black women out there to be themselves," she says.

At her clothing ceremony before receiving her habit, she put on an African dress and turban. "Not that I'd ever worn that before. But once I put it on, I thought, *Gee—I wish I had!*" She laughs. "I had to come to a Benedictine abbey with all these white women to find a way to be black."

I ask how making a natural-colored cheese will actually help black women whom she's never met to be themselves. She says, "That's the leap of faith. That's the work of prayer. Everything we do here is a form of prayer."

Gregorian chant, she says, is a major expression of prayer. Because the chant evolved before the use of harmony, the women must sing in unison—hitting the same notes in the same rhythm and often breathing at the same time. "The chant itself has a lift and fall. Like your moods, like everything you do—it's upbeat, downbeat, lift and fall. When you feel that wave, you're singing in line with the rhythm of all creation. And you're singing with a group where everyone is doing her part and breathing together and totally present. Man, there is nothing better!"

She pauses. "But on the other hand, 'R-E-S-P-E-C-T' ain't so bad either!"

AFTER I LEFT THE ABBEY, I LEARNED that in the past it had attracted not only admiration but controversy. During the eighties, there were allegations reported in the press that the chaplain, Rev. Francis Prokes, and Lady Abbess Benedict Duss were taking the abbey in a "cultlike" direction, pressuring nuns and lay people to donate money and land, and advancing a bizarre theology that stressed the potency of female sexuality. The atmosphere was said to be psychologically damaging, prompting ten nuns to leave. In 1991 the Vatican ordered an investigation, and in 1994, Prokes was removed and the Reverend Matthew Stark, abbot of Portsmouth Abbey, was appointed by Rome to oversee Regina Laudis for three years.

The nuns will not discuss the investigation or its findings. Monsignor Thomas M. Ginty, chancellor of the Archdiocese of Hartford, says the abbey is "in excellent standing with the Vatican. Any woman who would consider entering the abbey would be entering a legitimate religious order in full communion with the Roman Catholic Church. They're not a cult, not disobedient to the Holy Father. They are very good women who may have needed to correct a few things and they have done that."

THE ACCUSATIONS OF THE PAST DO not jibe with the impressions I receive on my visit. Saturday afternoon I join the nuns on a work project headed by Mother Augusta, who has a dark beauty, like that of Andie MacDowell, and a playful humor. She says we're going to clear trees and brush at the edge of the cow pasture. She uses a chain saw to cut down trees and saw them into pieces, while three novices and I—like a fire brigade—carry and pass the heavy pieces across the field to a nun who feeds them into a chipper. It starts to rain, but no one misses a beat, lifting and carrying logs. I borrow a raincoat and check my watch every ten minutes. I have bad knees and a bad back and am recovering from the flu, and I just want to survive here with no injury.

When we finally stop at 4:00, drinking lemonade and singing a hymn to Mary, I'm relieved and feel that pleasant tiredness that follows exertion. Many guests like to join the work team because it's an opportunity to interact with the nuns and leave something of oneself on the land. Jim Palmer painted a porch. Mother Lucia sent him a note of thanks and assured him: "The material remembers."

MOTHER DOLORES HART IS THE ONLY nun in the Academy of Motion Pictures Arts and Sciences. She was a movie star at age 18, starring with Elvis Presley in *Loving You* and *King Creole*. In six years, she made ten films, including *Where the Boys Are*. She is still beautiful at 65, with flawless skin and enormous blue eyes. She looks glamorous in her habit; for a special procession after Vespers, she wears a jaunty black-and-white straw hat and dark glasses.

I ask her why, when she'd attained what so many humans dream of—stardom, riches, access to the most celebrated people—she was ready to give it all up at 24.

She thinks a moment. "If I were 24, could I do it again?" she asks. "I say, 'Please

> On my second night at the abbey, I fall asleep in an unaccustomed state of calm and awaken with quiet pleasure.

don't test me.' I thank God I only had to do it once, because it was so difficult humanly. Being able to do it was a gift of grace."

She began visiting the abbey while performing on Broadway in *The Pleasure of His Company*—a role for which she won a Tony nomination. After entering the abbey, she says, "I did have to join the human race." She learned to be a carpenter and made coffins so the nuns could "bury our own dead." Other nuns say she was instrumental in shaping Regina Laudis, and she presently serves as Mother Prioress, the second in command.

In 1997 Mother Dolores was diagnosed with idiopathic sensory neuropathy, a torturous disease of the nervous system that made her feel that her feet were on fire and sent shooting pains to all parts of her body. The challenge of the illness, she says, is to "go beyond my own pain," to develop greater love and wrestle with the question of why people suffer.

When a bell rings for prayer and we end our parlor, she takes my hands in hers and kisses them.

PEOPLE VISIT THE ABBEY FROM ALL parts of the country and different fields—politics, science, the arts—to learn from the nuns and deepen their spiritual lives. A notable number come for a retreat on their birthdays. The Benedictine Rule is that all guests are to be received "as Christ." No fees are charged.

Many visitors cannot help feeling the pull of a community that has love at its core, and begin to ask themselves, *Could I live here?* What I find most difficult to imagine is giving up physical intimacy. When I question the nuns about this, they say they still have sexual desires but they work with them, each in her own way.

The nuns do not speak of altered states or mystic visions. They talk about the freedom they have to become themselves and the exhilaration of living with extraordinary women, which is also a challenge, particularly for those who've lived alone. Mother Lucia says, "People get angry, depressed, jealous, down, just as anybody does. The difference is that you're in a community that's oriented to keep moving—to reach out, to pray, or sometimes to just let the darkness be."

When I tell her some of the guests feel transported, she says, "We don't go in search of that experience. But the gift will be given. It could be in the dairy, it could be with the animals or when we pray in the middle of the night." She smiles from across the grille. "You wouldn't stay in this life if you didn't have the assurance of that love from time to time."

A SIGN IN THE GUESTHOUSE ASKS US to change our linens before we leave. I find clean sheets in the cupboard and start to yank and tug at the antique bed. Frustrated, trying to hurry and get the job done, I stop and think: *The nuns put love into the cheese, the flowers and fruit they grow, the animals they care for, the shawls they weave, and the honey they make. Why not put love into the linens, for the next guest who arrives feeling shy, uncertain, and expectant?* I slow down and smooth the pillows gently, "tenderly," as Mother Margaret Georgina had suggested handling the cheese. The material remembers. ●

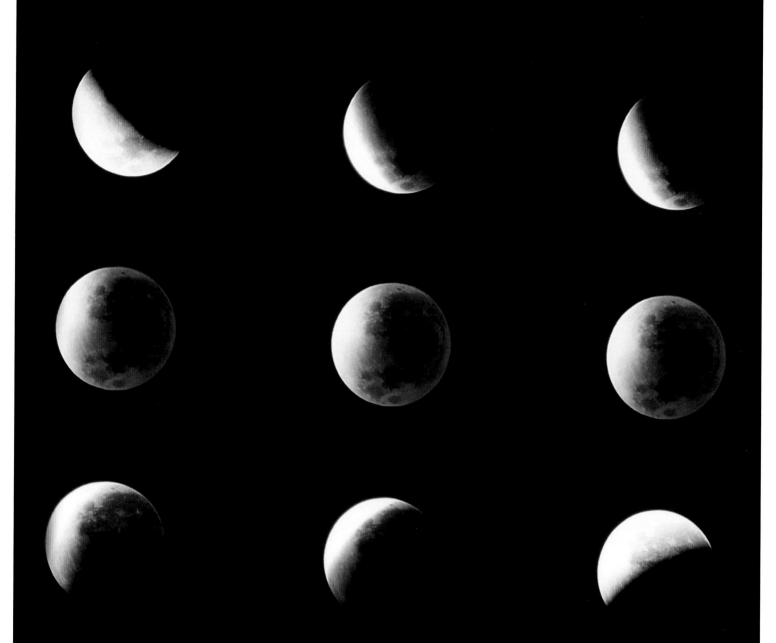

The Cure for
Craziness
There's only one way to save your sanity in this speeded-up, lunatic world. Patience, says **SHARON SALZBERG**.

Take a cue from the unrushable rhythm of nature.

ONE AUTUMN I TRAVELED TO A bookstore in western Massachusetts to hear Stephen Batchelor, a Buddhist scholar, speak about his recently published book. As the evening went on, I found myself distracted by a demonstration making its way down the street toward us. Clear shouts rang out: "What do we want?" The chanted response came through only as *mumble mumble mumble.*" I tried to go back to listening to Stephen's lecture, but the mumbles were soon followed by a yell: "When do we want it?" And then a roar: *"Now! Now! Now!"*

No matter how close the demonstrators came, the object of all that passion, that unyielding demand, remained a mystery. But each insistent cry of *"Now!"* crackled in the air as though shooting off sparks.

In some ways, I find the idea of calling out "now" beautiful. As a child facing the trauma of my mother's death when I was 9, and my father's mental illness when I was 11, I was often met by a wall of silence from adults, a postponement of any overt grief to a time when it might be more manageable. Most of us have had a well-meaning friend address our freshly broken hearts with "You'll see things differently later. You'll feel better in a while." Whatever their intentions, that "later" can seem like a callous judgment that our present understanding is inadequate. A "now" erupting from within us would, in many cases, feel wildly satisfying.

Our willingness to insist on "now" honors our conviction that we have a right to be happy, to be safe, to be heard. Our "now" may recognize that others deserve an end to abuse or oppression. Many situations of loss, exploitation, or injustice are deplorable, and our heart's demand for a better world is expressed in that "now."

But there's also something beautiful and deeply wise in being aware of the rhythms of life, the rhythms of nature. All of us know the mind-set that says our desires must be realized immediately. It's easy to forget that, no matter what we'd prefer, dreams come true one step at a time. A journey isn't just a vacancy between one place and the next but is worth paying attention to for its own sake. To be tyrannized by time, with its pressures of anticipation, expectation, comparison, and judgment, will not make our goals any easier to accomplish.

When my teaching colleague Joseph Goldstein was a child, he had a garden in which he grew carrots. He was so excited when the first green fluffy shoots came out of the soil that he pulled them up to look at the carrots that were growing and to help them along. We needn't be in a hurry to reap the results of our efforts faster than the world can bestow them. Being alive means doing the best we can and then letting nature take its course. We plant a seed, nurture it, water it, and let it be. Knowing there's a bigger picture than what we see in front of us, even if it isn't perfectly clear, allows us to be more peaceful, to learn as things develop.

Knowing there's a bigger picture allows us to be more peaceful, to learn as things develop.

If we can be quieter, more in the moment with what is actually happening, a world of perception opens up for us based on where we are, not on where we one day hope to be. "Nobody sees a flower, really; it is so small," said artist Georgia O'Keeffe. "We haven't time, and to see takes time, like to have a friend takes time." If we learn to take a little more time and be more fully aware of just where we are, we might see many new flowers and have many more friends.

ONE WAY OF DESCRIBING an ability to hold our convictions without drawing premature conclusions, feeling automatically defeated, or losing sight of what goodness life might be offering us today is the old-fashioned virtue patience. Despite the common misconception, having patience doesn't mean making a pact with the devil of denial, ignoring our emotions and aspirations. It means being wholeheartedly engaged in the process that's unfolding, rather than yanking up our carrots, ripping open a budding flower, demanding a caterpillar hurry up and get that chrysalis stage over with.

True patience isn't gritting one's teeth and saying, "I'll bear with this for another five minutes because I'm sure it will be over by then and something better will come along." Patience isn't dour, and it isn't unhappy. It's a steady strength that we apply to each experience we face. If the situation calls for action, we must take it—patience doesn't mean inertia or complacence. Instead, it gives us a courageous dedication to the long haul, along with the willingness to connect with the multi-layered truth of what is right here.

Are those of us not naturally blessed with patience doomed to yell at our children or our forgetful parents, litter our office floors with disemboweled computer parts (or at least threaten to), or berate ourselves each time we fail to live up to our own expectations? Or can we cultivate a new way of responding?

Anytime we're waiting—for the checkout person to ring us up, for the doctor's office to call, for a friend who has hurt us to apologize—we can remember we're alive right now. We can be determined to use this moment as a vehicle for paying attention, for growing, for opening.

Whenever we're pushing against what is, as though if we tried hard enough we could force the tempo of change, we can take a breath. Whatever our vision for how things should be in the future, we can make sure we do the very next thing we need to do today.

And whenever we're in a fury of impatient resentment because our companion is walking too slowly or the mail came too late or we're being ignored or we can't concentrate or we can't name what we want...or any of the countless everyday things we find hard, we can remind ourselves of what is good right now. Then, as we work to redress what is wrong, the belligerence, agitation, and frustration will drain out of our "now," and the word can become a declaration of purpose and strength, supported by the gentle, developing power of patience. ●

·SAYING GRACE·

It's at home in pizza joints and great restaurants. It stops time (and overeating).
LAUREN F. WINNER on the pleasures of an old-fashioned ritual.

Grace helps you take a moment to notice that you're lucky.

In my kitchen, we begin our meals by holding hands and bowing our heads. We usually say the short and sweet grace found in the Episcopal Book of Common Prayer:

"Bless this food to our use and us to Thy service."

Sometimes, when my husband is out of town, I experiment a little bit. Lately, I've offered this haiku by Basho, the 17th-century Japanese poet:

*In the twilight rain
These brilliant-hued hibiscus—
A lovely sunset.*

I don't have hibiscus, but saying Basho's poem helps me notice, and be thankful for, the magnolia tree out my window, the slow sunset, the pretty table linens. Whether you recite a Zen poem or a Christian prayer, saying grace does good work at the table. On the simplest level, saying grace means offering thanksgiving—*grace* comes from the Latin *gratiarum actio,* "act of thanks." To say grace before meals is, among other things, to remember that it was God, not my credit card, that provided my meal. But whether or not you're a believer, a pre-meal thanksgiving recognizes the dozens of people who did hard work to get food to your table—the farmers, the grocery store clerks, the friends or relatives or restaurant chef who transformed a pile of raw vegetables into a bowl of delectable soup.

I'll admit to a certain squeamishness about saying grace in restaurants. Praying at home is one thing, but bowing my head at Wendy's or Jean Georges is quite another. (I never know what to do when a waitress appears as I'm praying. Interrupt myself? Ignore her?) And yet increasingly, I try to overcome my discomfort and boldly say grace at restaurants precisely because I find it so easy, when I go out to eat, to take for granted the low-paid folks who set the table, wash the dishes, and generally make my night on the town possible. To pray before my meal, even if it's awkward, is to remind myself how privileged I am, how much I owe.

Saying grace suggests not only the *grazie* of thanksgiving but also the calm, gracious elegance of living fully and well. You don't find grace said when people are rushing around, scarfing food, eating over the sink or in the car, polishing off a meal in ten minutes flat.

You find grace offered at tables where people sit still, where they're trying to pay attention. Indeed, doctors will tell you that there are physiological benefits to saying grace before meals. People who do it tend to eat more slowly, aiding digestion, while speed eaters don't give their bodies time to register that they're full.

Sometimes I forget to say grace. I fail to say it when I'm ravenous and also when I'm distracted, when eating has nothing to do with intention and everything to do with fueling my body. These hasty meals are probably the times when I need to say grace the most—when I need to pause, feel lucky, and purposefully create a space of repose and awareness in my hectic day. We can't always eat on fine china or by candlelight, but grace is portable. In an age when we so often eat without thinking about it, saying grace can transform a mere meal into an act of celebration, focus, and gratitude.

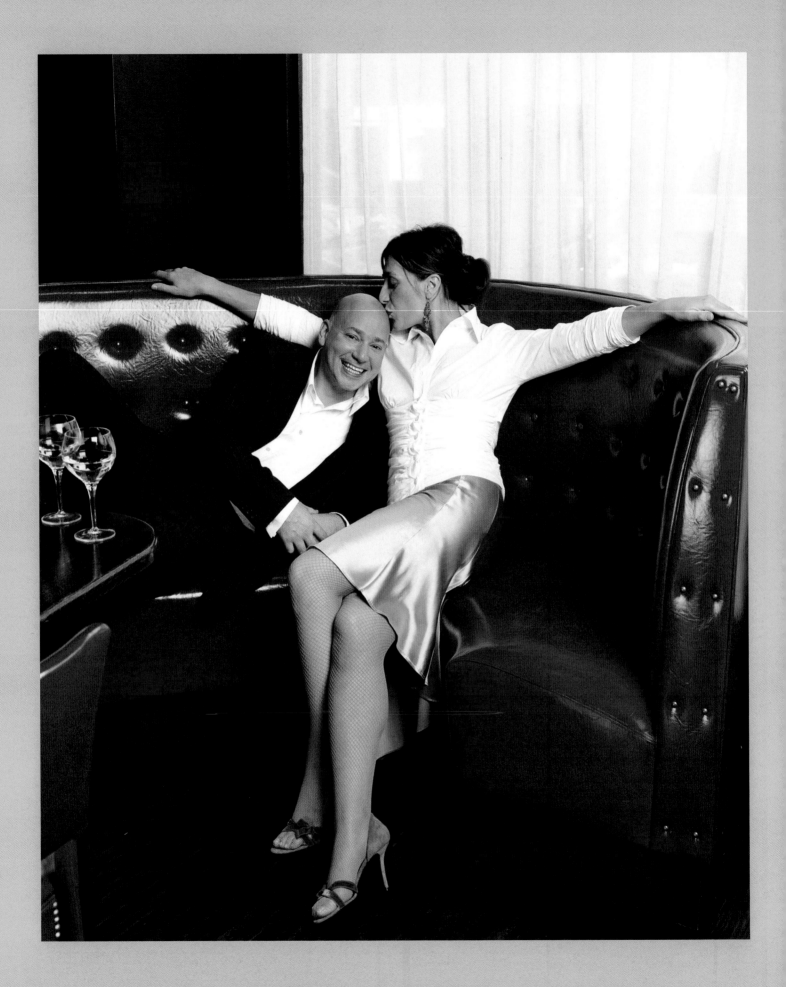

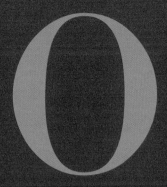

Relationships

The people in your life sustain you, revive you,
comfort you, and may even keep you healthy.
They can also drive you completely crazy. Here's help.

Dating 120

Couples 131

Marriage 157

Sex 175

Talking & Listening 187

Family 201

On Being a Parent 219

Friends 239

O
Dating

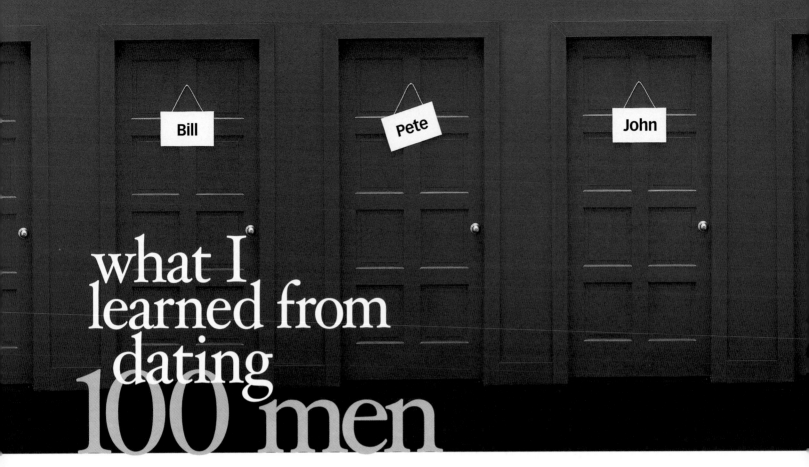

Bill   Pete   John

what I learned from dating 100 men

She was 34 and she meant business, so she placed an ad with an online dating service and

LAST YEAR, IN UNDER SIX months, I dated more than 100 men. I dated on beaches, on hiking trails, on the back of a Harley-Davidson. I told more than 100 men about my work, my family, my years in Czechoslovakia. I weathered personal-revelation fatigue and relied on pep talks from girlfriends to see me through. I didn't kiss any of these men, reserving physical contact for the one—I might as well say it—who would eventually win my heart.

After years alone, on the cusp of my 35th birthday, I was serious. I'd learned that letting myself kiss the wrong guy set in motion a sort of unwitting hormonal bonding stronger than rational thinking. If I was going to meet the right man, I decided, I needed to remain chemical-free, to think clearly, to get to know him first.

I didn't understand this in my 20s. Back then, I'd followed the Hollywood movie model wherein men and women tend to tumble into bed, then into love, and finally into marriage. The string of breakups I endured demonstrated that, for me at least, this strategy wasn't working.

My frequent experiences with the Wrong Man also taught me what I wanted this time around. I was looking for someone who could see my best self despite my imperfections. A gentle but strong man with the capacity to become as deeply devoted to me as I would be to him. In a word: available. I suspected it might take awhile to find him in greater Los Angeles, and I was right.

To get started, I posted an ad on an online dating site. I asked a girlfriend to take a picture of me bathed in late afternoon sunlight and wore the most glamorous smile I could muster. I stated that I wanted a man who "somehow manages to strike that tricky balance of being both dependable and spontaneous. Or who can happily tolerate both of these aspects in me."

I got a lot of responses right off the bat. Some were ludicrous, like the 50-something guy in a Hawaiian shirt who offered to fly me to Vegas for the weekend. I deleted far more than I answered. But Week One still found me on dates with 14 men at local coffee shops. In Week Two, I slowed down to seven. I shook hands with a Danish architect and an hour later zoomed across town to meet a swoony soap opera actor. The next day was tea with an airfreight handler, followed that evening by a walk with a real estate lawyer. I dated aerospace engineers, entrepreneurs, doctors, an oceanographer, film animators, a romantic man who lived impecuniously on a boat, and a self-proclaimed gazillionaire who resided atop a mountain.

"Are you insane?" my astonished girlfriends said, laughing.

I was overwhelmed but exhilarated. And I overdid it. At the end of Week One, I startled friends and myself by bursting uncontrollably into tears. A lifetime of pent-up loneliness came unglued all at once. Then I hit a groove. No matter how the date went, I reminded myself I was taking a stand for what I wanted.

And I tried to relax. I steadied myself right before each new hello. Nothing was worse or more exquisite than my date's first

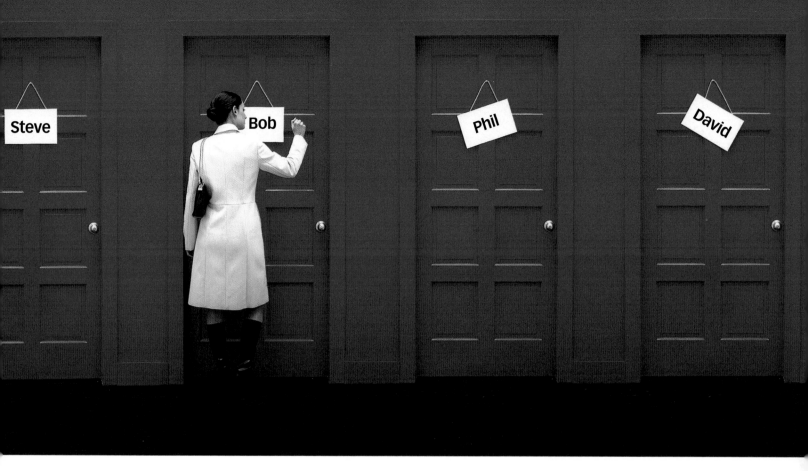

let the e-mails roll in. **ANN MARSH** on panning for the date that was worth waiting for.

flicker of disappointment or approval. If he clearly wasn't interested—like the swing-dancing entertainment lawyer or the Harvard-educated wine expert—then he was simply another woman's catch. I got out of her way. I knew I'd meet someone else tomorrow. Even if a first date wasn't fantastic, I tended to accept second dates to make sure I hadn't been too hasty in my judgment. About four or five men survived through fourth or fifth dates before I said goodbye. The thing I liked best about my whole dating project was that it validated that nagging sense I'd had for years: Every Saturday night I'd spent alone or with girlfriends, I'd believed there had to be several thousand potential dates out there for me, somewhere. It turns out I was right.

To date so many men, I needed to be honest in a new way. In my 20s, when the wrong man asked me out, I usually lied. I was either (a) busy, (b) dating someone else, or (c) moving to Siberia for a year. Sensing my fib, some men refused to let go. A few talked me into dates or, worse, relationships. I marvel to think I left the nest with-

out ever learning how to verbalize my own needs and desires.

One of my earliest electronic dates taught me about honesty. "It was really nice to meet you," the tall, good-looking athlete wrote me in an e-mail after Date Number Two, "but I didn't feel that indescribable something that would tell me we're a match."

I sat there looking at my computer screen. He had found the words to describe my own sentiments. I didn't feel rejected. I felt liberated by his courage. Better yet, I stole his line.

A handsome telecommunications executive I met over a drink at a restaurant one evening looked and sounded far less alluring to me a few days later in the sober light of day. In a subsequent telephone conversation, my whole body tensed while I told him that I didn't get the sense he was the right one and that I didn't want either of us to waste precious time. I wished him well. He sounded a little startled. But the discomfort was short-lived. We were both free.

It's embarrassing to admit that I was

learning the very basics about personal boundaries at the age of 34. But it was also a thrill. Like a suit of comfortable, lightweight body armor, my newly declared boundaries kept me safe.

At times my faith flagged, like when the well-spoken National Guard pilot bought me a single California roll for dinner and called for the check. Phew. Rejection in a bit of raw fish. The best remedy was always the next date. When the soap opera actor or the triathlete didn't call—both of whom had looked deep into my eyes and proclaimed their attraction to me—I did nothing. I let them go. I wanted a man whose actions matched his words.

The initial frenzy mellowed to a couple of dates a month, and one sunny Sunday afternoon in late summer, I met Johanne. I had, by this time, trained myself to listen closely to what my deepest instincts said in the first nanosecond of meeting a man. Hmm...maybe, I thought when I spied him waiting across the Art Deco lobby of a seaside hotel. With every subsequent date, the voice grew surer.

I never expected my man would come from a faraway continent where he was raised on a tea plantation, but he does. We can talk and play and work things out together. We have each finally found a home in the other.

Johanne says he's more confident in my feelings for him, knowing I looked long and hard to find him. He's right. The parade of men who preceded him helped me know myself better. They repeatedly tested my ability to speak up or to stay quiet when I needed to. They certainly taught me to appreciate the man who, in the end, answered not only my ad but my dreams. ●

personal ads: the dos, the don'ts, the absolute musts

Should you mention your snoring, your dexterity with the flute, your knobby knees? **LESLEY DORMEN** tells us how she got the guy.

Twelve years ago, I took a chance and wrote a personal ad. Meet men without leaving the house! What could be bad? I wrote my ad thoughtfully. I considered every word. My finished product reflected my attitude at the time—a combination of "you have to play to win" and "hey, why not?" I ended up meeting my husband. Did I get lucky? Sure. But I had prepared the way.

Here's what I've learned about writing a good ad:

1. PUT ON LIPSTICK. Or a cowboy hat. Or your coolest T-shirt and stilettos. Play your favorite CD. Props that make you feel soulful, frisky, and fascinating help you make those claims for yourself in your ad.

2. POST A TERRIFIC PHOTO OF YOURSELF if you're using an Internet dating service. If he likes the photo, he'll read the ad.

3. IF IT'S A PRINT-ONLY AD, AVOID OVERSELLING YOUR APPEARANCE with dubious claims like "Sharon Stone look-alike." I started my magazine personal with: "Curvy, almond-eyed writer, fit (good shoulders)...." My husband says he was attracted to the soft sell of the description and the quirky confidence of the assertion. More to the point: I wanted to attract a man who appreciated subtlety.

4. SHOW YOUR PERSONALITY, DON'T TELL IT. Create a persona and your ad stands out. Instead of saying you're funny or well educated or caring, demonstrate that. What are your interests? Paintings? Which ones? Your garden? Why? Try an ad that consists entirely of your favorite movie dialogue or a list of beloved fictional characters. Your essence shines through the details. Be specific. Be surprising. A woman I know snagged a boyfriend when she described her ideal job as a combination of circus performer and archaeologist.

5. SERIOUSLY AVOID PERSONAL-AD SPEAK. Don't "like fine dining" when you can be passionate about Memphis barbecue, don't "enjoy movies" when you can declare your enthusiasm for Mel Brooks.

6. INCLUDE THE BASICS: your age and occupation, whether or not you have children, whether you're looking for a date or a life partner.

7. DON'T LIE ABOUT YOUR AGE—OR ANY-THING ELSE. If you're 42 but look 32, say so (or let your picture do the talking). "Mid-30s" or "early 40s" is fine, but assume he'll round up.

8. UNLESS YOU KNOW FOR SURE that you only want to meet, say, a nonsmoking Portuguese-speaking dentist, go easy on the list of qualities he must have. My ad requested a man "financially stable, kinda handsome, who can slow dance, make me laugh, read between the lines." Cast a wide net and edit out the responses. You never know.

9. IT'S LOVE, NOT BRAIN SURGERY. You can do it over. You can do it again.

are we having fun yet?

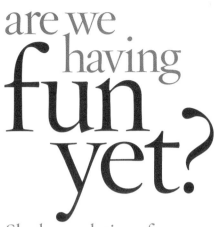

She knew dating after a divorce would be nerve-racking. But courage producing? Compassion building? **LISE FUNDERBURG** gets back in the game— this time playing by a whole new set of rules.

PEOPLE WHO SAY DATING was fun either don't remember or are simply wrong. When I plunged back into it, four years ago and freshly divorced, I was stunned by how hard it all was—knowing what to say, where to go, what to order off the menu, whether I was having a good time. Decisions I could make hundreds of times a day without thinking were suddenly excruciatingly difficult, freighted with the weight of the world, with the possibility of affecting my destiny. This was not—how do I put it?—fun. So I radically revised my approach to the enterprise: I began to use the world's most awkward social situation to practice the art of being me.

Successful dating—defined as anything better than an evening of *Seinfeld* reruns— required soul-searching and habit-breaking. I had to come clean with myself and admit the stakes were high. Time to discard the casual stance (I don't care what happens.... I'm not nervous.... I do this all the time) that was more armor than authentic feeling. I recognized the importance of seeking love and also that the chances of finding it were unbelievably slim. Such low probability was oddly comforting:

I had the long shot's permission to run the race my way.

Like many women I know, I had always been more concerned with being liked than with liking. What would happen if I stopped arranging my behavior around attracting the other person? I changed the way I dressed for a date—still choosing clothes that looked good but not more revealing or frilly than I would normally wear. I tried not to fill the pauses in the conversation, thinking instead, *This is uncomfortable—for both of us.* I fully answered questions about my work (*I write about community and race and identity and...thrift shopping!*) and my interests (*I garden and dabble in masonry and...thrift shop!*), including those parts that I imagined might not appeal to my dinner partner.

I also reconsidered the way I looked at my dates. It's hard to see a person accurately when there's even a sliver of a chance that he might turn out to be the person with whom you share children and utility bills and a bed for years on end. What you *want* so often blocks what's actually there. And what's *there* on the table between you is two luggage racks full of baggage—a Samsonite sundae piled high with hopes, dreams, disappointments, losses, and long-held ways of understanding the world. We're all products of a particular time and place, family and religion, history and culture, coincidence and physical attributes. To listen with openness and say what you mean across that mass takes concentration and presence of mind. No time left to worry about whether you should have worn the Manolos.

One of my vision-clarifying exercises was to reexamine how I perceived my date's imperfections. (This was tricky because I had the capacity to find fatal flaws before the bartender took our order or the latte got its foam.) Some of the faultfinding was accurate, but most of it was defensiveness and anxiety. So I began to practice grace and charity, to give these near strangers a wide berth, to allow them the sincere, complicated, and glorious humanity that I, too, was working so hard to let out.

Even if nothing resulted between us— the usual scenario—we had shared a reasonable attempt to make a connection.

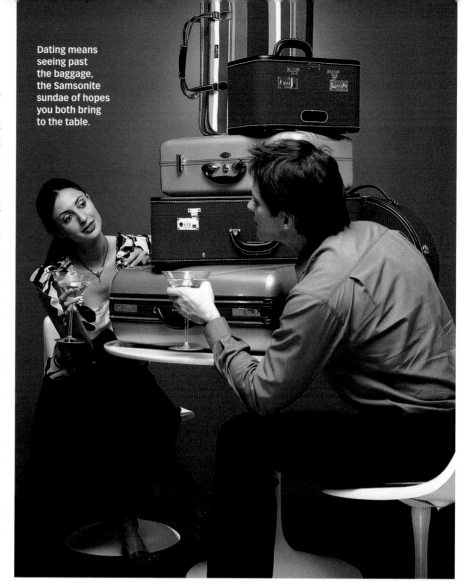

Dating means seeing past the baggage, the Samsonite sundae of hopes you both bring to the table.

Here's what I learned:
For dating to work, stop trying to make it work.

Thinking of us as colleagues and not adversaries helped me relax, and I often enjoyed myself even when no sparks flew.

Just when I was getting the hang of being myself and disentangling nervousness from neurosis, I went on a date that ended my need to date...possibly forever. I didn't automatically write him off just because he got the time wrong and seemed a tad pessimistic and repeatedly pronounced Europe absolutely superior to the United States—in everything from transit systems to architecture and motorcycles. I was cautious but not condemning. I talked to him about my work (all of it) and my hobbies (all of them). He was interested in some, not in others. By the third date I knew which of my first impressions held up (the good ones) and which didn't (the not-good

ones). Fate played a part: We were lucky in our timing and fortunate in having great chemistry. But we each made the choice to be ourselves—to be aggressively true to our own strengths and weaknesses, our hopes and disappointments, our clarity and our murk—and that has made the deepest impression of all.

Here's what I learned: In order for dating to work, stop trying to make it work. I don't mean to suggest that you'll suddenly be having the time of your life. I found dating—my three-year bout of it—difficult and challenging and sometimes heartrending. But I was determined to approach it with a gentleness toward myself and the other sorry sot across from me, and to breathe, breathe, breathe through it all. What a difference that has made. •

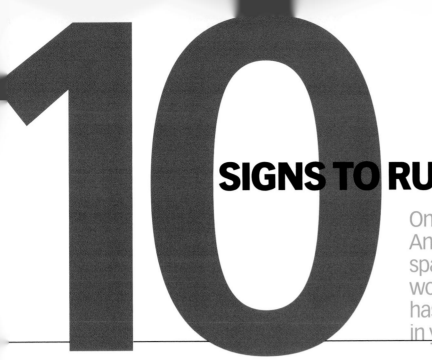

10 SIGNS TO RUN FOR YOUR LIFE

One guy is needier than quicksand. Another is jealous of your cocker spaniel. A third quietly hates all womankind. **Pam Houston** has a list of men you should put in your rearview mirror, ASAP.

❯Joe No-Show

YOU MEET IN A CITY WHERE NEITHER of you lives, at a convention or a wedding. The calls and e-mails are making the phone lines sweat; two months later he's begging you to visit. You tell the woman next to you on the plane that after years of searching you think you've met The One, and the two of you giggle with anticipation all the way to baggage claim. Thirty minutes later, when the carousel stops going around, she looks at you with deep pity and asks if she can give you a ride somewhere. That is the moment to go straight back to the ticket counter. Do not wait two hours until his father, whom you've never met, walks up to you with a browbeaten expression and explains that the man of your dreams got caught in an argument with his ex-wife — and will try to meet you later. Understand that this situation can only get worse before it gets better. Save yourself two or three of the best years of your life.

❯Mr. Jealousy

AT FIRST HE'LL GET A LITTLE SHORT with a waiter who flirts with you. Then he'll be exasperated by how long you and the postmaster discuss the rising price of stamps. When he points out that you and your brother hug too long to be appropriate, or that your gynecologist is a lesbian and obviously has the hots for you, it's time to give him his walking papers. However flattering his jealousies may seem the first five minutes of your relationship, they'll get old and confining more quickly than you can imagine, and when you do finally break up with him, he will hang the scarves you left behind on your trees like nooses and follow you and the next man you date all over town.

❯The Bully

THIS IS THE MAN WHO SITS YOU down, grabs your arm, pulls your hair, or pokes your chest. While most of us know better than to let ourselves get socked in the mouth the way Ralph Kramden was always threatening to do to Alice (but even then never following through), there's a whole universe of more "minor" infractions in the violence department that should disqualify your new beau instantaneously but all too often does not.

❯The Two-Timer

FOR THE FIRST TIME SINCE YOU'VE been dating, he's too sick to make a date. You try to ignore the fact that it happens to be your birthday, and you assemble the ingredients for your famous chicken soup. You drop it off inside his door. Two days later, he's still sick, but you've been invited over. You ask if you can heat up some soup for him, and he says, in a small congested voice, that would be wonderful. You pour the soup from the Tupperware into the pot, and you see that there are mushrooms in it. *Your* famous chicken soup doesn't contain mushrooms. Conclude that this man has another source of soup and will continue to cheat on you for as long as you give him the chance.

❯The "Liberated" Man

I USED TO HAVE A FRIEND WHO said, "I seem to have a very liberating effect on whatever man I'm dating. We go on three dates, and the next thing I know he's moved in with me, he's quit his job, and his car is up on blocks in my yard." Certain men are more prone to this type of liberation than others, I have found: Carpenters, river guides, and flamenco guitarists all fall into the category of men who are perfectly willing to hand themselves over to the care of a good woman, as well as visual artists, stage performers, and racers (ski, bike, boat) of all kinds.

❯The Betrayed

I SEEM TO HAVE DATED AN INORDI-nate number of men who have just been left by a woman for a woman. In general, these men are angry beyond all reason, no matter to what lengths they may go to disguise it, and if you date one, be ready to give up all your girlfriends or you will be accused of being a lesbian, too.

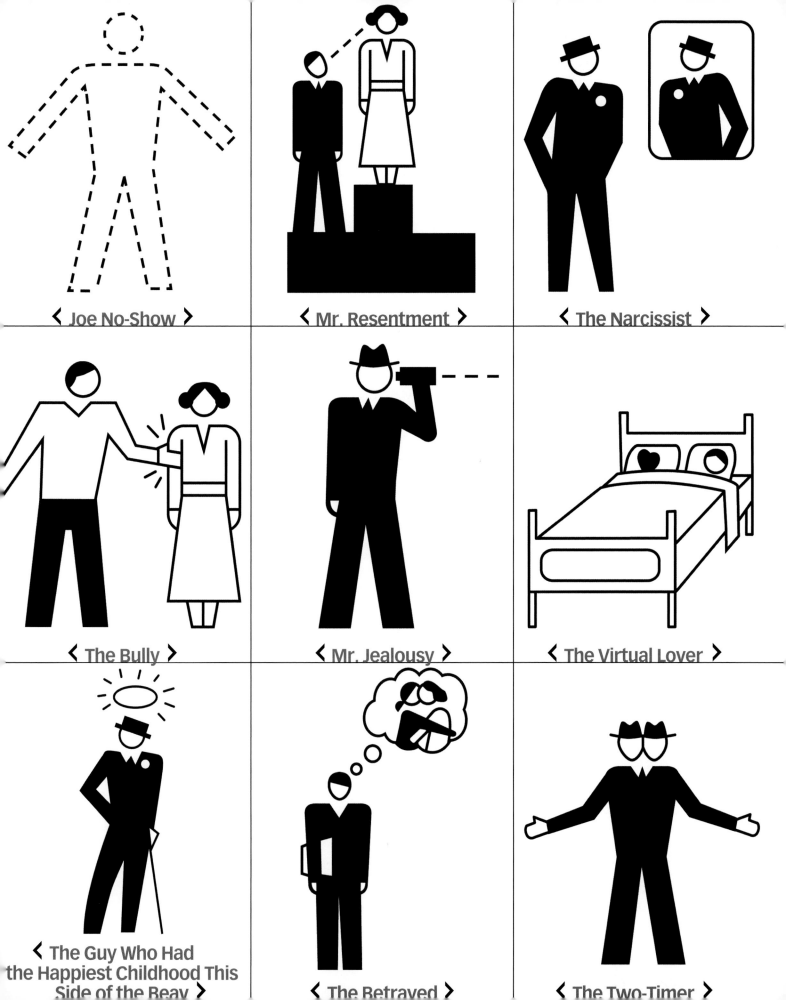

‹ Joe No-Show ›

‹ Mr. Resentment ›

‹ The Narcissist ›

‹ The Bully ›

‹ Mr. Jealousy ›

‹ The Virtual Lover ›

‹ The Guy Who Had
the Happiest Childhood This
Side of the Beav ›

‹ The Betrayed ›

‹ The Two-Timer ›

The Narcissist

HE DOESN'T LIKE YOUR DOG? DO we even need to talk about this one? Put it at the top of the category that includes he won't make eye contact with your kid, he doesn't want to meet your sister, and he whines the first time you make plans with your girlfriend. A man threatened by the love you have for the dog you sleep with is going to be threatened by more things than you can name. Dating him is inviting the type of conflict into your life that will make you tired before you even get up in the morning.

Mr. Resentment

PAY CLOSE ATTENTION TO HOW he handles your accomplishments. If you get a promotion with a raise and he breaks it down to show you how it really only amounts to six dollars a day after taxes, that's the first strike. When he uses any expression like "your little project," count that as two. Just because men are having a hard time adjusting to the idea that women are capable breadwinners doesn't mean you have to martyr yourself into helping them make the transition. There are men out there more than happy to bask in the glow their women cast and to consider your talents a positive reflection on them.

The Virtual Lover

WHAT A RELIEF IT IS WHEN A MAN doesn't try to force you into bed on the first date. How charmed you are when, on the third date, he says he wants to wait until "you both can't stand it anymore." How sympathetic you become when, on the sixth date, he tells you how badly he was hurt by your predecessor. How confused you are six months later when you've realized his pager goes off every time you get naked, but he's still sending you roses and talking teddy bears. A surprising number of great romancers out there never get around to having sex. To the date-weary woman, this can seem like not the worst combination, but beware. Eventually he will blame his problems on the smell of your breath or the size of your thighs.

The Guy Who Had the Happiest Childhood This Side of the Beav

HIS MOTHER WAS PERFECT; HIS father never smoked or drank or cheated. He hates the way his friends blame their parents for everything, when he and his seven brothers and sisters had love pouring down on them from the moment they woke in the morning until they went to bed. However refreshing this might sound the first time you hear it, listen carefully for a voice that is trying to convince itself, listen for the creak and crack of a personal mythology in the throes of shattering. When it comes crashing to the ground, it's going to make a very big noise, and most likely your relationship will come crashing down with it.

How to Recognize a Good Guy When You See Him

He listens, rubs your feet, comforts the dog, and says yes to whipped cream. What are you waiting for?

You want a man who can make you laugh when you're down and who laughs with you when you're up, a man who listens and asks questions and responds. A man who rubs your feet to put you to sleep and who goes out for café mochas when you have to stay up and who knows that on those working all-nighters the answer to any question involving whipped cream is yes.

You want a man who'll wash your hair, who'll cook you dinner, who'll talk to your father on the phone when you can't bear to, who'll read to you on trips, and who's happy when you read (or sing or dance) for him.

You want a man who when he finds out that there are $199 fares to Kona suggests you go with your best girlfriend while he stays home and takes care of your dog. You want a man who will drive that same dog around all night when he is hallucinating and howling after the vet gave him too much postsurgical morphine, because you are up for promotion and have an interview with the dean at 8 A.M.

You want a man who loves many things: his work, his landscape, a sports team, his friends.

You want a man who knows that love is not a pie, that sex is not a sport, that faith (in the world, in each other) is a little like a full-time job.

You want a man who knows that women have a secret, and even though he can't know what it is, he is smart enough to want to live in its light.

Most important, you want a man who can continue to surprise you, for a week, a month, a year, a lifetime, which is to say a man who has a big imagination, and who is willing to use it to win your heart.   —P.H.

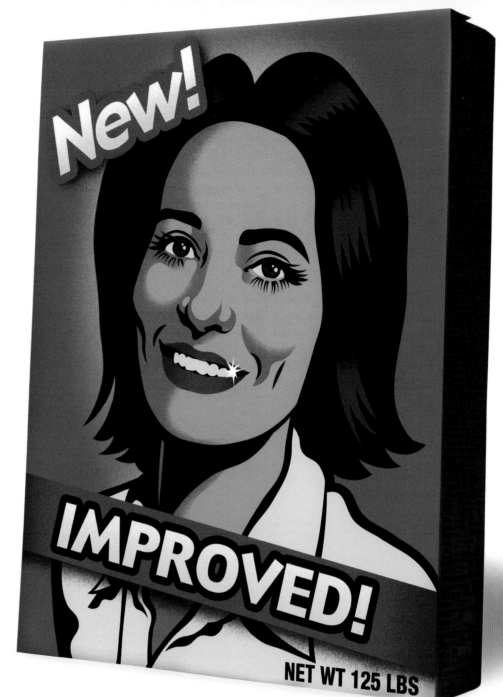

New!

IMPROVED!

NET WT 125 LBS

Okay, you're not a box of detergent, but you feel you've been left on the shelf. **MICHELLE BURFORD** meets a marriage consultant with a Harvard MBA and a 15-step program aimed at altar-ing your life.

Getting Married: The Strategic Approach

ALL SINGLES IN SEARCH OF A whinefest should roll right on past this train stop—anyone who gets off at Rachel Greenwald's station will be served a particularly strong shot of truth. Her book, *Find a Husband After 35 Using What I Learned at Harvard Business School,* makes zero allowances for always-the-bridesmaid brooding. But for the woman who's ready to vault to the altar, Rachel has a promise: Put yourself on a 15-step plan she calls The Program, and you'll have one foot in that Vera Wang gown.

Five years ago, Rachel launched her consulting business, findahusband after 35.com, in Denver and began teaching clients the same principles she'd used in packaging products such as Evian water (she once served as that company's marketing manager) and Carolee jewelry.

Merchandise yourself, says Rachel Greenwald.

"I'm treating singleness as a marketing issue," says Rachel, who calls her program a "strategic plan" in which the woman is the "product" to be advertised. "My program is for the woman who is sick of wallowing in why she's single. The point is that she is—and what will she do about it? What I'm offering her is an objective business perspective." But doesn't it seem a tad contrived to market a human being? "If you were looking for a job, you could call it 'contrived' to put your résumé online, ask friends for leads, and buy a new interview suit," she writes. "But you'd do it—because you'd be more likely to find a job.... Why is it different with trying to find a husband?"

This from a wife (and now mother of three) who met her husband 11 years ago using her own step number 12—"Event Marketing: Throw a Program Party!" which means creating a "strategic networking event" to showcase yourself. "I felt so fortunate to have found my husband and to be so happy, I wanted my single friends to have the same experience," Rachel writes.

AS HER COMPANY SUCCEEDED— "at least 80 percent of my clients have gotten married within 12 to 18 months of hiring me," she says—word spread. She then took her act on the road with seminars (topic: Marriage 911) and now claims that while a husband is not a panacea, she can tell you how to find a good one faster than you can spell *Tiffany princess-cut diamond.*

The day I catch up with Rachel at Manhattan's Harvard Club, I've come to see whether she can convince me, the former chubby chick with the Afro, that her techniques will work. I sashay in wearing a fire-engine-red dress (in her chapter titled "Packaging: Create Your Best Look," she suggests ditching all that black for a color that will differentiate me from the 32 million other single women my age—30—and older). Perhaps because she's already married, she can justify her black suit, Jackie O chic as it is. Our quick phoner the previous day—we were two strong gusts of energy spinning toward each other—immediately becomes, upon meeting, a whirlwind exchange of chatter and laughter that draws glances from a few blue bloods around us. Rachel, who enunciates each of her syllables with English-teacher perfection, oozes intensity with every gesture she uses to punctuate her rapid-fire statements. She whisks me to an empty sitting room, seldom shifts her gaze from me as she listens to my dating history, then insists, as the pitch of her voice climbs, that The Program can rescue me. "When you sign up 100 percent for anything—whether it's losing weight, finding a job, or quitting an addiction, I have no doubt that it becomes a challenge you can rise above," she tells me. "I've seen what the power of focus can do for a woman who's committed not just in words but in action."

"I give you the tools to attract the highest number of men quickly and efficiently."

Me, too—which is why Rachel is my kind of gutsy girl: all the kick of Cheddar on rye, minus any trace of baloney. As in this bit of bluntness she delivers in her chapter "Telemarketing: Bring Out Your Rolodex": "Let me tell you right up front that you're *not* gonna like this step!" she writes. "But trust me, it can yield very good results.... You are going to call everyone you know and directly ask them to fix you up." That means all human life forms currently listed in your Palm V—landlords, lawyers, grannies, hairstylists, florists, stockbrokers, long-lost gal pals from summer camp, former colleagues, and even old boyfriends you're still on good terms with.

Oh, exhale: This approach needn't make you seem desperate. "Each person will probably think you're calling two or three friends, not two or three hundred," Rachel says. She estimates, based on her experience with clients and her business school training, that you'll score one blind date for every ten calls. "Why go through this torture?" she writes. "This statistic says it all: 'Fifty percent of people now married or living together were introduced by good friends or family members.'"

After poring over the 15 steps—everything from "Make The Program Your Number One Priority" to "Pump Up the Volume" ("My approach gives you the tools to attract the highest number of men quickly and efficiently")—I decide to test-drive creating a "personal brand." "This is what sets you apart from your competitors—and to be effective, it must be memorable and specific," she explains. "Madonna's brand might be 'outrageous, sexual pop singer.' We're all multifaceted, so you need to give your friends who'll set you up on blind dates a shorthand way of summing you up." This, she says, derives from the business principle that a well-defined brand is essential to the success of any product, be it Jo Malone fragrance, the U.S. mail, or you. Not only should your brand ring true to your "customers"—the people you'll ask to scare up dates for you or the countless men with whom you'll click Cosmo glasses—it should also be designed to attract the kind of partner you're looking for.

Rachel has me draw up a megalist of my most appealing attributes, like "resilience" and "playfulness." Then I choose three ("writer," "warm smile," and "grew up in Phoenix") as a basis for a brand—"sunny girl from Arizona." On the two Web sites where I've posted a profile, I update my photo (in the old one, we agree, the bad lighting doesn't exactly say "sunny girl"). I then begin "advertising" by calling every girlfriend I have and asking for a setup. This move alone nets me three dates.

For those who snatch up Rachel's book, I suggest enlisting the help of a supporter (in step two, she suggests you find a "program mentor," preferably someone married) who won't be any less shy than Rachel about delivering the hard news straight. (After seeing my potential online photo, in which I'm sitting on a bed, she asks, "Do you want a husband or a one-night stand?") In this program, the truth is the essential bottom layer upon which your entire five-tier wedding cake will stand.

Within two weeks of trying Rachel's strategies, I, the girl who once spent Friday nights booting up TiVo for an *American Idol* marathon, am now juggling so many suitors that I've started a "man-agement" diary. One of my dates has even led to a second, a third, and a fourth. What a difference a brand—and perhaps 12 to 18 months—can make. •

O
Couples

Dr. Phil's MANual

You probably have one of these at home, or you're considering acquiring one—an adult human male. Here, **PHILLIP C. McGRAW, PHD**, provides a consumer guide to your model's inner workings. Don't start him up until you've read these instructions fully.

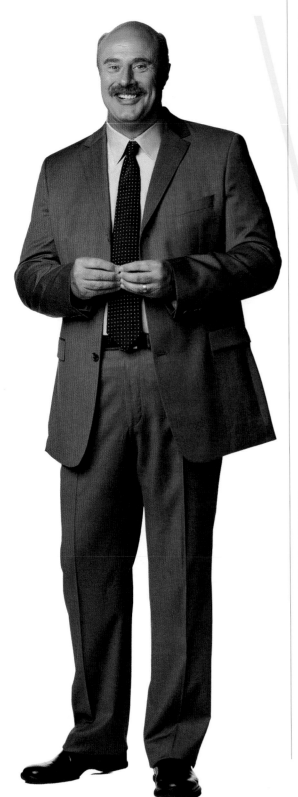

WOMEN, HOW MANY TIMES HAVE you looked at the man in your life, shook your head, and wondered, *Can he really be that stupid/insensitive/tuned out/selfish/clueless?* The answer is, No, he's probably not that bad. But he is, shall we say, *different.* And some of the things that cause you to question his mental or emotional acumen are pretty easy to explain. I'm going to give you the inside scoop that will help you get more of what you want and less of what you don't from your Y-chromosomed partner.

You've told me what you want: a confidant, a connection, a caring supporter who's plugged into your life. You want safety, fidelity, and—last but certainly not least—intimacy. Here's the problem: The level of intimacy you want is, for many of us males, totally foreign and unnatural. Hold on, now—don't shoot me yet! I'm not making excuses; I'm just being honest. I'm not saying we can't, I'm not even saying we aren't kind of, sort of, maybe, actually achieving intimacy now. What I'm saying is that to many men, behaving how you want us to behave feels as bizarre to us as it would to you if we asked you to stand out in the yard scratching your crotch, burping, and spitting every 30 seconds.

Before you judge the man in your life, figure him out. Anyone knows that if you're going to train bears, you need to understand bears. If you're going to train penguins, you need to understand penguins. So let's take a peek behind the curtain of maledom. Let's look at what makes these boys tick, what makes them do what they do and not do what they don't.

Understanding a man will be easier if you keep in mind a few core male characteristics that probably drive his behavior. Please understand, I recognize that there are a million exceptions to the following observations. Nevertheless, if you're looking for a "sensical" explanation for what seems like nonsensical male behavior, I promise you that you'll find some important clues in this list.

MEN EXPRESS THEIR FEELINGS THROUGH THE CURRENCY THEY VALUE

Currency is what matters to people. It's the reward that motivates people to act in a particular way—to engage in certain behaviors and to avoid others. If you want to influence a man, you need to know what he treasures. Maybe it's money, time, his car. Maybe it's his daughter from a previous marriage. Maybe it's some secret or fear he has guarded closely all his life. If you want to know how a man really feels, pay attention to how he treats what he values. Whatever it is, if he gives you what is precious to him (whether you value it or not), he has performed an act of love that may mean much more to him than any words he might say.

How this affects you: When people expect A but get B, they're upset. When they expect B and in fact get B, they're not upset. Exactly the same outcome, yet two very different reactions. So many women

are upset about what their men do or don't do—not because what they do or don't do is wrong but because it is different from what the women expected. Women express emotion verbally, and men express it by using their currency. The result is the same; the reaction is different.

What you can do about it: Start by answering this question: Do you want your man to really love you, or do you want him to love you the way *you* would love you?

If it's the latter, you need to recognize that in many ways, you're dealing with an alien life form. If you insist on measuring him with your yardstick, he hasn't got a chance.

Now ask yourself:

■ Am I wanting and expecting the wrong thing?
■ Am I failing to recognize that he is giving me what I want?
■ Am I asking this man to give me something he just doesn't have?

If you answered yes to any of those questions, part of your solution may be very much under your own control, if you'll just recognize it.

I once gave my wife, Robin, a card that pictured a male and a female cat sitting on a fence, looking lovingly at each other and the moon. The male cat says to his girlfriend, "If I had two dead rats, I would give you one!" Bingo! In a man's world, that's love. He wants to give her what he values. It's also true that in a man's world, talk is cheap—very cheap. A man can say "I love you" and mean nothing. But if he gives you what he values, that counts.

The point is that a man may be show-ing his love in a way that means something to him, even though his technique isn't exactly the one that you would choose. If he's doing that, then you'd be cheating yourself if you overlooked it. I'm not saying that you can't teach him to speak your language. What I am saying is that he may be expressing his feelings in a foreign tongue, one that it would comfort you to learn.

The lesson here is twofold: Identify what he values, and determine whether he is sharing that with you. Watch what he does with his "personal accounts." If his currency is his time, is he sharing it with you? If it's his car, does he let you drive it, or are you instructed to stand ten feet away? If his currency is his daughter from his previous marriage, does he encourage you to interact with her—or are you excluded from any kind of relationship with her? Either way, you can be certain that he is communicating his feelings by deeds rather than words. You need to hear what isn't being said.

MEN MAKE CHOICES IN A RELATIONSHIP BASED ON FEAR

Men invariably protect themselves. If they believe that they are in some way inferior, inadequate, or undesirable, they will do anything to avoid having that deficiency highlighted.

How this affects you: Men adopt a "get them before they get you" mentality. They definitely believe in the old saying from sports that the best defense is a good offense. Result: If they suspect that for some reason they're not your Prince

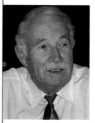
Charming, they will actively seek to alienate you so they can say it was their choice and not your rejection that created distance in the relationship. Bottom line: It stands to (his) reason that if he doesn't put himself—his feelings, his ego, his desires—on the line, then he can't get hurt.

What you can do about it: The best strategy you can undertake to deal with a partner who is motivated by fear and self-protection is to talk about this fear openly. Be warned: Men will jump through fire to avoid this conversation, because their egos won't stand for them to admit that they fear something. What you can do is deal directly with their fear of rejection.

To prepare for this conversation, you need to ask yourself some important questions:

■ Are you in fact rejecting him?
■ Are you sending him messages that say "You are inferior and undesirable"?
■ Are you making him so low on your priority list that he has no choice but to conclude that he is undesirable and has been rejected?

Please understand, I'm not recommending that you just admire your partner unequivocally or encourage behavior that isn't worthy of admiration. I'm saying that you must consider whether or not you are playing into his worst fears. His worst fear is that he's not good enough for you, and that you are going to dump him.

Reassure him that while there may be

What Men Want from Women

▶ Men are definitely the weaker sex; your admiration is a huge deal for them. They need external validation, and validation from the woman they love is the kind they value most.

▶ A man needs to know that his partner is proud of him and of what he does. He knows he's not the president of the United States, he knows he's not saving the world every day, he knows that he is probably just a cog in the machinery. I don't care if he is a doctor, a janitor, an architect, or a garbage

collector—he needs to know that you are proud of how he does what he does. He needs to know that you are proud of how he protects, provides for, and relates to his family.

▶ He can bluster all day long, he can brag till the cows come home, but make no mistake, when you look him in the eye or put your arms around his neck and say, "Have I told you today how proud I am of how you did such and such?" it will be worth its weight in gold to him.

issues that need to be discussed, you're not putting the relationship on the line over those problems. If you let him know that you have no intention of withholding your love, affection, attention, or sexual interaction in a punitive way, you can reduce his fear of rejection.

MEN HAVE BEEN RAISED TO LIVE OUT A MALE STEREOTYPE

A lot of the disconnect between men and women has to do with the fact that men have been socialized in a way that runs counter to the way women do things. This "masculine code" is something that women simply have to be aware of to interact effectively with men. Think of these beliefs as deeply rooted rules of behavior, part and parcel of what it means to be a man.

■ Big boys don't cry: We hear it at football practice—"Get up and shake it off; that's not a bone sticking out, so get going." It takes some men a lifetime to learn that maybe big boys don't cry, but grown men do. It's an incredibly difficult lesson for us to learn.

■ Linear thinking is all: Most men tend to insist on a rigid chain of logic from A to B, B to C, C to D, and so on. By contrast, most women are more intuitive. They're more likely to say, "Something ain't right here," even though they may not be able to identify specific, logical steps that point to that conclusion.

Dr. Phil's MENtors

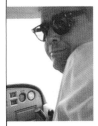

WHO: *Bill Solomon, my flight instructor.* He was a "flying cowboy," certainly one of the most down-to-earth, no-nonsense people I've ever known. He taught me, "When you are airborne, what you've got is yourself. You'd better depend on who you are. If you're in trouble, some guy 30 miles away in a radio room on the ground won't save you. It's you and the airplane. You'd better know yourself, and you'd better depend on yourself."
BEST ADVICE: "There ain't nowhere you gotta be tomorrow that's worth dying for today. Don't push it!"

Dr. Phil's MENtors

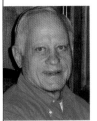

WHO: *Jim McCoy, one of my best friends and a lifelong tennis partner.* Jim is probably the single smartest person I've ever met. He invented and patented something called the Echometer, which measures and analyzes the performance of an oil well. It's one of the most significant technologies in the history of the oil field. His philosophy has always been "Be fair. If you can't get up the hill without beatin' the horse, then you need to get a different horse. You don't grind people in this life." He's incredibly successful, and he never loses balance. He always keeps focused and does the right thing.
BEST ADVICE: "Don't be a hardhead. If what you're doing is not working, change it, and change it now."

■ It can always be fixed: The male's reaction to conflict is usually something like "You got a problem? Here's how you fix it." Whereas the woman involved may not care anything about the fix. For her, knowing that the problem has been recognized and that her emotional circumstances have been acknowledged may be all the fix she desires.

■ Power + Control = Success: Men are socialized to measure their own value in terms of how much power and control they have—not how sensitive they can be or how deeply they can connect with another person.

How this affects you: Every single way in which the world makes a man is at odds with most women's definition of intimacy. Relationships in general, and intimacy in particular, are all about taking down your defenses. Intimacy means trusting people enough to give them the power to hurt you. And that is absolutely contrary to a man's nature.

There's no doubt that you need an active participant in your relationship. The problem is, the person you're trying to get to jump in the water with you is scared to death of what will happen if he does. As a result, you spend your time pursuing your partner, rather than interacting with him. You're looking at the back of his head and

yelling from a quarter-mile back (men can be really fast when they're scared). You are relegated to the behavior that men tend to label as nagging. Men say, "You're on me about this all the time; you're always after me." The truth is that of course you're after them all the time—because they're running all the time.

What you can do about it: To help a man overcome his fear of vulnerability and intimacy, you have to demystify the whole area for him. He knows that his emotional self contains information that could potentially be used against him, so you have to convince him that he can trust you with it. Teach him that when he allows himself to be vulnerable with you, he can be assured of a good outcome.

A lot of men run from an intimate topic because they think there will be no end to the discussion. They react so badly when you say "Can we talk?" because they think it's a life sentence, an interminable assignment to the hell that is vulnerability.

You can handle this whole subject much more effectively if you let your partner know there's a light at the end of the tunnel. Tell him, "We've got thirty minutes here; let's talk for that period of time." When the time ends, stop.

Also, you tend to get what you give. If you're open and honest, and you reveal true things about your intimate self, you're

What Never to Do

▶ The biggest mistake you can make in a relationship is to be entrusted with potentially hurtful information and to use it as leverage in an argument. If your partner opens up to you about his fears, needs, desires, and other secrets, and you turn that on him, you've gone to a place from which there is likely no recovery. You must be a good steward of his private revelations.

▶ If you take a judgmental attitude and are always ready to condemn a man's every move, you may be right, but you'll also be lonely. Decide right now that your goal is to be successful rather than to prove yourself right and men wrong. Focus on understanding *how* men think, rather than *why* they do, and I promise you'll get a lot more of what you want.

much more likely to have that behavior reciprocated than if you simply demand that he do so.

MEN TEND TO BE HIGHLY COMPETITIVE

I've heard so many men talk about this lately, true to that masculine code that we talked about earlier: They need to feel that they're in control. It's as if men have never stopped wanting to be the knight in shining armor who saves the damsel in distress.

How this affects you: A lot of men will tell you candidly that they are indeed threatened by women's competency. An ambitious, bright young male in corporate America will be identified as a go-getter; he's labeled as a young lion on the move. A woman who demonstrates exactly the same degree of ambition will be labeled as a hostile, aggressive bitch.

What you can do about it: You can let your man know that just because you are a successful, independent, financially self-sufficient woman, you haven't stopped being vulnerable. A woman has to be willing to show her needs and not be afraid of them. If his attitude is, I've got nothing to offer you, let him know that he does. You need him to be a partner and a soft place for you to fall.

MEN ARE HUNTERS

As a result of the substantial differences between men and women when it comes to sex—differences that are psychosocial, biochemical, and neurological—trying to get a man to function according to female standards is like trying to get a pig to fly. It's just not going to happen. That old but often accurate notion that men are hunters seems especially applicable here.

How this affects you: Men have less of certain hormones and more of others than women do, and that fuels us to respond in different ways. For most women, sex is primarily an emotional thing; for most men, it's primarily physical.

A man often fails to see how sex and other aspects of the relationship are intertwined. I have always counseled women that there are times you make love, and there are times when it's purely recreational: Wham, bam, thank you ma'am—

just a complete physical release, and cover me up when you're done. Men and women both need to recognize that there's a range of feeling when it comes to sex. If you don't acknowledge that range, the two of you are going to have a problem.

I've been asked why men almost always interpret physical affection as a signal for sex. My answer? Because if physical closeness has gotten scarce, men take whatever encouragement they can get. See, here's the problem: Women say, "You can't hug the SOB or he'll want to take you to bed." Well, that's because you haven't hugged him in two weeks! If men believe that they are deprived sexually—remember, they are hunters—they will start constantly hunting for sex. If you go into the wild, you can walk right past a well-fed lion, you can walk right past a well-fed bear. But if those beasts are hungry, you're in danger. It's the same thing with men. If men feel, *I am deprived, I am hungry,* then yes, they're spring-loaded for sex. They'll jump on you if you just walk by slow.

There is definitely a double standard with men when it comes to fidelity. If they are having an extramarital affair or an extra-relational affair, they'll probably look at it as if they are going and taking some-

How to Find the Good Ones

I hear both men and women say, "There aren't any good ones left!" Since both sides say it, it can't be true.

▶ First ask yourself, How are your recognition skills? Do the qualities that initially attract you to a man make him a good long-term partner? If your answer is no, then change your selection criteria. They say that nice guys finish last. It may be that the ol' boy who's hustling you may not be the person you want raising your children or being there for you when you're sick.

▶ If you just get up, go to work, go home, go to bed, then start the whole thing over the next morning, a guy would have to throw himself on the hood of your car to meet you. Lift up your head, broaden the criteria, and don't be too quick to eliminate candidates.

Dr. Phil's MENtors

WHO: *Viktor Frankl, Austrian psychiatrist.*
Frankl survived a German death camp during the Holocaust. He then wrote *Man's Search for Meaning,* a book I've read probably 50 times. While in the death camp, Frankl realized that other people can sometimes control everything about your life, but *not* the attitude you take toward what happens in your life—we have a choice about how we react to events. This truth affected me as a cognitive behaviorist. I've read everything he's ever written. He's had a profound influence on my personal and professional philosophies.
BEST ADVICE: "Create meaning to your suffering."

thing from a woman, not giving something of themselves away. There's no emotional investment there.

Men are visually stimulated, which means if they are in a target-rich environment, they may well become aroused. This is not just a maturity issue; their brains are actually wired that way, which is very different from your own wiring. Take the orientation as a hunter, bring immaturity into the mix, and you end up with a man who will misguidedly measure his worth at least in part by his conquests. But this is not some involuntary reflex action over which he has no control. It is a choice. Men can be amazingly shortsighted on these issues, often failing to project ahead to the consequences of their actions on their wives or children.

What you can do about it: Discussing the matter of fidelity, before a crisis occurs, is crucial. Couples need to talk about what fidelity means to each of them so there's no confusion. Understanding that men fear rejection and therefore thrive on acceptance and are easily visually stimulated, you can program out a considerable risk of unfaithfulness by investing energy in what may seem superficial: your appearance and the level of sexual activity in your relationship. Please don't write to me objecting! I'm not saying this is fair, only that it is effective. Let the training begin. ●

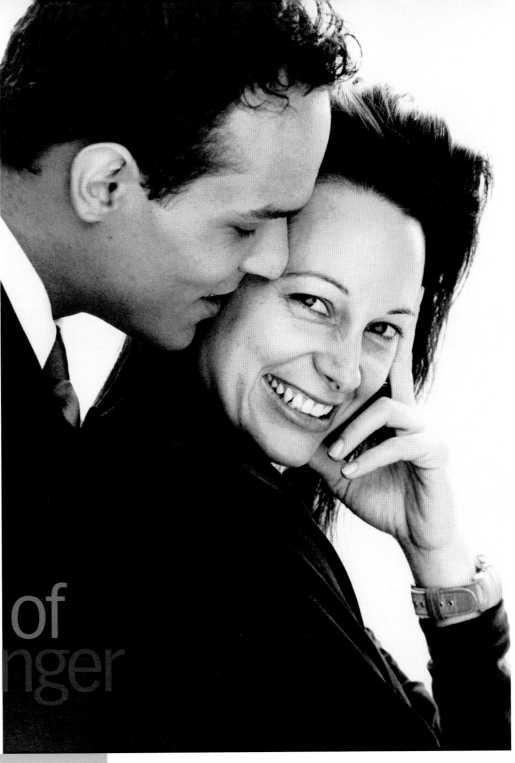

When **LYNN SNOWDEN PICKET** was graduating from seventh grade, her husband was in diapers. But that was then, and this (life with a gorgeous, healthy, appreciative, sexually fired-up man) is now.

In Praise of Younger Men

"THIS IS NOTHING COMPARED TO THE long lines during the oil crisis," I say to my husband, Bronson, as he pulls into a particularly crowded Mobil station near the Holland Tunnel. "Gas rationing! Remember that?"

"Actually, no," he says, smiling. I look at him, stunned that he could forget such a big part of 1973. People were siphoning fuel from their neighbors' cars in the dead of night! Then it hits me: He was born in 1971. I was born in 1958. Riiiight.

We've been together for seven years now, and I'm so used to considering Bronson my peer that I often forget about our 13½-year age difference. This wasn't always the case. In the beginning, if I wasn't thinking, *Is he too young for me? Am I too old for him?* someone else was thinking it for me—and blurting out, "Hey, have you seen *How Stella Got Her Groove Back*? You'd really dig it." Or "Susan Sarandon and Tim Robbins! She's older than he is, you know."

Does our culture's collective discomfort with a reversal of the usual younger woman–older man dynamic come, as scientists suggest, from a

deep-rooted evolutionary instinct that drives women to choose the wiser, older, more powerful alpha male over the untested young buck? Or could it be caused by something as shallow and immediate as a woman's not wanting anyone to think her date is her younger brother or, God help us, her son? Maybe women feel that because girls have a head start on maturity back in the seventh grade, our emotional and spiritual equals must forever be at least five years older than we are. Whatever part of the conventional wisdom they buy into, American women find it easy to summarily reject younger men. Too bad. They could be denying themselves the most wonderful relationship of their lives.

I was married once before, to a man five years my senior. After 12 increasingly dreary years capped by a wrenching divorce, I couldn't imagine why women in my situation (childless divorcées) complained about the prospect of reentering single life. Wasn't that the good news? Wasn't finally having some laughs, romance, and excitement the way to take the "crisis" out of "midlife"? Parties, rock concerts, nightclubs—I dated the way I should have when I was younger: for fun, without an eye toward marriage.

During that time, when I was in my late 30s, I made an important sociological discovery: Men over 40 are profoundly different from those under 35, and it's not just their hairlines.

AS MUCH AS WE'RE LOATH TO ADMIT it, we base most of our expectations about a relationship on the one we observed, for better or worse, growing up at home. A man who came of age in the 1960s, before the women's movement exploded, when his (more likely than not) stay-at-home mom did the cooking and cleaning, might have to work hard at accepting the fact that his life won't be just like his dad's. A man who came of age in the 1970s or '80s doesn't think twice about being married to a woman with her own career, or splitting the household chores with her. He probably grew up having to pitch in and help with dinner (if only to defrost it); he knows his way around a washing machine, and maybe even had to change a diaper or two. When it comes to gender roles and the division of labor, you're better off with a man whose mother has already fought the big battles for you.

The fact that a younger man's very busy mom probably didn't have time to whip up many culinary delights for the family can also work to your advantage. Anything you serve, however clumsily, is going to be greeted with unbelievable enthusiasm. Home cooking was something Bronson always hoped to experience, not The Way Things Used to Be. He'd walk a mile for my chocolate Kahlúa cheesecake, and he immediately bragged about my spaghetti sauce to his friends, who were envious of anything that didn't arrive by delivery boy. Staying over at a younger man's place may mean a breakfast of cold pizza and Mountain Dew, but at least you won't be offered Mylanta and Metamucil with your OJ. The reason for this is that he's Scarily Healthy. Open up a younger man's medicine cabinet, and you will see shaving gear, hair gel, a toothbrush, perhaps a squeezed-out tube of pimple cream, and, if he's something of a sophisticate, moisturizer. Of course, he probably won't have any first-aid supplies such as aspirin or Band-Aids, but before you curse his lack of preparedness, consider what else you won't see in his medicine cabinet: Di-Gel, minoxidil, Preparation H, Grecian Formula, Sominex, or Doan's pills for back pain. An empty medicine cabinet can actually be a beautiful thing.

> Women who reject younger men could be denying themselves the **most wonderful relationship** of their lives.

AN OLDER MAN, YOU MAY point out, has learned much from life and benefited from years of accumulated experience. What he may also have accumulated is an ex-wife (or two), and perhaps a child (or two), which means you get to be Daddy's New Friend. Or perhaps he never married but has in his past a nightmare of a long-term girlfriend who cheated on him with his former best friend. While years of relationships may teach a man to be a better partner, there's also the danger that he's learned to view women as gold-digging, untrustworthy sluts, parasitic leeches, or nagging harpies.

Younger men carry far less of this bitter emotional baggage. (Maybe he's carrying a grudge about one woman who done him wrong, but it's probably his mother.) They see women as wonderful, exotic creatures with many treasures to offer. They're not so far past the years when they pined to hold a real, live, naked woman that they take for granted what a terrific thrill and holy privilege it really is.

When I was in my 20s, my first husband and I went to three weddings in ten years. The vast majority of couples we knew simply lived together. The serially cohabiting older man sees dodging the bullet of matrimony as a badge of honor. His condemnation of marriage as a bourgeois convention makes him more of a tired, sad cliché than the ones he's using to describe matrimony. Since I've been with Bronson, we've averaged three weddings a year. This rush to the altar in the under-30 set has been denigrated (mostly by the over-30 set) as a spate of "starter marriages." Ultimately, I think the divorce rate will probably be the same as the break-up rate of the "just living together" generation, but I must say that it's infinitely more pleasant to listen to men who don't consider commitment to be a dirty word.

AS CREEPY AS THE DONE-IT-ALL, Warren Beatty type of older man is the one who hasn't done anything. This is the guy who's missed so much in his years on the planet that being with him makes you feel embalmed. I stopped dating a 48-year-old television executive when he labeled me a "maniac" because I said

I sunbathed topless. (In France.) Another guy old enough to have danced naked at Woodstock stared incredulously at my alternative rock CD collection ("I've never even heard of any of these guys," he said, waving around a Pearl Jam CD) and asked if I had any Kenny G or Jimmy Buffet. A guy who has spent the past 20 years in a well-insulated rut will make you tell his astounded buddies about the time you were in "a whaddya call it? A mosh pit?" You may have the feeling that your relationship now qualifies as his official Walk on the Wild Side. A younger man finds you fun rather than wild, interesting rather than threatening. He surprises you by showing up with a copy of that CD you liked at his place ("Queens of the Stone Age! Thanks!"), and he likes listening to your old Charlie Parker records. He offers to reorganize your computer's hard drive while you go out and get the wine. Sure, there are older men who can pull this off, but a 30-year-old guy was fooling around on a home computer (and programming the VCR and watching MTV) while he was still in grade school. The fact that you have three holes in one earlobe isn't even worth a comment from a younger man, whose last girlfriend may have had a pierced tongue.

DATING SOMEONE YOUNGER makes all the other men you know really, really nervous. Interestingly, the older men who exclusively date younger women are the most panicked and defensive. Because even if they're not interested in dating you, they won't relish the thought that you aren't interested in them for reasons that seem to spell out over-the-hill, no-longer-desirable, past-his-prime. (What is even worse for them to contemplate is the evidence that you're probably getting more action in the firm young flesh department than they are.) Men don't like the idea that women are thinking of sexy bodies (you know, the way they do), since it means that everything they hope is going to attract us—their salary, their Porsche—might turn out to be not so impressive after all.

There are some women who can't get past the fact that a younger man probably doesn't earn enough to take them to fancy restaurants on a regular basis. To that I say, you're missing the point. These same women are invariably the ones complaining about unimaginative guys for whom romance begins and ends with going out to dinner yet again. Where, they cry, are the afternoons spent eating bread and fruit and drinking a bottle of wine at the beach? Where's the touching, hand-presented little bouquet of daisies, rather than the predictable dozen roses delivered by the florist?

If you've ever said you'd rather have fun than dinner, dating a younger man offers you the chance to go have it. (And if you're in a corner office while he's still in a cubicle, you'll have the opportunity to put your feminist beliefs into action by picking up the tab the next time you crave a lovely dinner out.) But meanwhile, hike together through the woods. (Younger men can do this without complaining about their knees or their bad back.) Have him teach you how to surf. Spend all day making out at the beach. Stay in bed and order in Chinese. Thankfully, these are still extremely low-cost activities. A bonus: A younger man won't bore you with what an older guy might imagine is scintillating chat about his investments, his IRA funds, and his latest tax shelter.

And finally, yes, there's the sex. Some women—and nearly every older man—scoff at the idea that when it comes to sex, youth beats experience. Well, it does. First of all, the techniques necessary to please a woman are things that can be taught, and, more important, learned and mastered fairly quickly if one has a willing and interested partner—and a younger man is the very definition of willing and interested. Second, all the so-called experience in the world isn't going to help an older guy if after a meal and half a bottle of wine he's "too tired" to be able to show off these presumably stunning techniques. And consider this: If at first you don't succeed, try, try, try, and try again. In the same evening, if you like. And there's one area in which younger men have probably had more experience than their seniors: using condoms. Younger men came of age in the era of AIDS, and many have never (or rarely) had sex without a condom. This is definitely not the case with older men, who may be petulant and resistant about using them; they see themselves as being "spoiled" by the years and thrills of unprotected sex. And, worse, they may not really know how to use a condom—it's not quite as idiot-proof as the package instructions lead one to believe. A younger man may have learned condom basics in health class; he and his buddies may trade information about which brands are best. Ask yourself: This evening, would I rather trade memories of the Watergate hearings or discuss the merits of self-heating lubricants?

PERHAPS THE MOST STUNNING thing I've learned is that, eventually, any age difference ceases to matter. What I ultimately found in Bronson is someone who shares not only my interests but my values, none of which, ironically enough, have anything to do with age: friendship, fidelity, faith, a love of family, shared beliefs and priorities. It's a side benefit that he's made me proud of the fact that I remember watching the live broadcast of the first man walking on the moon, that he laughs when he hears how I kept murmuring "Shut up, Walter!" because Walter Cronkite had an uncanny habit of speaking at the precise moment an astronaut (on the moon!) made a comment. His interest in my stories and the way he values my perspective makes me feel sorry for the women I know who keep quiet when certain historic events come up, as if owning up to "being there" devalues them, and so is something they hide or lie about.

And for that, I say youth is not always wasted on the young. ●

THE GLASS EGO

Here's a closely guarded secret: Women have more influence over men than they think. Psychologist Jay Carter talks to **Michelle Burford** about male self-esteem, the criticism that could demolish a man, and what male intimacy is really about.

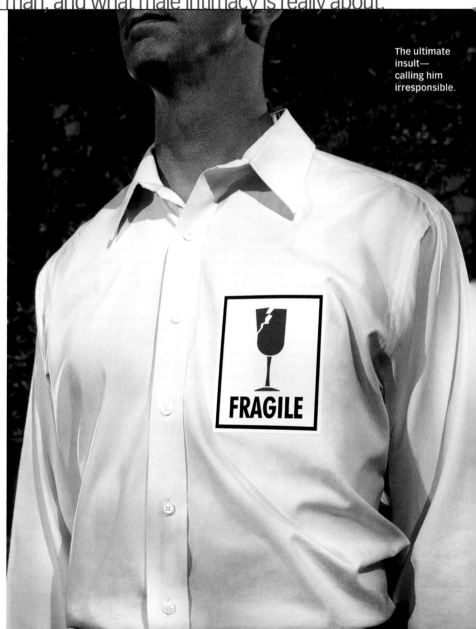

The ultimate insult—calling him irresponsible.

TWENTY-SIX YEARS OF COUNSELING men and couples has given Jay Carter an unusually clear window into men's hearts and minds. And his three books— *Nasty People, Nasty Men,* and *Nasty Women*— qualify him as an expert on, well, nastiness, and how to avoid it in your relationships. Carter's observations are so eye-opening that we asked him about everything from finding the key to a man's inner life to the best way to chew him out when you're mad:

FRAGILE

You've written that most women have no idea of their power to wound men. Where does this power originate?

During a boy's most important developmental period—his first five years—he usually gets his self-esteem from his mother. I think some of Freud's theories are hogwash, but I believe he was right about at least one: Whereas a girl might choose to grow up to become like her mother in certain ways, a boy tries to be *becoming* to his mother—to make her proud. Years later, when he meets someone he wants to spend his life with, he unconsciously gives her what I call his jujube doll—a kind of voodoo-like name I have for the part of a man's self-esteem that's vulnerable to a woman's opinion of him. If she sticks a pin in his doll, he recoils. Most women I talk with don't realize what kind of influence they have over men.

Men respect hopes and dreams. That's a language they speak.

In your book, Nasty Women, *you state that men are more word-oriented. But aren't women considered more verbal?*

Yes, but research on gender differences has proven that men tend to take words more literally and to hear them in more sweeping terms. Let's say a woman asks her husband to pick up a half-gallon of orange juice after work. When he arrives home empty-handed, she's irritated. She might offhandedly say, "You are so irresponsible." All he hears is the word *irresponsible*. He believes she's saying he's irresponsible in general. He thinks, *What about all the months I paid the mortgage? Does one slipup erase all my effort? And why is she overreacting?* With his self-esteem wounded, he may launch into a defense about what

convey her frustration without becoming a nag or know-it-all?

She can get his attention through action. If a man leaves his pajamas on the floor, a woman might get so upset that she'll accuse him of disregarding her feelings. Then for two days, he'll pick up the PJs to avoid an emotional outburst. But if two men were living together, one would simply say to the other, "Do you think you could put away your smelly pajamas before my girlfriend gets here?" The other agrees—but still leaves his PJs out. So his roommate finally says with a grin, "The next time you leave your pajamas out, I'm gonna burn 'em in the backyard." He does. When the other guy looks for his PJs, he finds a smoldering pile of cloth. That's how men operate. They don't call each other irresponsible or accuse each other of not caring about feelings; they simply burn the damn pajamas. For a woman to get a man's

"Most women I talk with don't realize what kind of influence they have over men."

Doesn't a woman likewise hand over part of her power to the most significant man in her life?

Yes, but she does it by sharing her most private feelings. The seat of a woman's soul is her emotions. A woman usually believes you know her when you know what she feels. But the seat of a man's soul is his intent or purpose. That's why when a woman bares her soul by disclosing her feelings, a man often doesn't recognize that as significant. He's been socialized to discount feelings. For him, baring the soul means sharing his hopes and dreams. He may say things that seem boring, silly, or outlandish: "You know what I'd do if I had $20,000? I'd invest it in lotto." But if a woman really listens, he'll share more. After a failure, a man might express his intentions by saying, "I know I've messed up, but here's what I wanted for our family." When a woman understands this, she can begin to share her own intentions as a way of drawing him closer.

it means to be responsible. She gets frustrated because he's so caught up in words that he doesn't acknowledge her feelings—and that's usually because he doesn't remember how important feelings are to her.

What if the man really is irresponsible? How do you communicate that without inciting a gender missile crisis?

If you decide you want to keep the man around, don't use the word *irresponsible*. You can call him a jerk or even an ass and it won't devastate him, because what is a jerk? That's not concretely definable. But what a man feels when you call him irresponsible is what a woman feels when you call her a bitch. It's the ultimate insult. So if you're angry at a man, just call him a bitch.

Suppose a woman tunes in to her partner's intentions but he doesn't reciprocate by hearing her needs. How can she

attention without bruising his jujube doll, she has to show rather than tell.

You've written that when a woman begins to care deeply for a man, he becomes her home-improvement project. Why?

A woman often marries a man for his potential. If women married men for who they actually were, there would be far fewer marriages. When a woman loves a man, she says to herself, *I could improve him. Once we're together, things will be different.* Since I began my practice in 1977, I've heard this refrain hundreds of times. I try to get it across to the woman that what she sees is what she gets. This is him. If he's drinking every Friday and Saturday night, look forward to a lifetime of weekend alcoholism. He may cut out Friday, but he'll still be a drinker. Men tend to resist change. In fact, one of the most prized characteristics of a man's friendship with other men is total acceptance. When a woman begins to encourage a man to live up to his potential, he misunderstands that as her overall dissatisfaction with him. What he feels is tantamount to what women feel when men don't hear and respond to what they say they need.

How might the relationship unravel when she expresses her disappointment?
The man may initially improve according to her recommendations—remember, he has a lot invested in what she thinks of him. But over time, he becomes slower to respond. Then there's the day when she inadvertently steps on his jujube doll with a spiked heel, and it's so painful that he snatches his self-esteem back. That's the day she loses significant influence. He tries to make himself not care what she thinks, which is why she begins to feel he's emotionally distant. He stops connecting. He

therapist can tell you is the most repeated phrase among men: "No matter what I do, I can never please this woman." While she's been genuinely trying to improve him with the best intentions, he's been feeling her efforts as a shot to his self-esteem. After all the work she has put into him—he finally eats with his mouth closed, he doesn't say ignorant things—he may run off with another woman. That's often because he's looking for someone who will think the world of him—someone who will see him as he thinks his wife once did. What he doesn't know is that he's bound to repeat the cycle because he hasn't done the work of understanding himself, the woman in his life, and the differences in how they communicate. He thinks his new woman is looking enraptured because he's the greatest, but what she's actually thinking is, *Wow—what potential.*

something like "It wasn't my intention to hurt you, but I have. I really do think you're a wonderful man." He may never admit that there are heel marks all over his doll, but if she approaches him this way, he'll slowly open up again.

How can a woman encourage her partner to reach his full potential without hurting his self-esteem?
By stroking the jujube doll before bringing the hammer down. Let's say a man leaves his McDonald's wrappers all over the car. The woman is angry that he's inconsiderate of her desire to drive without bits of cheese, pickles, and dried ketchup stuck to the steering wheel. What should she say? "I see how organized you are by the way you keep your desk, which is why I'm a bit surprised about the wreck our car is." Because she has first acknowledged the big

"A man will feel even more motivated to please a woman he loves if he knows that, in general, she already thinks the world of him."

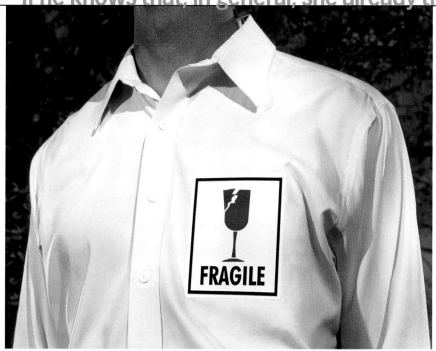

FRAGILE

doesn't look her in the eyes unless he's angry. When the marriage is on the brink of breakup, the woman drags him into my office. That's when I hear what almost any

Once a man has snatched away his jujube doll, can a woman ever get it back?
Yes. She can sit down with him and say

picture—"I know you're a neat guy"—the criticism doesn't sting. And if she keeps the whole thing light, she'll get a laugh out of him before he heads out to clean the car.

I'm not suggesting that women spend their lives building up men's egos. That's enabling and patronizing. This is not about telling a man he has the brightest gold chain or the biggest penis. Emphasizing a man's positive qualities is acknowledging the complete picture of who he is and what he has already done right.

After nearly three decades of counseling men, do you think most really want to please women?
Oh, yes! And I believe that a man will feel even more motivated to please a woman he loves if he knows that, in general, she already thinks the world of him. Once a woman tells a man how responsible and caring he is, he'll usually do all he can to live up to that image. Just to make her proud, he'll rise up and move mountains. ●

The ¢ents and Sensibility Quiz:

Suze Orman asks: Are You Two a Financial Match?

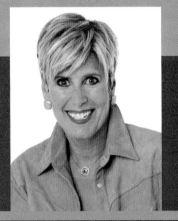

Financial disconnects are one of the main reasons relationships don't work. All the women who wrote to me recently could have avoided frustration and heartache if they had figured out ahead of time whether they were financially compatible with their partners. You and your partner should compare your answers to the quiz below. It will help you both identify where your financial patterns don't jibe and understand your money habits.

1 Lucy's take-home pay is twice as much as Jake's. They move in together and need help figuring out a plan for sharing costs. They should:

A. Split the costs 50-50.

B. Let Lucy handle housing costs and Jake pay the utilities.

C. Open a joint checking account into which Lucy deposits two-thirds of their combined monthly costs and Jake one-third, and pay the bills from that account.

2 Lucy and Jake are saving for a down payment on a house when their best friends invite them for a $4,000, two-week adventure in Thailand. They don't have the money for the trip, but they really want to go. They should:

A. Raid the down payment savings. Life is too short to pass up this opportunity!

B. Charge the vacation, then stop saving for the down payment for a few months to pay off the credit card bill.

C. Pass this time around, but ask their friends if they would consider planning a more modest trip in the future.

3 Though Lucy makes more money than Jake, she also spends more and has a large credit card balance. On Jake's smaller salary, he pays every bill on time and contributes to his 401(k). They get engaged and want advice on how to deal with their different money personalities. They should:

A. Deal with the money stuff after the wedding. The most important thing is that they love each other.

B. Split the living costs but keep their credit cards separate so each can spend what he or she wants.

C. Slow down! Their wedding will be a prelude to divorce if they don't take the time now to discuss how to get past their financial differences.

Answers:

Obviously, C is the soundest choice in each situation. Unless you and your partner agree on each point, use this quiz to start an ongoing conversation in which you strive to create a financially merged life that will help you achieve your mutual goals and dreams. Your payoff will be more than financial; the process of talking about these issues will bring more intimacy to your relationship. That's the real secret to a successful partnership.

Little Every Thing Every Thing He Does Is Stupid

Aw, you love the guy! *Except when he drives you completely mental.*

MARTHA BECK shows you what to do with a significantly annoying significant other.

R RECENTLY, I ASKED A GROUP OF ordinary American women to describe their significant others' most annoying characteristics. The responses were startling, not for their content but for the loathing I observed in these usually pleasant, well-adjusted people. If you want to see the red gleam of murder in someone's eyes, if you want chilling insight into the thinness and fragility of the civilized veneer that glosses over humanity's primal drives, don't read Greek tragedy or visit death row. Just listen to a few nice, normal folks talk about the way their spouses fake a Cockney accent, reuse unwashed underwear, or repeat every joke three times:

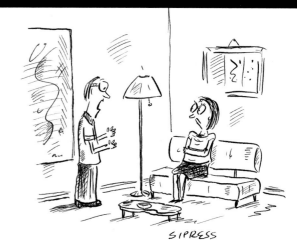

"Well, if it doesn't matter who's right and who's wrong, why don't I be right and you be wrong?"

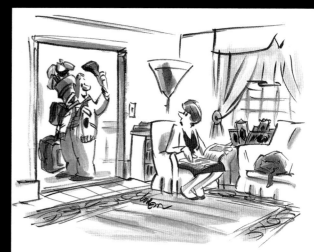

"Well, now that the kids have grown up and left I guess I'll be shoving along, too."

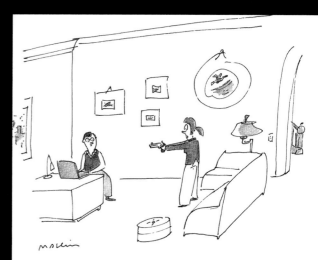

"O.K., step away from the laptop and hold up your end of the conversation."

"He's a wonderful guy, but after a meal he spends 20 minutes sucking food particles from between his teeth. He makes this whistling sound—ugh, I can't even think about it. I long to tell him those three little words: 'Use dental floss.'"

"My husband uses the phrase 'but yet' in every other sentence, and it drives me absolutely barking nuts. Say 'but' or say 'yet,' not both. It's like saying 'also too' or 'however although.' Where did he learn to talk, the Department of Redundancy Department?"

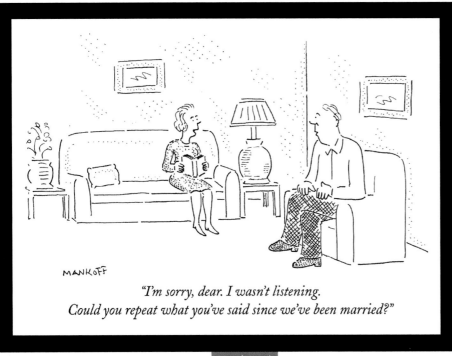

MANKOFF

"I'm sorry, dear. I wasn't listening.
Could you repeat what you've said since we've been married?"

Ignoring pet peeves is one option; behavior therapy, another.

"Mustard yellow. My boyfriend calls it gold, and, oh, does he love it. Everything he buys is mustard—furniture, clothes, even his car. I'm afraid one day he'll show up in another mustard yellow shirt, and I'll push him in front of a mustard yellow school bus."

HATING THE ONES WE LOVE

In order to sustain romance, and pledge our undying devotion to our partners, it might be wise to acknowledge the flashes of vile, indefensible hatred we occasionally feel toward them. Oh, don't look so shocked. If you've been in a relationship for more than six months, you've had those moments. We all have. Acknowledging them while they're still small can help us deal with them responsibly. Denying their existence allows them to grow until they overwhelm our social niceties, turning us into various manifestations of the Incredible Hulk.

Speaking of media images, consider the convict in the movie *Chicago* who got so sick of her husband's gum-popping that she fired "two warning shots...into his head." Or the woman in HBO's *Six Feet Under* who fatally clocks her salesman husband with a frying pan to stop him from droning on about his products (the morticians, to their own dismay, empathize with her completely). Think of Meryl Streep's deceased character in *Death Becomes Her,* turning to Bruce Willis and hissing, "Do you have to breathe?" Do you want to reach that point? If not, read on.

First:
Find the Meaning in Maddening Moments

Tom and Jerri were furious at each other. On their way to my office, they'd stopped for a cup of coffee. Tom had also purchased a newspaper and flipped to the sports page, holding out the front section and asking Jerri, "Do you want to look at this?" At that point, Jerri burst into tears, all communication ceased, and the couple were officially at war.

"He knows it makes me crazy when he does that," said Jerri, tears flowing again as she recounted the experience.

"What are you talking about?" Tom almost yelled. "I can't stand how you always get hysterical over nothing!"

Clearly, this had nothing to do with the newspaper. However, the coffee shop incident was an excellent "access point" for figuring out the core issues that were causing conflict. The key to this process is simply asking each person to describe, in detail, the meaning he or she gives to an event. I asked Jerri and Tom to tell me what each of them thought was going on during their coffee shop encounter.

"He never gives me his full attention," Jerri said. "He finds anything to distract him—traffic, the sports page, whatever. And then he gives me the rest of the paper, like he thinks I'm behind on current events."

Tom's jaw dropped. The motives Jerri had ascribed to his actions had nothing to do with his real intentions. "All I wanted to do was check the baseball scores—my dad and I used to do that. I gave Jerri the rest of the paper because my mom always read it."

Likewise, when Jerri began to cry, Tom knew that, as he put it, "she was accusing me of being a bad husband, trying to control me." This could not have been further from Jerri's intent. "I needed his attention for five minutes over breakfast. If I get that, I feel close to him all day."

Like Tom and Jerri, you'll often find that the behavior you don't like is triggering insecurities, fears, or unfinished grief. The next time you feel hatred flaring up, wait until you're no longer frothing mad, then calmly check whether the meaning you attach to events is the same as your partner's intention, listen to the response, and then suggest alternatives that might meet both your needs. This technique can turn a maddening moment into an opportunity for deeper mutual understanding and a significantly happier relationship.

Second:
Take Care of Your Share

Sometimes you'll search in vain for any deeper significance. Sometimes he's incredibly annoying, full stop. In that case, the easiest course of action is not to change him (though, as we shall see, this may be possible) but to figure out what you might do to reduce your own irritation. One of the following strategies may help:

1. Protect yourself from "social exhaustion."

Being around people is wonderful, but it also creates a unique kind of fatigue that can be alleviated only by privacy. Being intensely annoyed by a partner's quirks is often a sign that you've spent too much time together. Taking a few minutes to walk, sit, or lie down by yourself can dramatically improve your mood and resilience.

2. Ask yourself if your partner is doing something you'd love to do, except that it's against your rules.

Often people feel severely judgmental toward those who are doing the things they've denied themselves. Wanting your mate to eat healthy food is one thing, but if you writhe in fury whenever he munches a cookie, the issue may be that you're denying yourself too stringently. If so, don't beat him, join him.

3. Stay in your own business.

Byron Katie, author of *Loving What Is,* divides all business into three categories: mine, yours, and God's. Some people escape the content of their own lives by obsessing about the two other categories. Whenever you become intensely focused on changing someone else's behavior, you might want to check what part of your own business you're avoiding.

The first step is to accept that you're annoyed. Watch your mental turbulence without judging or repressing it. Then imagine that your loved one is suddenly whisked away to Timbuktu, leaving you with nobody to change—except yourself. What stuff is waiting for you? Is it frightening? Saddening? Unfamiliar? Observe your own resistance, offer yourself some sympathy, then commit to facing your problems. Better yet, enlist your partner. Tell him about the difficulty or scariness of your business. He'll probably listen and maybe offer help—and presto! Your need to get into his business will be replaced by increased love and gratitude.

Third:
Train His Brain

If the methods outlined above don't work for you, it may be time for some good old behaviorist training. This is a simple procedure, grounded in the fact that animals (including humans) will repeat behaviors that are positively rewarded and decrease those that aren't. I love behaviorist training because, in contrast to the noble approaches we've already discussed, it doesn't require all those tedious virtues (open communication, self-examination, authenticity, yada yada). It's just plain bribery, though invisible and, of course, well intentioned.

Begin by identifying small, easy-to-give treats your mate really loves: praise, chocolate, backrubs, shiny objects...list as many as you can. (I must admit, I myself have achieved thrilling results using only praise and chocolate.) Hand out these rewards whenever your mate does something you like, especially something that replaces the behavior you most hate. Don't tell him what you're doing, and don't react to the annoying behavior at all (carrots are much more effective than sticks). At first, reward behavior that goes anywhere near what you'd like to see. Then, as the positive behavior increases, offer the reward for more specific actions.

I once used this technique on a guest lecturer in one of my college classes. Before the professor arrived, I told my students to look excited and attentive whenever he walked toward the left side of the room. When he walked right, they'd simply drop their eyes. After 30 minutes, the scholar was crowding the far left classroom wall, unwilling to stray a step to the right—and he was quite unaware that he was doing it, much less why.

Likewise, I've seen sedentary people turn into exercise fanatics, slobs develop sophisticated manners, and undemonstrative louts become affectionately expressive, all because their mates rewarded them, consistently and judiciously, for the new behavior. This method requires persistence, like housebreaking a puppy, but if you're up for it, you'll find it highly effective.

REALIZE THIS LAST STRATEGY may seem Machiavellian, but would you rather shower your mate with kisses (real or Hershey's) or emerge from a mental mist to find you've strangled him for doing that weird falsetto humming thing?

I thought so.

This might be just the time to work on clearing out the fetid pockets of mate-hate in your relationship. Look for meaning in maddening moments, take your share of blame, and use gentle means of changing behavior.

Got that? Good girl!

Have a piece of chocolate! Keep this up, and by next Valentine's Day you'll hardly remember how it felt to hate the one you love. ●

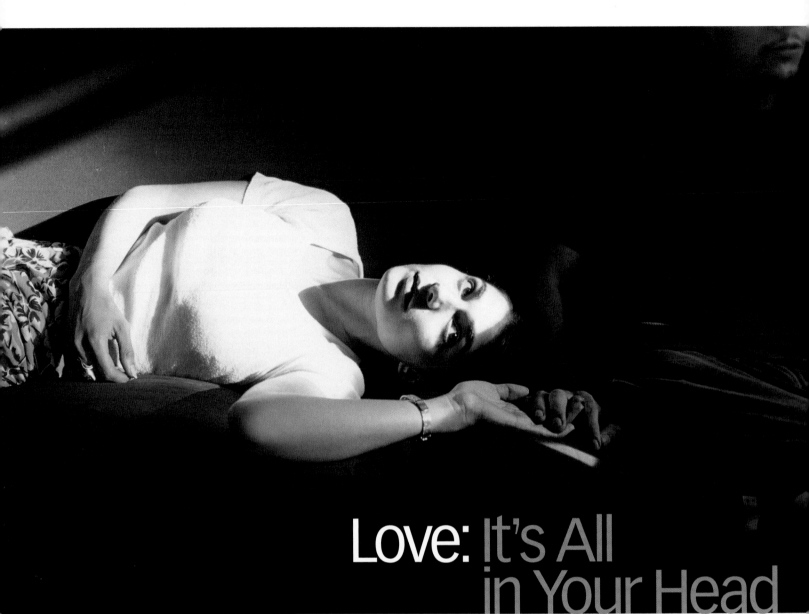

Love: It's All in Your Head

Is it possible to change another person's behavior—and transform a less-than-perfect relationship—simply by changing your own thoughts? Psychologist Henry Grayson's theory may very well revolutionize the way we look at love, friendship, and attachment. **MARK MATOUSEK** reports.

IN HIS HERETICAL BOOK, *MINDFUL LOVING,* HENRY GRAYSON, an eminent New York psychologist, relates a story that perfectly captures his mind-altering theory of love. A despondent patient had come to Grayson's office, complaining about being married to "the world's biggest shrew." As patients frequently do, Jon seemed to want commiseration from his loyal shrink.

Grayson isn't that kind of doctor. "What are you willing to do?" asked the therapist, turning the tables back on Jon.

"Anything," he replied. Grayson's instructions were oddly simple: The next time Jon became anxious over his wife's behavior, he was to focus on his own upsetting thoughts, replacing the inner wife-hating voice—*She's*

Couples therapy could be more effective *and* simpler, a maverick book says.

ruining my life!—with a tender memory of the woman he'd once loved. At first Jon couldn't recall such a woman; finally, a happy moment oozed up from the distant past. He promised Grayson he'd give it a try.

Jon was confused at his next appointment. He told Grayson his wife seemed more subdued somehow. "She must be coming down with a bug," Jon said.

"Try the experiment again," Grayson suggested.

At the following session, Jon was genuinely suspicious. He and his wife had spent their first tirade-free weekend at home in years. Perhaps she'd begun to see a therapist, Jon said, still failing to connect the dots. But a week later, Jon realized that the internal shift in his attitude had *created* the external shift in his wife's attitude.

The notion that relationships succeed or fail according to how we think about them may seem far-fetched. The science of relationships has tended to emphasize modifying outward behavior—which is why, according to Grayson, most couples therapy doesn't work. "It's like trying to clean up a river downstream rather than at its source," he says, settling his rangy, handsome self—think Mr. Rogers much better dressed—into the nook of a pale leather sofa. "We have to go upstream to what we're thinking—to the beliefs and behavior that come from our thoughts—instead of trying to change our emotions or, even worse, other people's behavior."

This principle applies to all relationships and not merely to the ones we call special. Specialness makes loving more difficult, Grayson claims—counterintuitive though that may sound—since casting people in the role of lover, mentor, spouse, or best friend raises expectations, which leads to fantasy, heartbreak, and pain. We suffer at the hands of those we love the most—that's the conundrum. "So much expectation," says Grayson, "blinds us to love."

There are two forms of attachment, apparently, both of which are known by the L word but which, in fact, are very different. "There's ego-based love," he tells me, using *ego* not to denote the Freudian sense of self that's indispensable to negotiating

daily life but to refer to the illusory armor that suffocates and cuts us off, the self-obsessed *me* that renders us so unspeakably lonely, stripped of the feelings of belonging and connection. "That's the irony," Grayson says. "First we imagine our separation from others, then we spend our precious lives trying, and failing, to bridge this false divide."

Spiritual love works on an opposite principle, he continues. Instead of the doomed attempt to "complete" ourselves through another person—the ego being chronically hungry, unworthy, unsatisfied—spiritual relationships hinge on the knowledge that each of us is already whole. "We're complete," Grayson insists, joining his fingers to form a circle. "We are made

"Once we're aware of who we are, there's **no difference** between giving and receiving."

from the very same energy as the rest of creation—love, as it is called in the gospels—in its myriad forms. Our essential nature is divine. In other words, we are already this wholeness, this love, that we seek outside ourselves."

TO APPRECIATE HOW AN agnostic scientist came to this mystical understanding, we need to trace Grayson's pilgrim's progress from choirboy to quantum clinician. Born 68 years ago in Alabama, he'd planned to become a Protestant minister till a few months in theology school convinced him that he had no faith—not of the church-approved kind, anyway. "I had stopped believing in the traditional concepts of a medieval, flat-earth 'sky God,' a deity that was far removed from us humans here on earth," he writes in the preface to his book. Grayson completed his studies nevertheless, earning

degrees in psychology and pastoral counseling, then worked briefly as a parish minister, struggling to reconcile traditional teachings with his desire to help his congregants feel God in "every aspect of their lives."

The strategy failed, at least for Grayson. Neither church religion nor advanced psychological studies satisfied his need to address what he calls the "massive problem of human suffering"—no less to enable our birthright of "indisturbable joy and peace." It was not until he found himself at a lecture in physics that a theory of how to heal the mind—and in turn solve the riddle of love—finally emerged in his thinking. "David Bohm turned my life upside down," says Grayson, referring to the innovative physicist who wrote, among other things, the classic *Quantum Theory.* "Bohm helped me understand that the reality we perceive is a tiny fraction of the universe as it really exists. At an invisible level, everything and everyone is interconnected in a most profound way, not only as human beings but as energy, mind, and matter."

With the barriers between inner and outer, self and other, cause and effect expanded in this prismatic light, Grayson came to see all relationships as being, in large part, an "inside job." Our core beliefs lead to thought constellations, which lead to perceptions, give rise to emotions, and cause, domino-like, outward behavior. What's more—and here's where Grayson's theory requires thinking outside the box—the behavior stemming from our own thoughts *may manifest in the people around us.* Jon's wife acted differently once he'd found a new way of viewing her, proving Heisenberg's principle that objects, including human ones, are changed somehow by the very act of being seen.

Lofty as this may sound, Grayson is a pragmatic man for whom ideas matter because they help people. "This means," he says, "that everyone is our soul mate. We share the same last name, which is God." In his popular tape series, "The New Physics of Love," as well as in his book, he offers advice on how to apply this cosmic law to our everyday lives. We start, he says, with awareness of our own minds and the development of the inner "witness," either through formal meditation or simple self-reflection. By stepping back from our thoughts, noticing how they tumble toward feelings, trigger opinions, and cause knee-jerk reactions, we learn to interrupt this sequence, to crack the ego's prison so that love can pass more freely between us. By learning to better navigate our mental terrain, we're better able to choose how we think about the world around us, to alter the frame through which we perceive our lives, ourselves, and our challenging loved ones.

What's more, there are reliable litmus tests for distinguishing counterfeit love from the real thing, Grayson says. Infatuation, the need to control, confusing love with worry, ensnaring someone as "special"—these are signs that ego, rather than heart, is driving a relationship. This counterfeit path is marked by potholes most of us recognize all too easily—demanding that love be earned, trying to change another's behavior, becoming addicted to someone's presence, and wanting to punish the other for disappointing us. The big giveaway to ego-based love, however, is the spoiling presence of fear. "For the ego in love," he tells me, "the greatest fear is losing the other person or losing yourself." Terrified by the threat of loss, we often fulfill our own prophecies.

The only remedy is commitment to practicing self-awareness. This starts with realizing once and for all that we vastly underestimate our capacity for love and are more profoundly interconnected than we can possibly know. The only thing blocking our awareness of this is ego's self-protecting harangue. "Love never hurts," Grayson tells me, having arrived at this wisdom through his own two marriages. "When my feelings are hurt, it's nearly always my interpretation of what has happened that causes the pain." Just think of the last time you misread someone's innocuous action as *all about you*. "I've come to understand my wife as a kind of mirror of my inner life. She's far more likely to be critical of me when I think critically of her."

By turning attention away from our partners, over whom we have little control, and focusing on this inside job, we begin to make love a path of enlightenment. This is Grayson's primary goal. "If the purpose of relationships is understood to be cultivating our own true nature and supporting

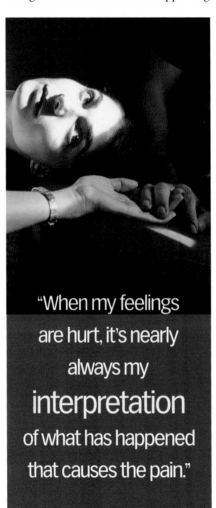

"When my feelings are hurt, it's nearly always my **interpretation** of what has happened that causes the pain."

our partners in finding theirs"—as opposed to sharing the bills, say, raising kids, or having a lot more sex—"then the label we place on the *form* love takes becomes secondary." Indeed, his chapter on "spiritual divorce" is likely to surprise some readers; according to Grayson, even "unhappy endings" can deepen—indeed transform—a continuing bond between once-married couples.

Knocking down more boundaries, Grayson claims that "once we're aware of who we really are, there's no big difference between giving and receiving. If I'm generous and attentive, it's because I want the best for you. This brings me joy and fulfillment rather than the drain that comes from a feeling of obligation. That's the kind of love that empowers, without desire for payback. If I want love," he says, "the best thing I can possibly do is extend this desire into the world as a loving thought—such as 'may all beings live in peace'—within my own mind."

THE SHIFT TO MINDFUL LOVing begins with acknowledgment that infatuation isn't real. "The bad news about 'falling in love' is that it isn't genuine love," he says. "It's based on an illusion, a fantasy of who someone will be. When the other person doesn't fulfill our dreams—which, of course, he or she never does—all sorts of bad things happen. You realize you've been living in a dream state, something you need to awaken from in order to love as your true self."

But, we protest, we want to find comfort in romantic love. Don't take *l'amour* away from us, we groan in adolescent despair. Love seems to be the last respectable place, in our too-grown-up lives, where we allow ourselves to be idiots, ridiculous messes, dramatic, impulsive, less than our p.c. best. Grayson's cure may seem bitter to the die-hard romantics among us. But one might ask, Do we need more grief and fear, more isolation, illusion, and heartbreak, in our love-starved world? Or do we need a change of mind, a liberated vision? Shall we whitewash the fences we build with our egos, or wake up to the glaring fact that love, according to every sage from every single wisdom tradition, is already here?

If Henry Grayson prevails over Hallmark, the answer will be clear as day. ●

If the Horse Is Dead, Get Off

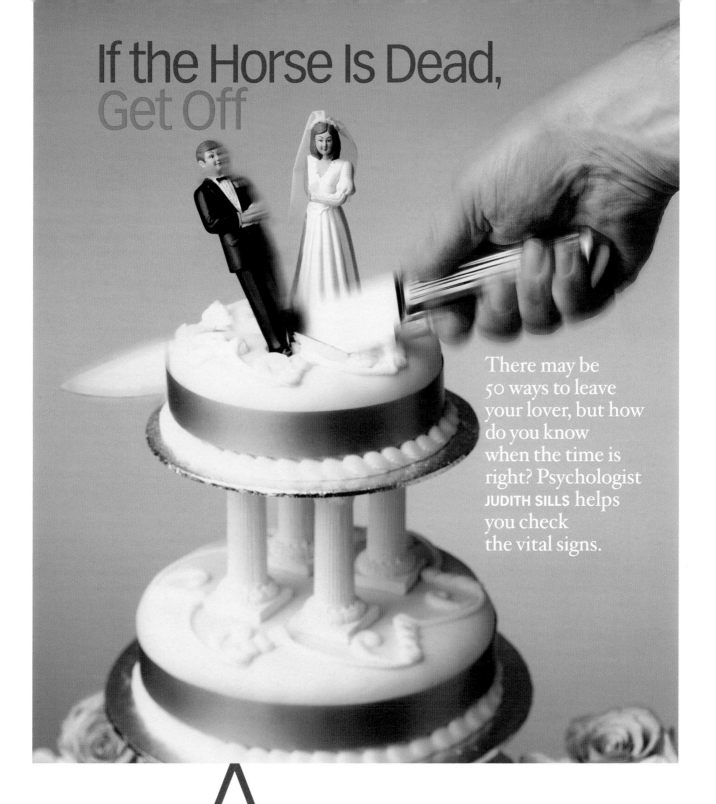

There may be 50 ways to leave your lover, but how do you know when the time is right? Psychologist **JUDITH SILLS** helps you check the vital signs.

A WOMAN SAT ACROSS FROM ME, FLATTENED BY frustration. "I've kept my marriage together by learning to choke down the ocean," she said. "For a while, it was easy. Lately, I'm suffocating. Is it just a bad patch? Or is it time to cut my losses?"

We swallow a lot to stay the course of love—more than we expected, sometimes more than we should. We absorb disappointment, wounding insults, and gusts of fury, and for long stretches our endurance is well worth it. Then—either all at once or with creeping

> Avoid going down with a sinking relationship.

awareness—we start to wonder: *Are the scales tipping against this attachment? Have I waited long enough for whatever it is I'm holding out for? Should I just let go?*

Love dies. That's a fact of life. But it also limps along, gasps for breath, and then weirdly resurrects itself—shocked awake by jealousy; recollected in a hospital room; revived after a separation, by a shared laugh, or just by the beauty of nature. Suddenly, there it is again, that heart tug of attachment. And besides, we may have other reasons to stay with someone: money, familiarity, duty, history. Add these hugely powerful forces together and maybe they *are* love, wearing a different mask.

OVER 25 YEARS OF PSYCHOtherapy practice and in the course of writing my book *The Comfort Trap or, What If You're Riding a Dead Horse?* I've seen how tricky it can be to leave someone. Often the hardest part of the escape is the decision to make it. We tell ourselves that even the best comfort zones—relationships, jobs, family life, or friendships—have unrewarding passages. Romantic partnerships, in particular, require perseverance and faith in order to reap the rewards of long-term love. So what's the difference between being a quitter and being a clear-thinking realist?

If a woman is lucky, she'll just know the difference, in her heart and her gut and wherever else intuition calls her name. We understand our partnerships in our mental underground. That's where we automatically measure our responsiveness to our partner's hand, the ease with which we turn to him for solace, and the anxious uncertainty or happiness we feel in his company. Through these and a hundred other cues, we recognize how strong or tenuous, how loving or toxic our connection is.

Your knowledge might reveal itself in images rather than words. One woman was troubled by the repeated vision of herself on a respirator. She came to believe this symbolized her fear that her unfaithful husband was as necessary to her as oxygen. The marriage was an esteem-eroding trap, but her frightened dependency kept her imprisoned. With her interpretation came a new image of herself outside the hospital. Six months of panic and planning later, she was in a lawyer's office, taking deep, reassuring breaths.

You might also have what I call a focusing moment, where your intuitive knowledge is spelled out in capital letters. "I finally got my paintings into a gallery," one woman said, explaining the instant she saw the end of a long romance. "I reached to call him and stopped. *He'll only be jealous,* I thought. *He'll bring me down.* I called anyway. He carped, as I predicted, and I knew."

A woman who is herself a therapist said, "In my work, I'm so used to seeing every

THE MOMENT I KNEW IT WAS OVER
A few anonymous stories from the trenches.

"We'd been together for four years when we went to see *La Bohème.* Two of the characters fall in love but then part company because, as I saw it, she was too needy and he couldn't be counted on. I cried through the whole damn opera, not because it was such a sad story but because their relationship seemed exactly like ours. We broke up the next day."

"I was taking a writing course and asked my then boyfriend to read my first piece. He responded, 'Don't show it to me until you can write like James Joyce.' It occurred to me that if I could write like James Joyce, I wouldn't ask him for his advice in the first place."

"We went to Europe together, and he was too afraid to try to speak a foreign language. I ended up doing all the talking until we arrived in London. There was something about his fear of trying, fear of adventure, fear of embarrassment — I just couldn't be with someone who was incapable of taking a risk."

"My boyfriend asked me to change the way I dressed because someone else didn't like how I looked."

"I literally ran out of grief. He had hurt me again—was it by not showing up or by ignoring my calls? No, this time, I'd actually caught him with someone else. Any other day, I'd have been reasoning with him and spilling tears on my clothes. I had swallowed so much pain for 18 months. But this time, finally, I sent that doggie back to the pound."

"I was really excited to be offered a sales job (I'd been miserable at work), but my significant other didn't support my decision to take it, saying it was too much of a gamble because it was on commission. He put money before my happiness."

point of view that I made more excuses for my husband than I should have. One day I heard him describe something that happened between us and I suddenly thought, *Hey, this is not just another perspective. He's lying. I'm married to a liar.* I never saw him the same way again."

Valuable as those flashes of insight are, most of us have to add to intuition the force of our judgment and will. In other words, we have to decide.

SOME SITUATIONS ARE CLEAR-cut: The relationship is bad because he's an unrecovered drug addict, alcoholic, or compulsive gambler. No matter how hard you try to lift him up, he will drag you down. If he is verbally or physically abusive, it's not just bad for you—it couldn't be worse. Get out.

From here the lines in the sand get softer. A relationship is bad for you when you yearn to get married and he won't marry you and you've given him all the time you have to give. ("But maybe I pressured him; maybe I rushed. How do I know I've waited long enough?" You don't know. You make up your mind.)

You face a similar crisis when you want to become a mother and he won't have a child. We can compromise a lot for love. But motherhood, for the woman who craves it, is too central a life experience to sacrifice. ("How do I know I'll find a better man in time to have a baby?" You don't. You choose to risk it. Or not.)

A relationship is destructive if it feels scary, cold, or flat-out unfriendly—and you're staying because you dream it will change or because "it's better than being alone." If tension has hardened into contempt, admit it: This isn't better than being alone. This is being alone but with a lead weight on your back.

MOST DIFFICULT OF ALL, love sometimes withers for no one reason. A relationship can be over not because it's bad for you but because it has ceased to be much of anything good. You're feeling flat or empty, sexually distracted or curiously

unaroused. Or you're inwardly angry, mentally scoring his offenses. Disappointment and frustration are hardy weeds, and they choke off fragile love too easily.

And yet he is your partner, your lover, your friend, a person in whom you have invested months, years, possibly decades. All of this you cherish, not to be discarded

> Don't pull the relationship life supports until you understand your role in the problem.

lightly. "I love the idea of him. I just can't stand the smell of him," one woman agonized, perfectly capturing our conflict between the heights of love and the daily chafing of intimacy.

If you don't have a strong intuition to light your way, how do you know when the not-so-great-but-maybe-good-enough relationship is kaput? The answer lies in what you want and need, in the compromises with which you choose to live, and in the hard choices you're able to make. You answer the tough questions by knowing

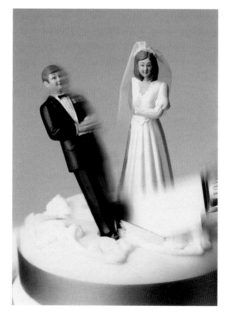

yourself, acknowledging your obligations, and living by your values.

Sure, you'll want to discuss these issues with him, but his responses are just one source of information. Your best decision will come from looking as deeply into yourself as you do the relationship.

Examine your history. If you usually want to back out at this point, you may need to stay longer and risk coming closer.

You might feel that the problem is all his, but it isn't. Don't pull the relationship life supports until you understand your role. Did the passion of motherhood divert your affections? Are you sexually restless, and has that made you more critical of him? Have you had a growth spurt that makes you less willing to tolerate what was acceptable before? If so, have you given him a chance to catch up?

WHEN YOU SEE YOUR PART, and you're either unwilling or unable to do what is necessary to improve things, or if your efforts are insufficient and he's not able to make up the difference, you know the romance is dead. Leave? Well, maybe.

If you have children, the obligation to provide them with the stable scaffolding they need to become solid grown-ups with rocky romances of their own may mean that you'll never openly declare this union over and gone. Your decision to go or stay will reflect your core beliefs about parenting, money, family, social status, a permanent New Year's Eve date, and all those other difficult issues that we iced over with the buttercream of being in love.

If you decide to cut your losses, I suggest you create a vivid, positive vision for your future. See it, say it, meditate on it, write it down, flash on it at every red light. When you catch yourself thinking you're too old, too poor, too weak, or too needy to make a change, laugh in your own face.

Letting go hurts.

But staying, once you've decided the relationship is really over, means being buried alive. Face your decision with courage, kindness, and a galloping leap of faith. Joy is waiting. ●

EXTREME BREAKUPS!

It's emotional agony, but for these five women, breathtakingly bad endings led to new connections, new wisdom, and new beginnings. Love and learn, says **Lise Funderburg**.

OST LIVING, BREATHING adults endure multiple romantic fractures in the course of a lifetime, but only one actual heart-splitting, Richter-scale breakup. In its aftermath, devastation tucks you in at night and wakes you up in the morning. Your day-to-day world is thrown out of whack, not to mention the past you thought was fixed and the double-occupancy future you assumed lay ahead. Sounds awful? Yes. Lonely? Excruciatingly. Invaluable? Perhaps.

What follows are the stories of women who went through heart-shredding breakups, the kind that left them absolutely sure, at one point or another, that they would never get out of bed again. But while none deny the palliative powers of a fling here or a pint of Godiva Chocolate Raspberry Truffle there, they all chose a risky and perilous road to full recovery: facing this nasty, low-down time head-on. No skirting the chasms of melancholy. No burying the doubts under a shiny, happy face. In the end, these women came out confronting a new, reality-based happiness.

But first came pain.

What kinds of breakups are we talking here? Consider Jill Bernstein, a public relations executive in New York, who was completely blindsided last spring. She went away for the weekend to celebrate her sister's 40th birthday and came home to an apartment with all the lights on and fresh flowers in a vase. Oh, and a note in the foyer announcing that after 11 years together (during which he referred to her as his wife and gave her a "ring of life"), her boyfriend, David, had moved out. His closets were bare, but every gift she'd ever given him was left behind: The Limoges decorative boxes had been lined up on a living room shelf and the polo shirts she'd brought him from a department store in her hometown of New Orleans were stacked neatly in a closet. He had paid the next month's rent and garage fee, removed his belongings from their joint storage space, and moved her things into a smaller unit, all of which he outlined in the note.

"It was like walking in on a suicide," she says, and she swears, even after months of scrutiny and super slo-mo replay, that she never saw it coming.

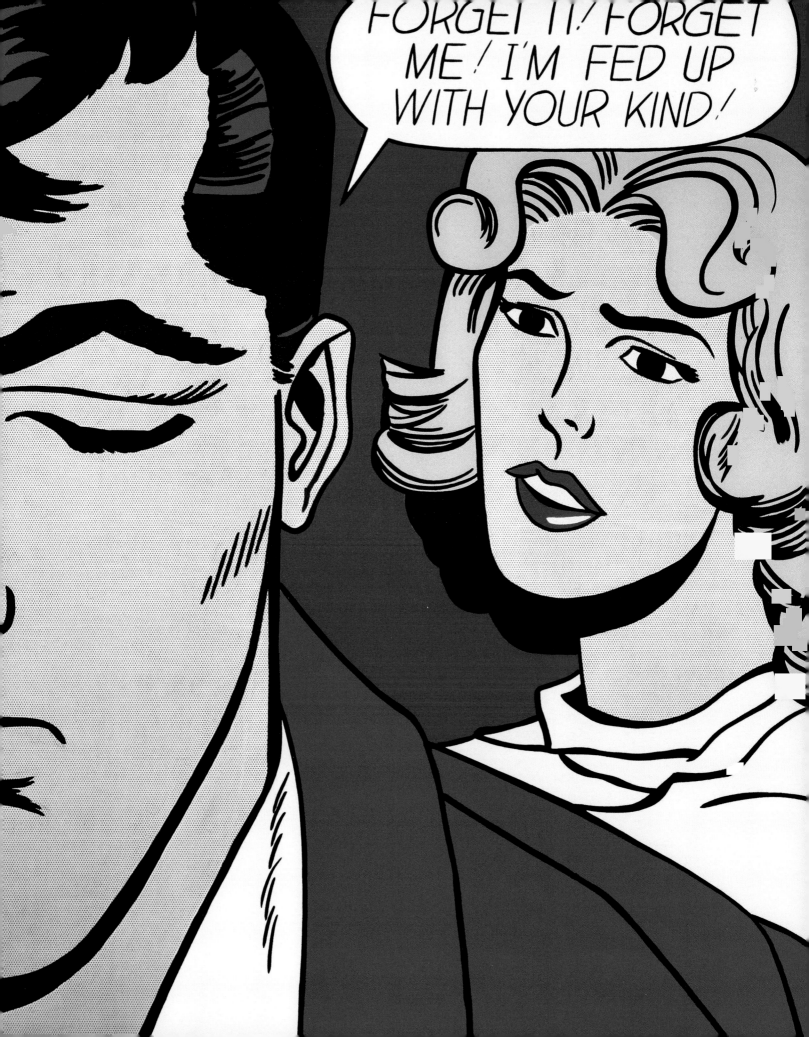

In the wake of a lover's departure, the wreckage looks like this: There's no one else to make coffee, get the paper, or warm up the bed. Couple friends don't call as often, or if they do, the newly single are less inclined to accept invitations where they'll be the odd woman out. Weekends stretch out as vast, uncharted oceans of solitude. And even when the woman was the one to call it off, sadness bounces off the walls like whispers in an echo chamber.

Grief can be stunning—literally—and yet you still have to go on business trips, unload the dishwasher, and face people. Within a month after Jill Bernstein's boyfriend left, she found a new apartment, removed him from her insurance policies

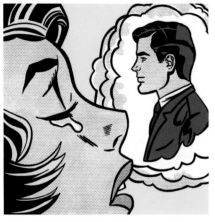

and will, and contacted a lawyer to help settle the last few details of the separation. She leaned on family members and a few close friends, and upped her therapy appointments to twice a week. Beyond that, she simply tried to put one foot in front of the other. "I never missed a day of work, and I never missed a facial appointment," Jill says, "but there were plenty of times in between where I was just digging in and holding on."

She didn't tell people at work, and she limited her number of confidantes to those she could trust. "I kept the circle small," Jill says. "It wasn't out of humiliation, it was to avoid sensory overload—I couldn't be bombarded with messages of consolation and compassion from hundreds of people. I needed a core group."

In the month following David's departure, Jill hated being alone. Her mother came up and spent a week, her sister and brother each came into town for a weekend, and local friends would stay overnight.

Calling on one's support system is essential not only for survival through the rough times but for keeping the loss in perspective. "By getting therapy, joining a religious community, creating a new network of friends, and finding safety in ongoing relationships, women realize that their whole emotional life is not just about that one person," says Abigail Trafford, health columnist for *The Washington Post* and author of *Crazy Time: Surviving Divorce and Building a New Life.* The emotional threads that still connect you to the world, primarily through friends and family, turn out to possess amazing tensile strength, she says. They also serve as a reminder that your capacity for loving relationships is much broader than one person. "You're in for some wonderful surprises," Trafford says. "You see how much people care for you."

On what would have been Jill and David's anniversary, one friend insisted

IN THE WAKE OF A LOVER'S DEPARTURE,
There's no one else to make coffee, get the paper, or

that she and Jill go out to a posh restaurant. When Jill arrived, she found a beautifully wrapped candle on her plate. The small gesture, so thoughtful and loving, overwhelmed her, and she burst into tears. "I felt important when I had been made to feel vaporized," she says.

AH, THE VAPORIZATION FACTOR. Of course we should all stand on our own two feet, identity-wise, but some feelings of emotional amputation are inescapable, as is the accompanying desire to cauterize the wounds by any available means. Succor comes in many forms: Drinking, overeating, and shopping are classics. Some women flit from one relationship to another, sucking out the romantic nectar and flying away when disappointment arises—what Trafford calls the hummingbird phase.

Franny Gottschal (a pseudonym) felt as though her husband had stopped seeing her years before they started couples counseling. One day Franny told their therapist about a dream she'd had the night before, an explicit scenario of her husband walking into a room, meeting a stranger, and having sex.

When Franny finished, her husband said, "I'm really freaked out." He admitted that something like that had happened just the day before. Franny took a deep breath.

"I said, 'I don't care that you had sex with someone else,'" Franny remembers. "'I care about being able to look our children in the eye and say we did everything we could to save our marriage. But you have to stop seeing her while we try.'"

Her husband returned to therapy a week later and said he wouldn't stop.

"I said, 'Fine, then you have to move out.' He did—and moved in with her. We'd been together 13 years." Six months after he left, she started dating with a vengeance. "I had nothing to lose. I wasn't looking for a relationship. I wanted to see what having fun would be like. Plus I was catching up on all the sex we didn't have in the marriage." She had a variety of interludes: long distance, rekindled past relationships, younger men, younger women, the trainer from her gym, the science teacher at her kids' school.

After another six months, life started to even out. The divorce was finalized, and when she took her kids on a vacation by herself for the first time, they all had a blast. Romance was still important to Franny, but increasingly so was reconstructing a family life.

She allowed a friend to write a personal ad on her behalf, and the man who responded was also a divorced parent, also someone still sorting out life as a single person. They've been dating for more than nine months. "We each put our children first, which puts us on an equal footing. There are things about him that I'm not crazy about, but I don't live under the illusion that there's one perfect person for you. He's not as funny as I am. He can be brash. I like late-night chats; he doesn't. He can withdraw while we're in social groups—I don't know what that's about. But right now, I don't feel a need to figure it out. I trust him. We have fun. And we have great sex."

Jill Bernstein realized early on that

there was a lot she did need to figure out. "I don't want this man and this situation to affect the rest of my life," she says. So far—and the process is still under way—she's identified a serious disconnect in her life. "I work hard, I love what I do, I ask questions, I'm a very confident professional—but I'm discovering that confidence has not always existed in my romantic life." She's grappling with tough questions: "What is it about me that put me in this position? What was I getting out of this relationship that did not allow me to see where the hairline fractures and broken bones were? That's the work I'm doing now."

The line between introspection and beating yourself over the head is, most of us know, filament thin, especially where love is concerned. In our culture, says Maxine Schnall, author of *What Doesn't Kill You Makes You Stronger: Turning Bad Breaks*

was talk about problems, and over time the tension filled their lives like white noise. It wasn't screaming fighting, she says; it was bad-vibe fighting. "So much was unspoken; you couldn't have a frank and honest conversation. We were both out of touch with how we really felt.

"If somebody had looked in from the outside, they would have said, 'Oh, man. Sharon, get out.' From inside, though, trying to figure out how I felt was like trying to get out of a deep, deep swamp. But I grew up thinking you just stayed together forever."

Eventually, she and Peter moved into separate apartments ten blocks from each other but tried to keep their relationship going. One night over dinner, he said to her, "How do I know you're the one?"

"Steam came out of my ears," Sharon says. "If he thought I wasn't the one, we should have broken up before seven years

New York designer Stacey Greenwald and her producer boyfriend, Hank, decided to marry. "If there was anyone on the planet I thought I could live with," she remembers, "it was him. I didn't believe I'd ever find a soul mate before him. I come from a family of achievers, I'm kooky and artistic, and he matched me in those ways."

Only after they got engaged did they begin to discuss what their marriage would be like. "Then things fell apart," she says. "Hank wanted to pursue his career at any cost. He wanted to move to Mexico and Brazil and expected me to live with him and have children in these transient settings. And I wondered, *What would I do? Would there be work for me?* He assumed I would follow him everywhere and in everything. Automatically."

They broke up four months after announcing their engagement. Suddenly,

THE WRECKAGE LOOKS LIKE THIS:
warm up the bed. Weekends stretch out as vast, uncharted oceans of solitude.

into Blessings, the tendency for self-blame falls along gender lines. "Women are relationship oriented. The guy will walk away and say, 'She was a bitch,' and the woman will say, 'What did I do wrong?' But blaming yourself is not going to help."

After Sharon Butler, a Connecticut-based artist and college professor, broke up with Peter, a freelance writer and film student, she felt the typical woman's remorse: If only she'd gotten along better with his mother. If only she'd been more domestically inclined. If only she'd had the same sense of family, the same social graces, the same love of the Boston Red Sox. But eventually she started asking the kinds of questions that would put her seven-year relationship to rest and help her move on.

They'd met in Boston after college. Peter was cute and funny and did a great impersonation of U2 singer Bono. They skied in Park City, Utah; weekended at the beaches near her Connecticut hometown; and after a year of dating, moved in together in Boston, where Peter was raised. Sharon loved exploring the city with him and through his politically and socially connected family. What the couple didn't do

passed. It was so incomprehensible. What was so hard for him? Did he have a checklist of pros and cons? You'd think when he said 'I love you,' it meant 'You're the one.'"

She walked out. After a few failed attempts at reconciliation, she moved back to Connecticut, and for the next few months, she painted, took long bike rides, and thought. And thought. In dissecting the past, she realized she didn't know Peter any better after seven years than after their first week together. They'd never talked about a future. They were both emotionally reserved, and though they had seemed compatible in the beginning, the more she committed herself to art, the more their paths diverged.

"Ultimately, I thought, *Would I have wanted to do anything differently to make things work?*" she says. "But that would have meant me making all the sacrifices and compromises, and frankly, I'm just not that kind of person." There was nothing wrong with either of them as individuals, she decided; the problem was with them together. As Abigail Trafford says, "No one person is completely in control—sometimes it's just life."

Stacey was without a future. She remembers allowing herself to be catatonic for a couple of weeks. One morning she sat by her kitchen window with a cup of coffee. "A bee flew into the coffee and stung me on my tongue," she says. It was like a physical manifestation of the breakup. "I almost passed out from the pain. But it was a wake-up call. I was so happy to feel that much pain. I swear it got him out of my system. I started to understand where I hadn't taken care of myself and had left it up to him. I had no skills in terms of making myself happy—I had no vision other than being under the wing of a guy with a big personality."

Once she started feeling again, she also started acting, determined to answer her own question: "What the hell am I going to do for happiness?" Over the next two years, she started working out, bought an apartment, got a new circle of friends, quit smoking, and got a better job. As she rebuilt her life to suit her tastes, Stacey came to see that she and her ex-fiancé weren't a good fit. "Despite the love, you've got to be able to coexist. He was wild and fun, and we liked the same things. He just wasn't ready for marriage. He was thinking for one person and not for two. But he was the one who came along at the time when I was ready to get married."

Inadvertently, Hank had given Stacey essential survival tools for life after him: a gym membership, a dog, and, after their breakup, critical advice on the apartment she ended up buying. More important, she was left to discover her own ambitions. "Some people might have taken it like any other breakup and moved on, but I saw in all that pain an opportunity to grow. It was a very, very intense time. The progress was emotional. The pain was bad. Yet I could still see everything was loaded with symbolism and depth and poetry."

These days Stacey is the poster child for dating at 40. "I'm really loving it," she says. "It takes a confident man to like someone my age: He has to be able to take a woman who's seasoned and has a personality. He has to like you for who you are—he's not going to get a big family or arm candy, that kind of stuff. And I'm in the perfect position to be dating and choosing the right people because I'm so much myself and so confident in who I am. So it's a very sweet time in my life. That's an unexpected gift."

When she thinks of Hank, she says, "I loved him, he did great things for me, but the aftermath of the breakup was as important—if not more—to my life than the relationship itself had been."

Embedded in the soul-searcher's aftermath is a shockingly wonderful moment: The fury, sorrow, and picture-shredding ire recede, supplanted by fond memories and sincere admiration. Seeing your ex as a villain is easy, but savoring his good qualities is essential to maintaining a balanced view of what happened, says Maxine Schnall. Witness Claudia Raab, a sustainable agriculture activist in Philadelphia.

After 17 years of marriage, Claudia's husband went on a separate vacation one summer while their teenage daughter was at camp. When he got back, he moped for days, napping frequently and hardly speaking. Claudia thought it was jet lag.

"Finally, I asked what the matter was," she remembers. "He said, 'I want a divorce.'"

Claudia was horrified. She went into physical shock: She was boiling hot, then freezing cold. They went to a counselor, but her husband's determination never flagged. "Looking back," Claudia says, "I can see that I was very depressed throughout my marriage. I was in love with my depression and not with my husband. I really respect him for confronting that, even though I felt I was probably going to die of pain and suffering at the time."

Since the divorce, Claudia has come to love and admire her husband more. "It took me about three years to get past it," she says. "I went into therapy, and I lost 20 pounds. I just submerged myself in my grief; it took a lot of self-examination, therapy, and willingness to admit that he was right. And that is not like me. That's what's changed. I liked having all the control at all times, and finally I was willing to realize he was right."

Claudia is still her ex's champion in the parenting department. "I realized I chose him for what a good father he would be—not necessarily because we would make a great husband and wife." Her intuition about him was right. "He's the best, the ultimate, a splendid father. I knew he would be. He fathered our daughter in a way I wish every woman could be fathered. And it's made for a pretty secure kid."

Claudia herself feels more secure, realizing that she can get through a life turned upside down. "The divorce was so cataclysmic," Claudia says, "but now I feel I could weather anything. I know I could."

With hard work and some luck, that's what women find as they muddle through the trauma, columnist Trafford says. They discover their own resilience. They've survived without closing themselves off to the world, which is a notable achievement. And they've learned a valuable truth, which is that mistakes are inevitable. "Relationships are the biggest trial and error part of life," says Schnall. "You learn by doing, and the mistakes go into the totality of who you are."

Sharon Butler has come to feel compassion for both herself and her ex, to see their relationship as part of how they each became adults. "We grew up together," she says. Four years after Peter and Sharon separated, she married a man whose personality better complements her own. They recently celebrated their tenth anniversary; their daughter is in preschool. "My husband, Dan, has a lot of the same qualities as Peter in terms of sociability and love of current events," Sharon says. "But Dan relishes confrontation; he doesn't mind saying what's on his mind. Sometimes that's hard for me, but it also makes me more willing to open up."

Claudia dates occasionally but is holding out for someone whose personality is as forceful as her own. "In my next relationship," she says, "I'll have to give a whole lot more. I'll have to be a lot more emotionally available and allow as much intimacy as there could possibly be. The act of self-discovery and all the possibilities are tantalizing. I'm curious about my potential to love."

One well-meaning friend of Jill Bernstein's has suggested she try a dating service, but Jill is otherwise engaged. "I can only be the great, self-actualized person I want to be once I've gone through this process," she says. "I have to try to understand more where the flaws were in the relationship and in my part of it. I will never have the answers from David. So I'm only left with me."

She's come far enough along, though, to realize that she won't wither and die if she's never part of a couple again. "What's important," she says, "is leading a full life. I've always wanted to go to Antarctica—and I'm finally going this month."

FIVE DIFFERENT HEARTBREAKS, FIVE healthier women. In other words, anyone with a shattered heart can win the prize—a happier life, a better relationship next time around—but only by making use of the mess right there in front of you. You have to think about it. Feel it. Mourn it. Miss him, resent him, and wish you could tell him the funny thing you saw that only he would understand because it reminds you of that market stall in Oaxaca from your honeymoon. And if you do all that, really breathe the sorrow, and let the sadness frame each beat of your heart, you'll not only be able to let it go, you'll find yourself arriving at a new place, in which you know more clearly what you want and need and what you have to offer.

So here are the real rules: Don't run with scissors, don't leave the iron on, don't cross against the light, and don't be afraid of a broken heart. •

Marriage

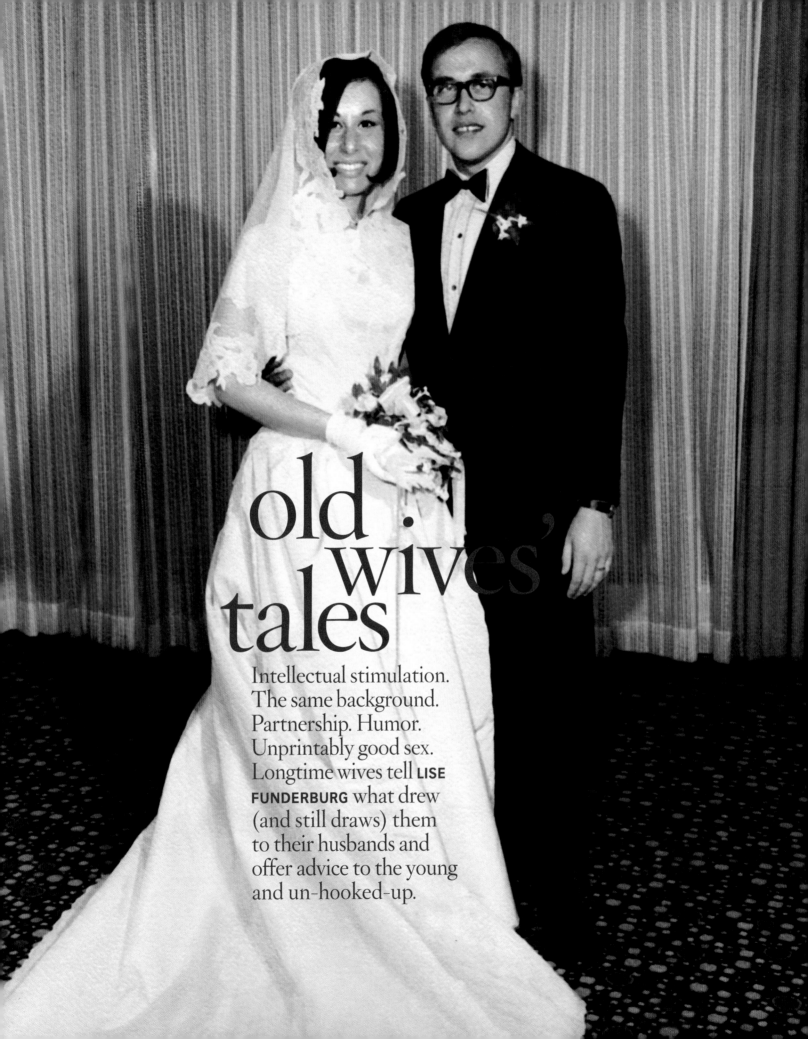

old wives' tales

Intellectual stimulation. The same background. Partnership. Humor. Unprintably good sex. Longtime wives tell **LISE FUNDERBURG** what drew (and still draws) them to their husbands and offer advice to the young and un-hooked-up.

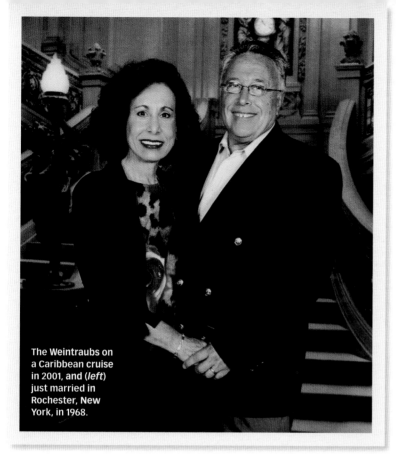

The Weintraubs on a Caribbean cruise in 2001, and (*left*) just married in Rochester, New York, in 1968.

Janice and Stanley Weintraub

Ages: both 62
Years married: 35
Occupations: part-time dental hygienist; realtor

How did you know he was the one? I believed in him. He didn't have a job, he wasn't a college grad and I was, but I saw his potential. I saw that he was loving, caring, and very interested in me. He had all the traits to be a good husband and father. He was a good salesman—he sold me!

What's made it last? Having a sense of humor. He taught me that, too, though I am still not a hundred percent there yet.

Advice? Choose your battles and understand that as you change, your mate also changes. You have to involve yourself in different activities and hobbies so you don't become boring, and you have to realize that you don't marry one person—you marry the entire family.

Yvonne and Harold Haskins

Ages: "We're both still working, so let's just say 'mature.'"
Years married: 33
Occupations: attorney, underwriter for Fannie Mae; senior administrator at the University of Pennsylvania

How did you know he was the one? It was a gradual process. I respected him for the work he was doing in the community before I fell in love with him. I was a police officer and he was a youth worker. I got to know his soul and his values and his thought process and how he viewed the world before I ever dated him. Then one summer, I was in the hospital and he brought me the biggest milk shake I'd ever had.

What's made it last? We're still stimulated by each other intellectually, and I still think he's the sexiest man in the world. He's as witty as the devil, and I appreciate that. We've always been partners, and we were always looking at the world and helping in our small way. He has a thousand kids around the world that he's worked with—he's gotten more black kids through the University of Pennsylvania than I can count. You hear the pride when I talk about him. At the same time, I hear from other people that he's proud of me.

Advice? I wish someone had told me in my young life that I didn't have to carry all the weight in the relationship. That was what happened in my failed first marriage. I was a "nobody can do it better than I can" person, but half the time I was wishing someone else would take it away.

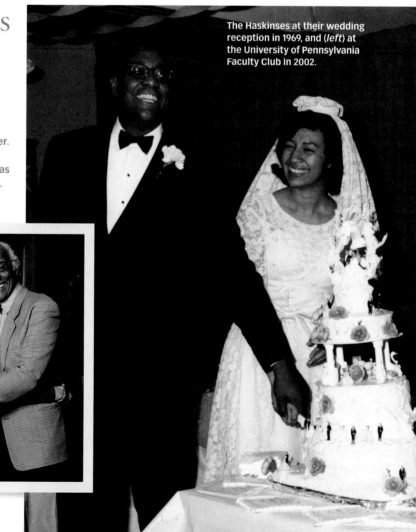

The Haskinses at their wedding reception in 1969, and (*left*) at the University of Pennsylvania Faculty Club in 2002.

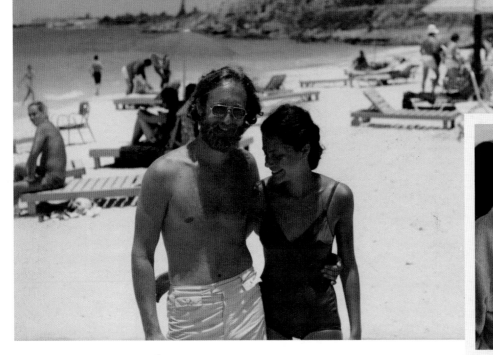

Liz Bien and Alan Gewirtz

Ages: 52 and 53
Years married: 25
Occupations: university administrator; professor of medicine

How did you know he was the one? We went to school together; he was one of my closest friends.

What's made it last? I always say that it's because he's slightly deaf and legally blind. That we're very different is helpful—when he's down in the dumps I'm up, and when I'm down he's usually optimistic. You also have to admire the person you marry. He has to be smart and funny. Alan makes me laugh.

Advice? Pick your battles. But it helps to fight, because it's good to get it out in the open rather than let it simmer. I don't believe in being passive-aggressive.

Aracely and Carlos Rosales

Ages: 45 and 49
Years married: 24
Occupations: health communications consultant; owner of a translation service

How did you know he was the one? We met young—when I was 15 and he was 18. I always thought he was special, more considerate than most men. He was very respectful to his family and to mine. And if I needed something, he would look for it. He was patient and he always made me laugh.

What's made it last? We come from the same background, so we have a lot of things in common, and because we met so young, we grew up together. We moved from Guatemala to the United States, faced the same issues—learning another language and culture, leaving everything we had, including our families. In order to survive, we had to support each other. From the beginning, we knew that we were going to get married and it was going to be forever. We were never thinking, *Let's try it and see how it works.*

Advice? Being in love definitely helps. Nurture the love any way you can. Work around the person's strengths and weaknesses. Did anybody else say anything about sex? Make it good. To do that you have to challenge yourself. Grow with it. When we go to weddings for young couples these days and they ask us to sign their book, we now write: "Solve any problem with sex."

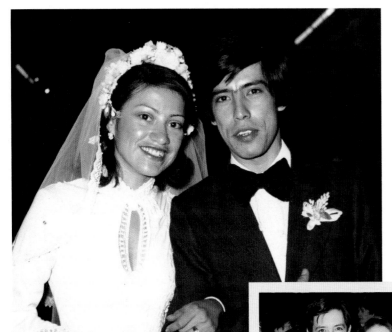

Above: The Rosaleses on their wedding day in Guatemala City in July 1978, and (*right*) at a Chinese New Year celebration in 2000.

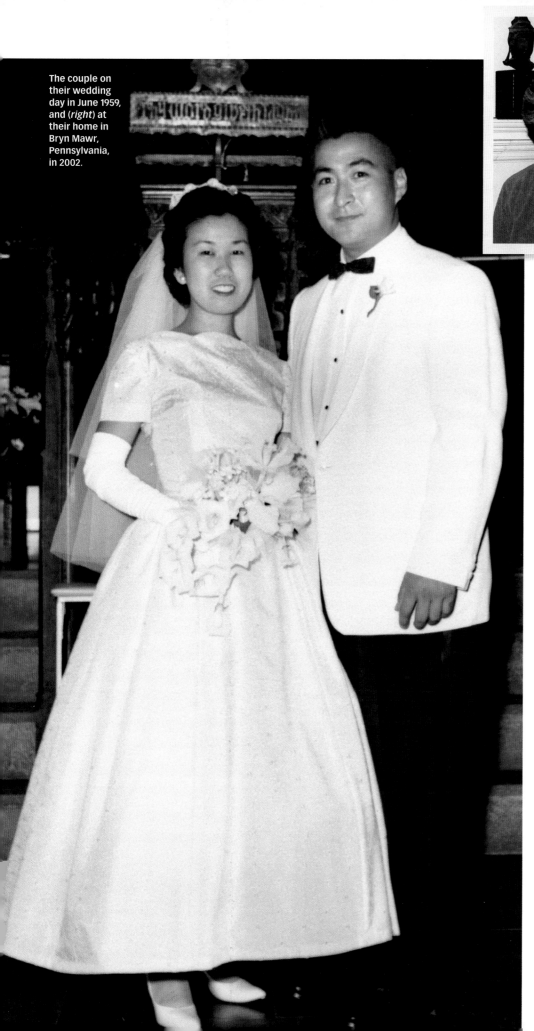

The couple on their wedding day in June 1959, and (*right*) at their home in Bryn Mawr, Pennsylvania, in 2002.

Miiko and Herbert Horikawa

Ages: 67 and 70
Years married: 43
Occupations: retired school librarian; psychologist

How did you know he was the one? I had a list of qualities in my mind. I wanted an Asian man. I wanted someone with a college education, a sense of humor, a strong character, and who was decisive and caring. I never thought I was going to find this man, but Herb qualified in all of those categories, *and* he was big, five feet nine inches tall. All my Japanese-American girlfriends were five feet or less. I was five feet two and felt like a horse. I wanted someone I didn't tower over.

What's made it last? In the first part of our marriage, we were like-minded in our focus on the family. Herb used to help me with the household chores so I wasn't stuck with the children all the time. He helped with the laundry; we shopped together because I didn't drive. And we'd have to take the kids because we were too poor to have a babysitter. We were together a lot and that really made the marriage work.

Advice? Supporting each other is really important. It's so easy to be disrespectful. I would sometimes be critical or snide, and he would call me on it. Now I know him well enough not to say things in ways that are going to hurt him. If it's important to me, I say it nicely.

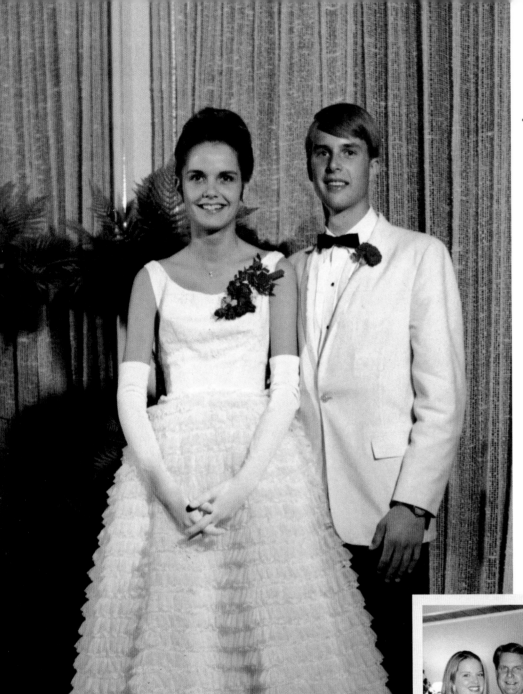

Georgia and Jerry Carter

Ages: both 51
Years married: 30
Occupations: wedding coordinator; advertising executive

How did you know he was the one?
That tingle. We were sophomores in high school, and I used to watch him come out of the boys' bathroom and go to the water fountain every day at lunch. I used to stare at him. We officially met at a formal school Easter dance, and we were inseparable from that night on. That was 1967.

What's made it last? You always have to have something to look forward to, and we're always on the go. Jerry walked in last night and said, "Want to go to Reno?"

Advice? Always be open. Don't be afraid to say what's on your mind. I used to keep it all inside, and then I'd get mad. I just didn't want to talk or tell him how I felt. I can remember my daughter saying, "Why are you keeping it in? That's so stupid!" That was about ten years ago. I don't do that anymore. Even if it hurts, say it.

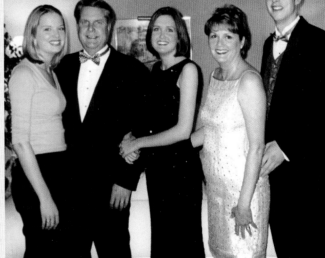

Left: The Carters at their 1968 junior prom in Phoenix, and (*above*) with their children, Jill, Elizabeth, and Ryan, in 2001.

Dee Ito and Marshall Arisman

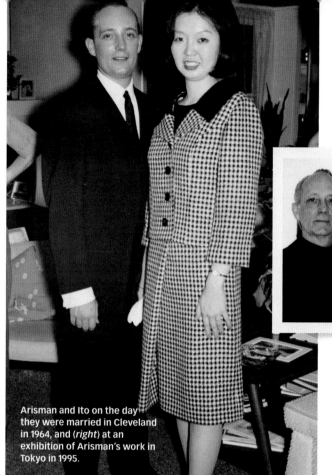

Ages: 65 and 64
Years married: 38
Occupations: writer; painter, illustrator, and teacher

Arisman and Ito on the day they were married in Cleveland in 1964, and (*right*) at an exhibition of Arisman's work in Tokyo in 1995.

How did you know he was the one?
We met when I was working on a children's book. I liked his illustrations, and he was really funny. I found out he liked his parents a lot, which was important because I liked my family. He was very direct. He was very good-looking, and that always helps. When we got married, there were very few racially mixed couples—I'm Japanese-American and he's Swedish-American—and when we walked down the street, people would look at us. But in a funny way we were oblivious, because we saw ourselves as so much the same: We both came from middle-class families and have one sibling; we both grew up in small towns.

What's made it last? The fact that we allow each other the space to do what we want to do is a major part of it.

Advice? Early on you want this person to know everything about you. You wait for him to recognize that you're in pain. It doesn't take long to figure out that people are *not* going to figure it out every time, no matter how sensitive they are. You have to ask for the attention you need. Also, you learn not to take everything as criticism; it's information. That means believing the other person loves you. That's no small thing.

Beth and Martin Johnson

Ages: 43 and 42
Years married: 20
Occupations: independent school admissions director; counselor for disabled adults

How did you know he was the one? We were working at Roy Rogers the year after high school. I saw him and got goose bumps. But it was more about who he was on the inside. He's a deep thinker. He's slow to anger. He wanted to be part of my life. He's got the greatest smile and the cutest butt; calf muscles to die for. He came down the steps recently, had on jeans and an undershirt with no sleeves, and leaned on the banister, and I was like, "Ahhhh. Take me, I'm yours." He still does it for me.

What's made it last? The truth? The sex is phenomenal. We can't keep our hands off each other. Our children tell us, "Get a room." The older you get, the better it gets. You know more. Your bodies change and you get a bigger bed. And you make sure it doesn't squeak. We're both more patient. There are things I've done I'm not willing to have in print.

Advice? Keep everybody else out of your business. That's huge. If you need counseling, get an impartial person—not someone on his side of the family or one of your girlfriends. When the deal goes down at night, it's just the two of you. ●

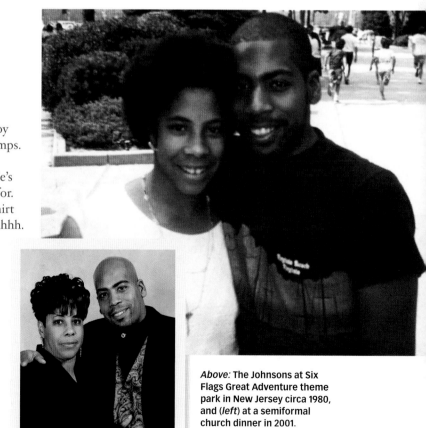

Above: The Johnsons at Six Flags Great Adventure theme park in New Jersey circa 1980, and (*left*) at a semiformal church dinner in 2001.

Marriage 163

Love Actually

Partnership isn't about his and hers, yours and mine, IOU and you-owe-me. It's a subtler form of math that adds up to magic.
By Amy Bloom

Photography by
Karen Hirshan

I LOVE WEDDINGS; I ALWAYS HAVE. I like old brides, for their guts, their seasoned optimism, and their fashion sense—a pale pink or navy silk suit is so much more flattering on most of us than Cinderella's clouds of white tulle. I like the young shiny brides who don't know anything about anything, except how much in love they are. I like Great-Aunt Frieda doing the mambo with the groom's recently rehabbed second cousin. I like the depths of gooey sentimentality that otherwise normal accountants, architects, and football players reveal when toasting their baby brothers. I like shockingly expensive bouquets, with exotic flowers flown in from tiny countries, and I like—maybe just a little bit more—a big handful of black-eyed Susans stuck into an old blue pitcher.

I like Steve and Bruce, abandoning their jeans for matching tuxedos, adjusting each other's bow ties before tying the big knot in the sanctuary of St. Luke's, and I like the rough, tough, crew-cut guy in his army uniform and gleaming shoes, blinking back tears as he marries his college sweetheart on her parents' lawn.

I like everything about weddings.

And they bear the same relationship to marriage as Fisher-Price ads do to childhood, as a bathtub does to the Atlantic. It takes something to get married: nerve, hope, a strong desire to make a certain statement—and it takes something to stay married: more hope, determination, a sense of humor, and needs that are best met by being in a pair. And beyond the idea of marriage, which some of us cannot do

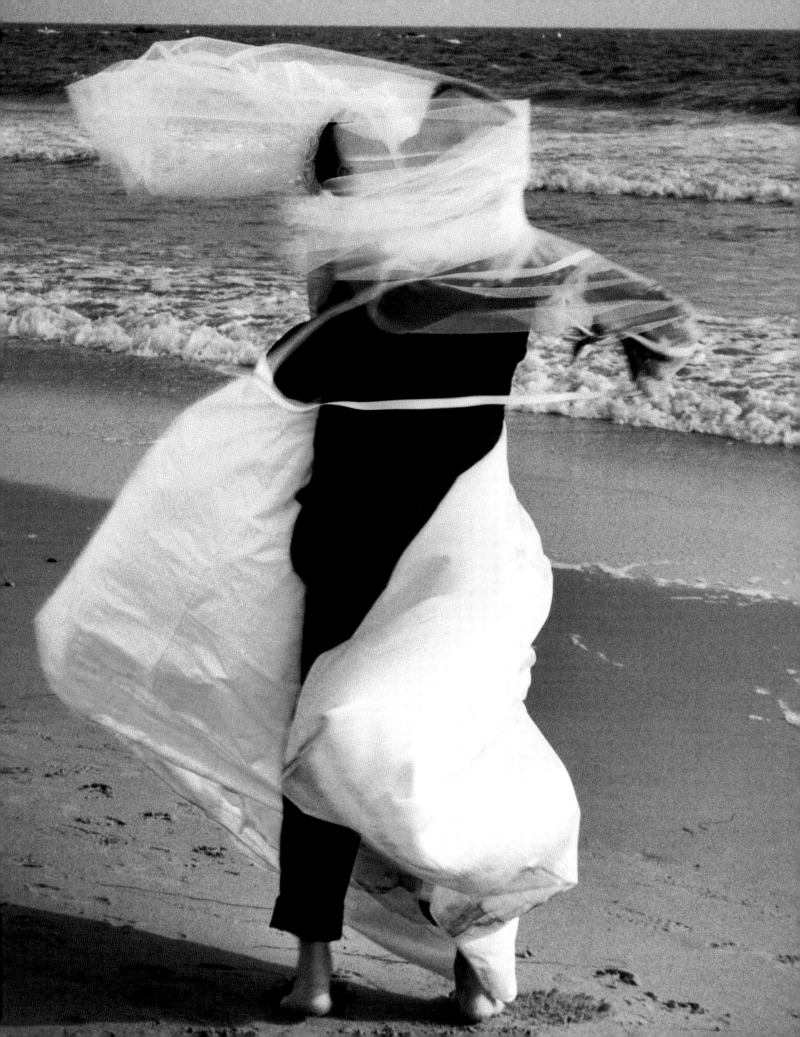

and lots of us would rather not, is the question of partnership. In the old days, for middle-class people, partnership meant He went off to work and did Outside Things, and She stayed home and raised children and other Indoor Things. In the even older days, it was Hunting and Gathering on one hand and Nursing and Cooking on the other, but at any point in history up until the very recent past, the meaning of the marital partnership was: The world is divided into two spheres, and I will take one and you will take the other. (I know, I know—a lot of ladies who would have been happy driving trucks or running countries had to darn socks, make dinner for six, and run errands, and the number of gentlemen who gave up Jobs and Outside Things in order to accommodate the lady of their choice was notoriously small.) But even in the somewhat skewed nature of those traditional partnerships, there was clarity. Like white-glove etiquette and pinching corsets and dress codes, the world is on the whole a better, fairer, more humane place without them...and yet.

And yet, in their absence, there is an awful lot of uncertainty and not a little unattractive behavior. The quid pro quo and you-owe-me of modern marriage, the lists that people make under the encouraging eye of the worst kind of couples therapists are not partnership.

It may be that three I-picked-up-your-towels equal one I-took-the-car-for-an-oil-change, and that everyone dutifully does their timed 45 minutes of housework, but that's not a partnership. Keeping track of every slight and misstep ("And in 1984, you told my mother you didn't like the tablecloth she made us!"), including the blockbusters ("Thanks for the nice earrings. They look like the ones you gave that slut I caught you with when we were engaged. What do you mean? I *have* let it go"), may help someone feel in control of life, but it won't enhance the life or the partnership. Putting all of your needs a mile behind the other person's is not what I have in mind, either. You can't have a partnership when

one person is an emotional dray horse and the other person makes a meaningful contribution or sacrifice once every 20 years; that may be a very strong relationship (and we've all seen them: two people both in love with one of them), but it's not a partnership. And suffering isn't what I have in mind, either, although some of that may be necessary. (You might have to go to hockey when you prefer the Mets; you might have to go to Holly Near when you'd prefer Blossom Dearie; and you will certainly have to

> The point is to make the other person as happy as we can, because their happiness adds to ours.

spend some time, at some special occasion, with some people you don't like, unless your spouse is such a friendless, sibling-less, childless orphan that you never see anyone but your side, which is also a problem.) To be a real partner requires the best of friendship, parenting, and lover, in such a combination and quantity that we can hardly bear to expect it of Him or Her for fear of being disappointed, and we certainly hope that no one will expect it of us.

I THINK WE SHOULD EXPECT MORE and give more, in the little ways as well as the big ones. Little things shape a life: He buys the jewelry he knows she likes, not the stuff he'd like her to wear; she wears the

nightgown he's crazy about and not her favorite T-shirt. I think of my sister, reading companionably on the couch while her husband, in the great tradition of husbands, channel surfs interminably. It used to make her crazy and crabby—and the remote-control mania will never make sense to her—but instead of berating him, she realized that not only does he like it better when she's near him, because he loves her, but she likes it better, too.

I think of an older couple who lived in the country in a house they had both labored on—mostly her, as is sometimes the case—until one day she announced that she wanted to spend her last years in her favorite city. He began to say that he hated that city and he hated change and he was damned if he was going to pack up his books one more time and at his age—and then he thought, *She makes me so happy and made us such a happy home, let me give this to her.* And now they live in that big city and take long morning walks along her favorite river, and it's become his as well. I think of two dear men, who have managed to put their very serious careers, as writer and doctor, always slightly behind their relationship. He wrote hard and the doctor worked hard, paying the bills for both of them. The writer hit it big and, with his loving encouragement, the doctor began to think that he might like to work hard, but in a studio, not an office.

They have balanced their needs and wants and given just a little more weight to the other's happiness, and that's what I'm talking about. It's doing your share, and then some.

In a true partnership, the kind worth striving for, the kind worth insisting on, and even, frankly, worth divorcing over, both people try to give as much or even a little more than they get. "Deserves" is not the point. "Fair" is not the point. And "owes" is certainly not the point. The point is to make the other person as happy as we can, because their happiness adds to ours. The point is—in the right hands, everything that you give, you get. ●

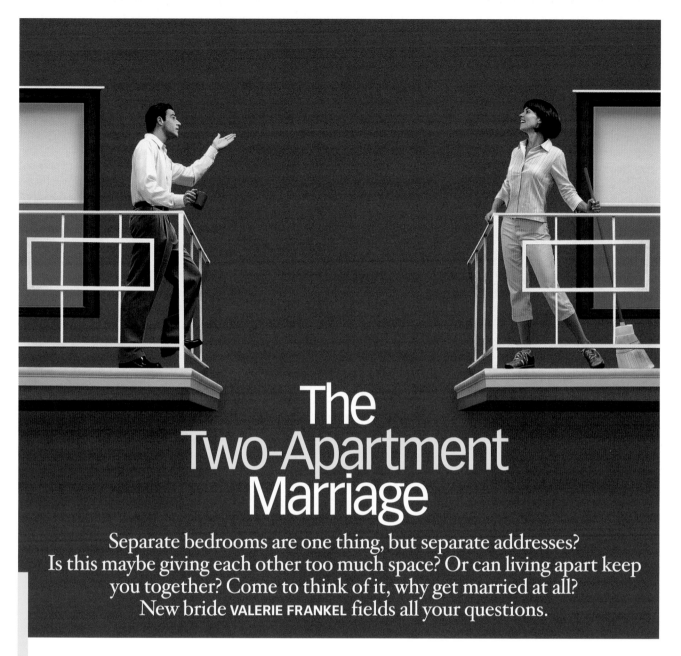

The Two-Apartment Marriage

Separate bedrooms are one thing, but separate addresses?
Is this maybe giving each other too much space? Or can living apart keep
you together? Come to think of it, why get married at all?
New bride **VALERIE FRANKEL** fields all your questions.

I GOT MARRIED! IT WAS A SMALL ceremony at my parents' farm in Vermont. Just family. My daughters were both flower girls and bridesmaidens. My groom played a love song for me on the French horn. We went to Maine for a brief honeymoon, then drove back to New York with the kids, where my new husband and I unpacked our suitcases. In our separate apartments.

When I tell people about the wedding, that last fragment—the "in our separate apartments" part—is when the jaws drop. I proceed to stammer something along the lines of "Steve will stay at my place in Brooklyn most of the time. But he needs privacy a couple of nights a week. He has lived alone for decades. The kids are exhausting. Unconventional marriages aren't

just for homosexuals anymore." Canned laughter (often only mine). And then, the reaction. I get either the diplomatic "Whatever works for you," the encouraging "Wish my husband would disappear two nights a week," or the judgmental "Why bother getting married at all?"

The judgmental reaction usually comes from never-married women, those who cling to the idealized version of postnuptial bliss and have limited experience with the frustration and suffocation of spending too much time with one person. And if I sound defensive, what of it? Maybe I am scrambling for justification. Our two-apartment arrangement doesn't match the fantasy I'd had—after my first husband died and before I'd met Steve—of a second

marriage. And yet this setup is the way it's going to be. For better or for worse.

Worse first. Catherine Cohan, PhD, a psychologist at the Population Research Institute at Pennsylvania State University and the woman who has conducted definitive research on cohabitation and marriage, says: "The overwhelming evidence is that couples who don't live together before marriage are happier and less likely to divorce. For your situation—a couple who doesn't live together *after* marriage—there's not much data to draw on. Studies do show that second marriages are less stable than first ones, and that stepfamilies have higher rates of divorce. Potentially, you're in the least stable situation."

Hardly a ringing endorsement from the

academic. Good thing I'm not marrying her. I'm the first to acknowledge that this arrangement isn't ideal. But I'm spinning the positive as fast as I can. I like having nights to myself to watch bad TV. I don't want his crap cramming my shelves. Sex is more exciting after a break. I'm not 22, entering a first marriage. I'm a grown-up, and I'm going to face this compromise with the requisite maturity. A model for my children's behavior, I'm not going to whine and stamp my feet and be a big baby when I don't get exactly what I want.

"You don't have to sell yourself," says Linda Carter, PhD, a clinical associate professor of psychiatry and director of the Family Studies Program at the NYU Child Study Center. "Separation is healthy. I recommend it, especially to couples who both work at home." Steve and I fit that profile, sort of. I write at home. Steve is an opera singer and musician who practices the horn at home and works some nights. We spend whole days on end loitering in my apartment together. "That can be intense," Carter warns. "If you're together too much, you may become supersensitive and lose perspective. Small misunderstandings become big arguments." In other words, being on top of each other can tear you apart. "What's also at stake is identity," she says. "Steve is going to be your husband, stepfather to your kids, spending the majority of his time at your apartment. He's had his place in Manhattan for, what? You said 20 years? He's attached to it. Most of his stuff is there. Keeping it is a way he can hold on to his identity."

So the recipe for our union calls for separate apartments, identities—and (you know you're curious) finances. Steve will continue to support his life, I'll continue to support mine (and the kids'), and never the twain shall meet. Our lawyers have sorted out the details. It was unsettling to plan for a divorce before we were even married. Carter thinks I'm being overly analytical about a practical matter. "Prenups are a responsible way to deal with the complications of remarriage and to resolve financial issues," she says. "Keep the finances separate, just as they have been."

Two other valuable marital assets, however, will not be contractually withheld.

In fact, if it weren't for my girls—ages 9 and 5—our marriage talk might never have shifted from "someday" to "August." My older daughter, Maggie, announced one morning that our quasi-engagement

Steve was the one who suggested marriage—and the one who imposed the two-apartment condition.

wasn't good enough: "I want to have a dad. A legal dad. We can go to city hall after school on Thursday. That's my free day." She told me to write it down in my planner. You wouldn't think legal status would matter to a kid as young as 9. But it does. I remember reading an article a year or so ago about the emotional relief felt by the children of gay couples when their parents were finally granted the right to marry. "Kids want what other kids have," says Janet Weisberg, PhD, a therapist in private practice in New York City who works with children in blended families. "She wants a dad to show off to her friends. But she also craves security. Having lost one parent, your daughters are vulnerable to losing another. An official marriage will be reassuring."

But how reassuring can it be if their official father doesn't live with us? It makes my heart sick when Lucy, my younger daughter, asks, "When is Steve coming back?" "It's not necessarily the living arrangement that provides a full father experience. It's the relationship," Weisberg says. "He should go to teacher conferences, school functions, birthday parties, and recitals." Steve already does that. Has for nearly three years. He also cleans my apartment, does our laundry, babysits when I go out with friends. He's patient and affec-

tionate, he draws endless princesses, he serves up the Bagel Bites. "This is a 50-year-old man who's never married and has no kids of his own?" Weisberg says. "And he does all that? I'd give him a lot of credit."

Carter raves about Steve's contributions, too. "Are you aware that many situations are not nearly as positive?" she asks. "Imagine a stepfather who is short-tempered and gets angry." I can't imagine entering that marriage, actually. Maybe those stepdads become short-tempered simply because they have no escape hatch. Carter wants to know, "Whose idea was it, the two-apartment arrangement?"

It was all Steve. He was the one to suggest marriage in the first place, just as he imposed the two-apartment condition. I wanted him to move in, help with the mortgage and bills. I also wanted to go to sleep with him every night, wake up with him every morning. I get lonely when work keeps him away (sometimes he goes on tour with his opera company for more than a week at a time). I have terrible insomnia when he's gone. And if I have a bad night, like last night when Lucy woke up crying with a stomachache, I wish he were there to calm me down once I've calmed her down. But he had an audition today, needed a good night's sleep. Like I don't have things to do in the morning?

You can see how this line of thought can get truly ugly, especially at 3 A.M. "Resentment, yes—that'll have to be dealt with," Carter says. She recommends, naturally, talking about it. And also planning as much as possible so the kids and I can anticipate Steve's movements. His absences should be mutually agreed upon. And, for the most part, they are. We do a rundown of the upcoming week every Sunday, see who has what social or professional plans, and figure out where he should be.

Steve agrees to everything. He's exceedingly amiable. And if this marriage is going to work, I'll have to be exceedingly understanding. This might be a challenge. But as I said, I'm a grown-up. And if I've learned nothing more in my 39 years, it's that you do what you have to do for happiness, at any cost. And the price I'm going to pay is two nights a week. Seems like a bargain. •

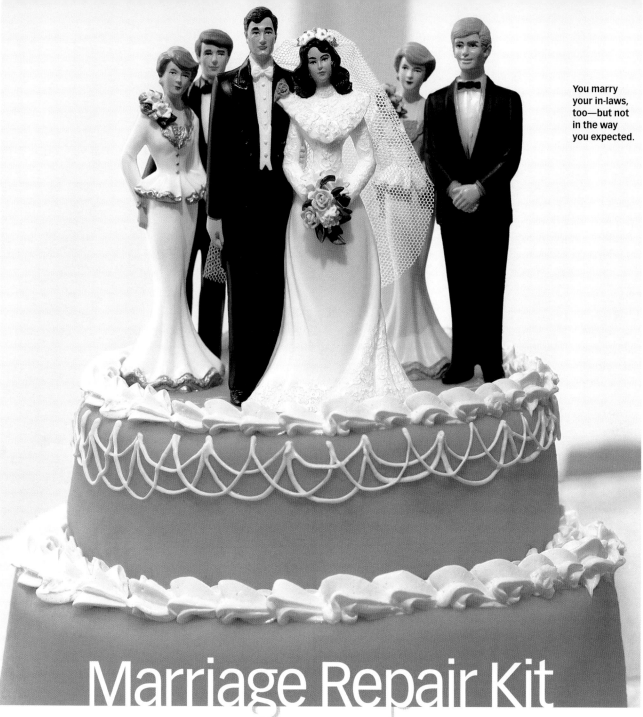

You marry your in-laws, too—but not in the way you expected.

Marriage Repair Kit

Disappointed in your mate? That could be an excellent sign. Couples therapists HARVILLE HENDRIX and HELEN LaKELLY HUNT write about the right kind of trouble.

WHEN WE FALL IN LOVE, WE SEE LIFE IN TECHNICOLOR. WE NIBBLE each other's ears and tell each other everything; our limitations and rigidities melt away. We're sexier, smarter, funnier, more giving. We feel whole; we're connected.

But inevitably, things start to go wrong. The veil of illusion falls away, and it turns out your partner has qualities you can't bear. Even traits you once admired grate on you. Old hurts resurface as you realize your partner cannot or will not love and care for you as promised.

Since he no longer willingly gives you what you need, you try to coerce him into caring through criticism, intimidation, shame, withdrawal, crying, anger—whatever works. The power struggle has begun and may continue for many years, until you split, settle into an uneasy truce, or look for help, desperate to have your dream back.

What's going on here? After reflecting deeply on this question, we've come to this conclusion: You've found what we call an Imago partner, someone who, we regret to say, is uniquely unqualified (at the moment) to give you the love you want. And this is what's *supposed* to happen.

The thesis is relatively simple: Although we think we have free choice in selecting our partners, our primitive brain has a non-negotiable agenda to find someone who resembles one of our childhood caretakers in order to complete unfinished business. No matter what our parents were like or how hard they tried, they weren't perfect. Invariably, they failed to meet some of our essential needs, which left us with an emotional wound.

Growing up, we instinctively developed a pattern of behavior to protect us from being wounded again. But at the same time, we continue to carry around an internal image, a sort of imprint of our caretakers' traits. As babies this imprint helped us distinguish our parents from other adults, much like a young zebra—whose mother circled it repeatedly right after birth—recognizes its mother's distinctive pattern of stripes. When, as adults, we meet someone who fits our emotional imprint, we fall in love. Our imperfect caretakers, freeze-dried in the memories of childhood, are reconstituted in our partner.

The romantic yearning we feel is the anticipation that our new love interest will meet the needs our caretakers failed to satisfy. But a problem arises immediately, because our partner, who also bears childhood hurts, enters the relationship with similar expectations and opposite patterns of self-protection. In the attraction stage, we're drawn to someone whose defense mechanism seems complementary to ours because it's so different. But before long, our differences create a core conflict. To complicate matters, though you'd think

instance, the anger you repressed because it was punished in your home, and which you unconsciously hate yourself for feeling, you "annex" in your partner. But, eventually, seeing your own forbidden emotions in him makes you so uncomfortable that you criticize his quick temper.

All of this seems to be a recipe for disaster, and for a long time it was a depressing state of affairs that puzzled us. How can we resolve childhood issues if our partners wound us in the same ways our caretakers did and we ourselves are stuck in patterns that wound our partners?

When you're unaware of the hidden agenda of romantic love, it *is* a disaster. You inevitably repeat your childhood scenarios with the same devastating consequences. But when you understand that you've chosen your partner to heal certain wounds, and that this healing is the key to the end of longing, you've taken the first step on the journey to real love.

It's crucial to accept the hard truth that incompatibility is the norm for relationships. Conflict is a sign that the psyche is trying to survive, to heal by stretching out of its defenses. It's only when you don't have this knowledge that conflict is destructive. (We believe that couples who claim never to argue are often shying away from intimacy; instead of sharing all of themselves, they may develop parallel lives.)

Romantic love is supposed to end. It's the glue that initially bonds two incompatible people so they can begin to do what needs to be done to heal each other. The good news is that the power struggle is also supposed to end. The emotional bond

become habitual. It means reconnecting through honest conversation and extending ourselves to give our partners what they need to heal. This is not easy, but it works.

Relationships aren't born of love, but of need; real love is born *in* relationships. You are already with your dream partner, but at the moment, he or she may be in disguise—and,

It's crucial to accept the hard truth that incompatibility is the norm.

we'd choose a partner with only our caretakers' positive traits, the negative traits are more indelibly imprinted on us. Unconsciously, we need to be healed by someone with the very deficits that hurt us in the first place. Since we don't understand what's going on, we're shocked when the awful truth about our beloved surfaces.

Our Imago is also likely to have the qualities—both good and bad—that we lost in the shuffle of socialization. For

created by romantic love evolves into a powerful organic bond through the process of resolving conflict.

With self-awareness we can correct what has gone wrong. But a conscious relationship isn't for the fainthearted. It requires reclaiming the lost, repressed parts of ourselves that we were told were dangerous. And it means learning coping mechanisms that are more effective than the crying or anger or withdrawal that has

like you, in pain. (If your partner is abusive, you need to recognize your part in the attraction and learn how to keep yourself emotionally and physically safe. Unless you're conscious of the dynamic, you might think divorce will solve your problems—only to select another partner with similar characteristics.) A conscious, honest relationship can restore your sense of aliveness and wholeness, and set you on the path of real love. ●

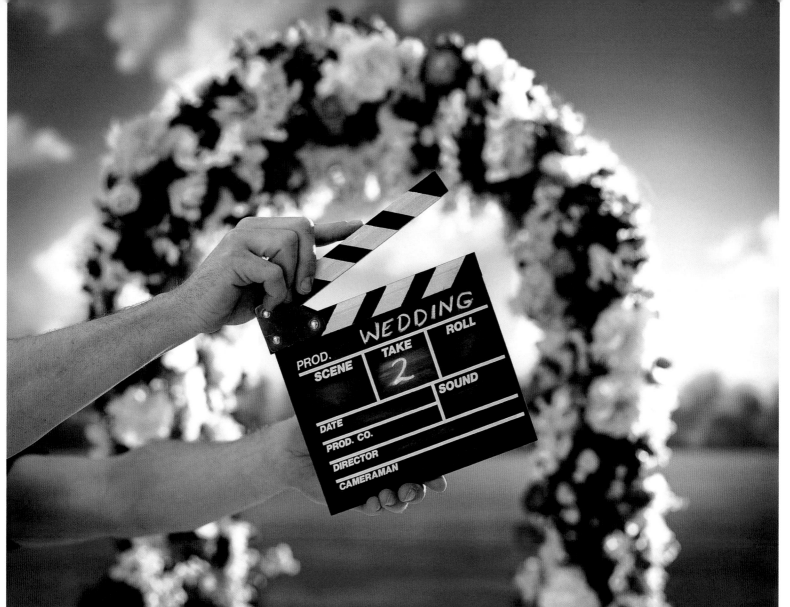

The Bride Wore Pedal Pushers

Older, wiser, and stunned silly by love, **MARION WINIK** and her new groom threw one hell of a party. A report on the wild charms of the second—or even third—wedding.

Vows can be even more passionate the second time around.

MY FIRST WEDDING REALLY WAS the happiest day of my life. Held at my mother's country club in the grand style of my girlish fantasies, it was orchids and lace and a half-dozen kinds of smoked fish. It was young people with moussed-out mid-eighties hairdos dancing to the Bronski Beat as my mother's friends looked on in wonder. It was a Jersey Jewish girl and a Philadelphia Catholic boy married by a mayor.

Thirteen years later, I married again. By then I'd been widowed and was raising two sons alone. In planning my second wedding, few of the frothy rituals that seemed so indispensable the first time made sense to me (and my mother would no longer be footing the bill). But my philosopher groom and I wanted something more romantic and personal than a quiet little trip to the courthouse. Not a gala but a flamboyant event in its own way, one that would involve our closest family and friends in our second attempts at lifelong partnership.

Like anyone who says the wedding vows more than once, we knew a few things about always and forever. For instance, things will always be more complicated than you think. And forever is a goal no mortal can claim. We knew by the broken hearts and families, by the funerals, by the trouble we'd seen, how little can be promised. And in light of all that, if we had the nerve to try again, if we were older and wiser and still stunned silly by love, shouldn't we throw ourselves one hell of a party?

We thought so, anyway. We decided to hold our ceremony in a glade in the woods behind our new house in rural Pennsylvania and then move to the backyard for what we'd begun to refer to as Woodstock III: the Love-In. I spent several afternoons with my 11-year-old stepdaughter-to-be, Emma, hand-embossing, tying ribbons, and dripping sealing wax on parchment envelopes for the invitations, which read:

Emma and Sam Sartwell
Hayes and Vince Winik
request the honor of your presence
at the marriage of their parents.

Like many second weddings, ours was as much about merging our families as forming a twosome. Emma was my maid of honor, 11-year-old Hayes was Crispin's best man, and the younger children, who were 8 and 9, walked us down the aisle. We all wore white: shorts for the kids, satin pedal pushers with a lace bustier for me, linen drawstring pants and a pullover for my curly blond husband, who played the wedding march on a Cajun accordion. In one of the few similarities to my first wedding, a mayor was on hand.

Combining two fully operational households, we hardly needed gifts. So instead of registering anywhere, we informed our guests that we'd be interning them as servants—we'd have a completely do-it-yourself wedding where the invitees were also the help and the entertainment.

The 35 adults and children who attended hauled rocks and rental equipment, decorated, arranged flowers, and prepared food. They brought in the crawfish feast from New Orleans for the rehearsal dinner and the tomato pies from Philly for the wedding lunch. My children's grandmother—my late first husband's mother—baked our wedding cake and drove down with it from the Poconos. The highlight of the whole event was a talent show in the cornfields that went on into the evening with music, poetry, lip-synched dance routines, and trampoline demonstrations.

One lingering question was answered for me that day: You can make those promises with just as much passion the second time around. Such is the regenerative power of the human heart.

STARTING AROUND THE TIME of our ceremony, in predictable generational lockstep, I've been invited to or heard of a whole raft of second weddings. I've been struck by the individuality and romanticism they share with ours, yet each expresses so differently. Released from their frozen positions atop the third tier of the cake—and from parental controls—brides and grooms are dreaming up celebrations that reflect their personalities and their approaches to marriage. (Remember John and Yoko? Second-wedding pioneers.)

One pair of friends remarried in a frescoed palazzo in Venice, then took the wedding party into the countryside for a few days of feasting and winetasting. Two newspaper editors we know rented out a lodge at Mammoth Lakes near Yosemite and invited 46 people for a weekend that included a five-mile hike on the morning of the ceremony. A designer friend whose first wedding involved not one but two enormous, rococo events—one in Mexico City and one in San Antonio—married the second time in a handmade minidress at the home of the elderly friend who had introduced her to the new guy. The couple served cake and Champagne to a party of four.

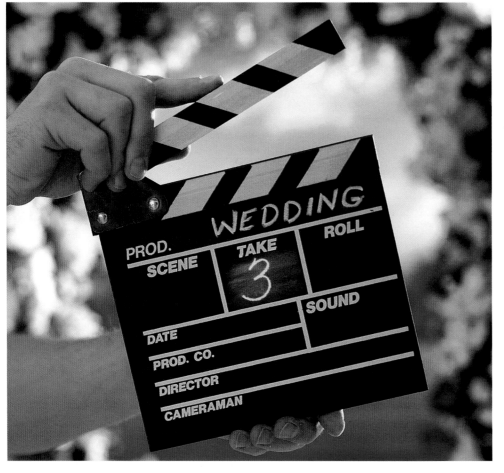

Last summer I received an invitation to a surprise 45th-birthday party for my friend Dubravka. People thought her boyfriend and her 14-year-old son, who were throwing the bash, were out of their minds. Dubravka is just not the type of person you throw a surprise party for. She's the type who takes care of everything and tells everyone else exactly what will be going on. One thing she had clearly told her friends was that she and Terry saw no need to get married.

On the night of the party, Dubravka acted astonished as one group of friends after another showed up. But shortly after cocktails, her son, John, mounted the stairs, thanked everyone for coming, and explained that, actually, the joke was on them. This wasn't only a birthday party, it was a wedding. Dubravka and Terry were married in front of the fireplace then and there. ("I thought that peach satin formal was a little much for a birthday dinner," my friend Ellen said later.)

People who knew I was collecting interesting second-wedding stories told me to call Harriette Cole, the author of *Jumping the Broom: The African-American Wedding Planner.* Ironically, and somewhat painfully, Cole had been asked to write the book while in the middle of a divorce. But she decided to go ahead with it anyway. "I wanted to focus on traditions that were not just pretty but substantive," she says. "Things that had helped people stay together." As it turned out, the project was the place where she buried her first marriage and found her second. She began dating George Chinsee, a photographer with whom she'd worked, and married him one month after the book's publication.

"We consulted Brahman priests for a date that would be good astrologically," says Cole, who is a devotee of Eastern spiritual traditions. They chose 11 o'clock on a Tuesday morning and found a beautiful spot—the Tea Garden in Loch Sheldrake, New York, near the couple's ashram. While Cole's first wedding was a Methodist extravaganza, her second marched to a world beat. She wore a gold and red form-fitted sheath, a crocheted cap, and golden sandals. Honored female relatives and friends were draped in hand-dyed scarves, honored men received vests, and all were served ginger beer and sorrel tea from the groom's native Jamaica.

The climax of the ceremony was jumping the broom, the African-American slave ritual that gave Cole's book its name. Because slaves couldn't legally marry, the act of jumping over a decorated broom—easily accessible as well as a symbol of homemaking—became the commitment ritual. "I'd written and talked so much

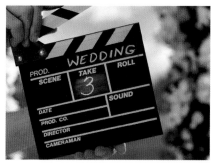

> Like anyone who says the wedding vows more than once, we knew a few things about always and forever.

about it, but it was another thing to do it," Cole says. "As we prepared to jump, there was a crescendo of drums meant to invoke the grace of the ancestors. Everybody stood up and started cheering. Then, the moment we jumped, I saw my dead grandmother's face. She was 101 when she died, right around the time I met George."

Finding a way to evoke the presence of those who have died is a common thread at second weddings, perhaps because those who have been around longer have more loss in their lives. My friends Bob and Vicki found a way to combine gift evasion with the theme of remembrance.

BEFORE SHE MET BOB, 56-YEAR-old Vicki, a nurse and hospital administrator in Baltimore, had raised her sons, given up dating, and thrown herself into marathon running and law school. So when she bumped into an old friend on the running trail and he wanted to fix her up on a date, she had to be convinced. "He's an amazing man," her friend said. "He was my English teacher in high school." It wasn't until the night of the date that Vicki thought, *His high school teacher? He has to be, like, 70 years old.*

He was. But doubts about her date dissolved as Bob started the evening by buying Vicki a tequila shot. Not long after, they moved in together and decided to be married at a French restaurant. "At my first wedding I saw no one because we were so busy taking pictures, and at my second wedding I ate nothing because we were so busy making sure friends were taken care of," Vicki says. "So I planned my third wedding with no cameras and lots of hors d'oeuvres." In lieu of gifts, guests were asked to donate to the cancer center where Bob's first wife had been a patient—both in memory of her and in honor of Vicki's older son, who had survived leukemia. The thousands of dollars raised meant a lot more to the couple than a barrage of new sheet sets and food processors would have.

I think Vicki and Bob would agree with the sentiment expressed in an e-mail I received when Sue Jernigan, the friend who introduced me to Crispin and whose own second marriage preceded ours by a year, heard of our engagement. We quoted her on our invitation: "This is the ephemeral and elusive happiness that you can't even look for because it doesn't have a name or a site. It floats and soars through luck, karma, destiny's twists and turns. If you are very blessed, you turn around and it grabs you tight around your heart. And you have the intuition to grab back, smiling and breathless, stupid and brave." •

The Un-Hollywood Wife

Mavis and Jay Leno go their own way, do their own thing, and have one of the happiest marriages in the world. What gives? Mavis Leno does the math. **By Michelle Burford**

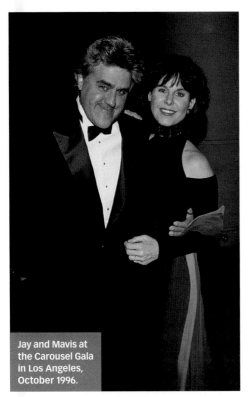

Jay and Mavis at the Carousel Gala in Los Angeles, October 1996.

QUESTION: *Jay says one reason your marriage has lasted is that you don't try to stop him from working so hard. True?*

ANSWER: One of my beliefs about a happy relationship—whether it's a marriage, a friendship, or a business—is that you let people go their own way. I always want to communicate to Jay that as far as I'm concerned, he can stop everything tomorrow. In fact, he can do any damn thing he wants and it's okay with me. Within reasonable limits, you have to mind your own business. If Jay's schedule becomes grueling, I'll just say, "How are you feeling? Don't you think you should cut yourself some slack?" And if Jay says to me, "I'm anxious about you doing this or that," I'll listen and address his fears. But if I decide I'm going to do something, I do it.

Q: *Does Jay still crack you up?*

A: He kills me! Jay has a lot of the attributes of my favorite uncle, Hugh. It wasn't conscious, but somewhere in my childhood, I decided Uncle Hugh was a good model for

what I wanted in a man—someone really funny and a bit mischievous. Many blue-eyed, black-haired men later, here I am with the man who has the best of those things.

Q: *Are you an "I love you" kind of couple?*

A: Oh, yes—he's extremely affectionate. And I come from a family where my father would tell my mother he loved her a hundred times a day. I don't know how many millions of times my dad said to me, "You just don't realize what an incredible woman your mother is. I'm the luckiest man in the world." It's natural for me to tell Jay he's handsome, to smooch him when he's sitting down and reading.

Q: *What's the greatest gift Jay ever gave you?*

A: The year before we married, we bought a house that took up most of our money. He mentioned an engagement ring, and I said, "Look, I don't need it. We've got the house." On our 16th anniversary, he asked me, "If you had it to do all over again, would you marry me?" I said, "It was the best thing I ever did. Why would you even ask?" He then whips out this spectacular diamond ring. I never thought I'd care about a diamond, but it really is fantastic.

Q: *How else does Jay show he cares?*

A: He's willing to do anything to support my ambitions—and to offer help before I ask. He's a real grown-up. My father was the most darling man in the world—but he was an actor, and for all intents and purposes, he was 12 all his life. I got used to being the designated grown-up in every relationship. When Jay says he'll take care of something, he does. We know we can lean on each other.

Q: *I know Jay has supported you in your fight to end the mistreatment of women by the Taliban—an issue you took on long before it was in vogue. Why this cause?*

A: Bias against women is just another form of bigotry, and bigots always have the same modus operandi. First they declare you inferior; then they systematically make it illegal for you to prove you're not. In their hearts, they know you're not inferior—they

just want a huge slice of the pie. The Taliban cut off all communication from other countries. Women had essentially been put under house arrest and had no way of knowing whether anybody saw this. When my dad was a teen, he did hard-rock mining to bring in money. One summer he lived through a cave-in. When he was rescued after a few hours, he said the most terrible thing wasn't thinking he would die; it was believing no one even knew he was in there. That's how I thought these women must have felt. I was frantic to let them know their plight was seen by the world and to bring them hope.

Q: *Weren't you nominated for the Nobel Peace Prize?*

A: Yes. My organization, the Feminist Majority Foundation, and the campaign I head—the Campaign to Stop Gender Apartheid in Afghanistan—were nominated in 2002. I couldn't be prouder than to lose to former president Carter!

Q: *In terms of gender equality, what change would you most like to see happen during your lifetime?*

A: Universal education for all women—for all human beings, really.

Q: *I've heard you read 10 to 15 books every week. If you could give me only one book to read, which one would it be?*

A: *The Fountain Overflows,* by Rebecca West.

Q: *One last question: What word best characterizes your relationship with Jay?*

A: *Joy.* I don't just love Jay—I'm madly in love. And I say this as someone who didn't think that state could persist. To my astonishment, it has—and that makes me feel a little silly about myself. There's a poem [in the movie *Roman Holiday*] that I've always used as a measure of whether I love somebody or am just kidding myself: "If I were dead and buried, and I heard your voice, beneath the sod my heart of dust would still rejoice." If I were dead and buried and Jay walked on my grave, my heart would still dance. He is just all joy to me. ●

O

Sex

a shy girl's guide to sex

It's not that she doesn't like sex; it's just that she prefers subtlety, indirection, holding off. A shy girl gets hot and heavy about her sex life. BY ANONYMOUS

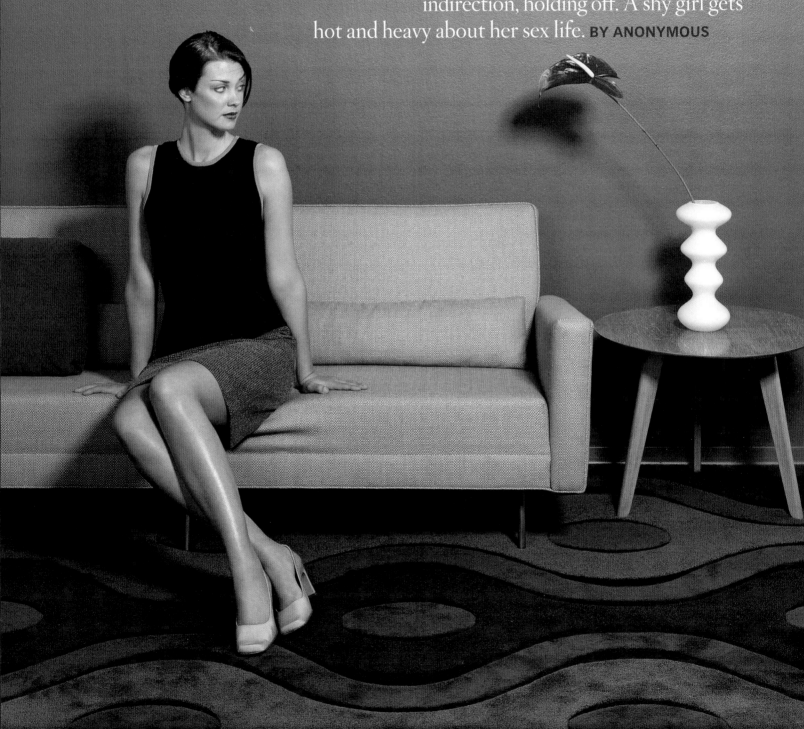

I AM NOT A PRUDE. I like sex. But I would never say that to your face, and I'm actually cringing here at my computer at the thought that somebody could walk in.... Well, you see where I'm heading. My own sexuality embarrasses me.

When I was a young teenager, my mother used to tell me that the world was divided into breast men and leg men, and that I would attract the leg men. I don't remember being upset. Or pleased. I remember thinking, *Well, that's it for shorts.* In college I wore flowing, ankle-length skirts and beginning in my 30s, long pants. I'm the only person I know who can imagine adding a burqa to my wardrobe. I never want to be obvious, so when I'm feeling sexy I try to hide it—to the point where my husband can't always tell that I'm turned on; he once asked if I'd consider holding up a sign.

Okay, so I'm a little shy. That wouldn't have seemed so strange 50 years ago, when Victoria still had secrets, a kiss was still a kiss rather than an IOU, and holding back was still a viable sexual strategy. Today you're supposed to tell your partner exactly what will satisfy you. ("Excuse me, could you pass the multiple orgasms?") The very thought of it makes me blush.

Please don't get me wrong: I admire a woman who is sexually confident. I love it when movie stars strut and preen—not Gwyneth Paltrow bending like a willow, but Catherine Zeta-Jones leading with her chest. If you show up in four-inch heels and a see-through dress, I'll think you're hot. But I'll be more intrigued by the woman next to you who smolders quietly. In grad school my Victorian literature professor read us a scene in which a woman rolled up her sleeve, revealing to her suitor a seductive white arm. I thought the professor would faint, and who could blame him? When the boy I was dating brought over his favorite hard-core porno books for me to learn from, I put them aside in favor of *A Man with a Maid,* in which the innocent virgin is outraged by her captor's lewd behavior. Of course I got bored as soon as the lady became a libertine. I liked the *Kama Sutra* because it made sex seem ornate, exotic; words like *penis* and *vagina*

the sex experts vs. the shy girl

Sparkly rouge on your nipples—or a gradual unveiling in the dark? You be the judge.

WHAT THE EXPERTS SAY:	WHAT THE SHY GIRL SAYS:
■ "Dressing for sex is a major part of fantasy role-playing." —*Orgasms for Two: The Joy of Partnersex*	■ If you're not a French maid, don't dress like one. Be yourself. Any piece of clothing can be sexy with a quietly passionate woman inside it.
■ "Part of talking hot is knowing what kind of language works for you and your partner." —*Sex Talk: Uncensored Exercises for Exploring What Really Turns You On*	■ Silence is rich. Use body language. Speak with your fingers and your eyes.
■ "If the two of you decide you'd like to make love outdoors, you might want to pack a picnic meal, making sure to include your favorite sex accessories." —*The 10 Secrets to Great Sex*	■ Leave a little to chance. Gravitate toward a quiet place (preferably a desert island), and let nature take its course.
■ "Find a sexy, R-rated movie. Have a movie night with your partner." —*Sex Matters for Women*	■ Watching perfect strangers have sex onscreen is overrated and makes you squirm. Find a movie—e.g., *The Remains of the Day*—in which everything is suggested and nothing shown. Let the sex come later, as a surprise.
■ "Spend some time writing down reaffirming statements about yourself, such as 'I am sexy,' 'I inspire others,' or 'I have beautiful eyes.' Carry these statements with you always, on cards in your wallet." —*Sexual Fitness*	■ Never write anything down unless you want to see it posted on the wall in the women's room.
■ "Outrageously flaunt the beauty of your erogenous zones. Wear...blush in your cleavage, red or sparkly rouge on your nipples." —*302 Advanced Techniques for Driving a Man Wild in Bed*	■ Show yourself gradually. Darkness is your friend. Draw the shades so you can let loose without embarrassment. Revel in your other senses for starters; then light a candle or two.

were clinical, but *lingam* and *yoni* came (so to speak) with a little mystery. Sex toys—always gifts from men who wanted to make me less inhibited—went to a top shelf and stayed there. Only last week my husband reached for something on the top of a wardrobe and came back with an ancient vibrator. Did I want to dust it off and try it? What do you think?

Sometimes I break through my shyness. Sometimes the sun shines in Seattle. More often, though, I accept the way I am and work around it because, to tell you the truth, I really don't want to change. I don't want to be more aggressive. I don't want to turn myself on. Pick up any sex manual (something I'd never do in public—what would the bookstore clerk think?) and you'll find instructions on learning to love your own body. Asks one guide, "When was the last time you took a good look at your vulva?" Um, never? The idea of lying on my

back, spreading my legs like a frog, and inspecting myself through a hand mirror has always seemed ludicrous to me. I don't have to look to know what's there, and if you tell me it's as lovely as a lotus flower, I won't believe you. (I wouldn't enter the penis in a beauty contest, either.) To quote the old Volkswagen ads, "It's ugly, but it works."

I guess getting naked can be fun, but I'd rather keep my body under wraps. I don't mind being secretly sensuous, the woman who lets down her hair when she wants to and afterward pins it right back up again. And if I'm buttoned up in bed, that's not indifference: That's being so turned on that I don't know what to do—yet. But I'm in no hurry. If I did hold up a sign (well, dear, you asked), it would say: GIVE ME TIME, AND SPACE. HOLD BACK A LITTLE, MAKE ME GO AFTER YOU. When a shy girl and a shy guy get together, anything can happen. ●

PHILLIP C. McGRAW, PhD, on what it takes to "put a little strut in your stuff."

Sexual Confidence

OF ALL THE THINGS THAT AFFECT our sexual satisfaction, the most important element is sexual confidence. By that I mean knowing not only that you're desirable but also that what you bring to a sexual encounter is likely to be highly valued by your partner.

Not surprisingly, sexually confident women seem to be more sexually active and have a whole lot more fun while they're at it. That doesn't mean they confuse quantity with quality. What sets the sexually confident woman apart is that she's relaxed. She experiences things fully because she isn't self-conscious. She doesn't obsess about rejection or failure, and as a result she enjoys success after success. But so many people speak of sexual confidence almost as if it were some kind of exotic potion, enjoyed only by a lucky few. They tell me they aren't certain they comprehend the concept, and they don't have a clue about how to get it.

If you're one of those folks, take heart and read on. The good news is that if this seemingly mystical characteristic is missing in your life, things can change. If you're sexually insecure or uptight, or just feel as if you aren't very good at it, all that can change—in a hurry. The *really* good news is that attaining sexual confidence is totally up to you. It's time for you to put a little strut in your stuff.

I'm going to focus on the female side of this topic, since most of you reading this are women. But many of the same principles apply to both sexes, so don't stop reading if you're a guy—you just might learn something.

A Little Help from My Friends

Although I've picked up some insight from 25-plus years of working with couples as well as sexually active singles, I was determined in preparing this article not to lean totally on my own understanding. So I sought the blessing of my wife, Robin, who was reluctant: She can't understand why *her* husband has to be the one who speaks to America about such private things. With Robin's okay, I made it my business to do some informal research. Now, out of 160 people who work on the *Dr. Phil* show, about 140 are women—a pretty big pool to draw from. Eight of my coworkers and I sat down for a roundtable discussion about sexual confidence. Their comments and observations have been invaluable—and in some cases, unprintable. I discovered that my very professional colleagues are pretty rowdy!

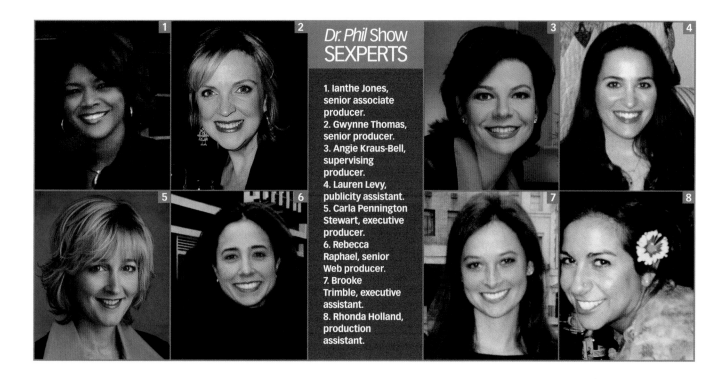

Sexual Confidence Defined

Clearly, there are some things that sexual confidence is not about. For starters, it's not about having a great body. Perhaps unexpectedly, older women describe themselves as much more sexually confident than younger ones. I say "unexpectedly" because younger women tend to be regarded as having more objective sex appeal. But older women have the extremely valuable benefit of experience. Carla, 41, put it this way: "If I took the confidence I have now and the body I had in my 20s or 30s, I'd be hell on wheels. But would I trade what I now understand about myself, my body, and sex just to have the body back? No way, no how!" When she was younger, her fear of rejection and insecurity caused her to be a people pleaser. She knows better now: It's not selfish in a sexual situation to please yourself. Think about it—what greater gift could you give your partner than to have a really good time? If you're having fun, your partner is going to have fun. And that's not a license for selfishness; it's a recognition that you can't give away what you don't have yourself.

Sexual confidence isn't something you need a partner to give to you or validate in you. In fact, if you're focusing too much on him, that can be a big distraction and erode your sexual confidence. Virtually all the women I talked to agreed that when they were younger, they were more inclined to let other people define their sense of self.

> Think about it— what greater gift could you give your partner than to have a really good time?

Women who know their bodies better—who know what turns them on—report enjoying sex more. They're more confident that their interactions will be successful. Rebecca, 29, though 12 years younger than Carla, endorsed her view. "If I had the confidence at 23 that I have now, I would have had a lot more fun," Rebecca says. "I'd have spent much less time worrying about what a guy was thinking and enjoyed myself more."

That's true of most of the women I've spoken to on this subject over the years. They tend to care much less as time goes by about what other people think. They certainly don't let men inhibit them. Older women, in particular, seem much more at ease with the prospect of being on their own, are more content with who they are, and feel far less desperation to be in a sexual relationship—which, in turn, allows them to relax and feel more secure in themselves. And that clearly boosts their sexual confidence.

This brings me to a point made over and over by the women in my little survey, a belief so widely shared that it's a core truth about sexual confidence: It is not all about sex. It is very much about power, the power that comes from liking and accepting yourself. A woman who is open-minded, wants to have fun, and isn't counting on getting an engagement ring within minutes of meeting a man has an ease about her that translates as power. By contrast, one who looks like she's on the prowl for Mr. Right and is deafened by the ticking of her biological clock sends a totally different message. And as any guy will tell you, that message is: *Run!* But if you're comfortable and genuinely happy, others sense it and want it. Women who like where they are in their lives exude an assurance that makes for some very positive vibes in the bedroom.

Getting Some

For all the media hype surrounding sex and the ways in which it's glamorized in our society, we're pretty darn rigid in the real world of Anytown, U.S.A., and it's difficult for many women to think of themselves as sexual beings, let alone enjoy that role. If your sexual confidence meter is on empty, here are a few ways to fuel up:

The key to unlocking your sexual confidence is to check your self-perception. Beauty is in the eye of the beholder—and you have to see yourself as beautiful before you can expect anyone else to. Yes, you need to feel good about your body. But as thousands of sensuous women will tell you, body image is far less important than just feeling good about yourself and your life overall. By deliberately steering your internal dialogue toward positive, empowering thoughts, you can increase your level of assurance. Maybe you need to replace your current internal dialogue with sexually confident messages like:

I'm happy.

I'm fabulous.

I've got it.

I'm beautiful.

Once your internal dialogue is playing the right words, pay attention to what you're saying nonverbally. You can use whatever words you like, but a huge percentage of what you communicate is coming through your body language, loud and clear. If a woman projects a sense of knowing that she's desirable, the man or men in her life will be drawn to her like bears to honey—and that's true whether or not she meets any notion of what a sexy woman "ought" to look like. The way she walks into a room, her posture, how she maintains eye contact, how she dresses, how much time she spends checking out other women and comparing herself to them—all contribute to the aura she exudes.

Before you can give off a confident aura, you need to be comfortable with your body. If you're one of those people who can't even look in the mirror when you're naked,

> Rent a video, read a book, buy a feather boa—but make it a priority to find out what works.

you need to get used to it. Maybe you need to start with lingerie. Maybe you need to begin with a snowsuit and work down from there. The point is, you need to feel comfortable with yourself, and then you can get to know your sexual self. Figure out whatever you need to do to get in the mood—whether it's lighting candles, playing music, or something else—and do it. Ultimately, a sexual response is much more successful when people lose their inhibitions. So you're going to have to learn to get comfortable in your own skin.

Now let's talk about technique. If you have knowledge about what works and what doesn't, you have power. Rent a video, read a book, buy a feather boa—but make it a priority to find out! And remember, something even more powerful than good technique is the willingness to surrender and immerse yourself in the interaction.

Someone who has good form but paints by the numbers isn't nearly as good a sexual partner as someone who is willing to throw self-consciousness to the wind and totally engage in the process.

Power, besides being highly attractive by itself, is the spice that lends an extra something to a woman's sexuality. Norman Mailer once wrote that Marilyn Monroe was so attractive to men because she looked "easy." Sorry, Norman, but I don't think that's exactly right.

For years, men have told me that they desire a woman who doesn't come off as looking like a sure thing. Approachable and unintimidating, yes, but not easy. "I think guys like women who might appear to be easy but who they know are not," says Ianthe, 31. Jennifer Aniston, for example, is viewed as the sexy girl next door; not too flirtatious—not easy—but not standoffish, either. There's power in her demeanor. Lots of sexually confident women, as different from one another as Jennifer Aniston and Marilyn Monroe, successfully navigate the fine line between accessibility and control.

As Gwynne, 42, says: "They give off an aura that says, *I've got it, you want it, and I'll decide if you can have it.*"

And, finally, you have to name it to claim it. It's not enough simply to say, "I want a sexually fulfilling relationship." Sexual confidence means being able to identify exactly what you like and dislike, and having the guts to express it. That may mean exploring your own body to find out what pleases you. Knowing what you want and what it takes to make you feel good will give you more confidence. That leads to more fun, which in turn increases your confidence, which creates more fun: Are you following me?

Good sex, healthy sex, is a kind of play. Be willing to get good at it, and find out what it's going to take for you to like and accept yourself. Know what makes you happy sexually. Acknowledge the power that you have as a woman. Then give yourself permission to be sexual and to enjoy it. ●

Why do we do it?

A young woman talks about the slow death of her mother. She has cared for her for many long months. Throughout all the arrangement-making, the tension, the sorrowful, relentless accretion of evidence of the inevitable, she doesn't express her fear or her sadness or her grief. She *talks* about it, but her feelings sit heavily as stones on her heart, and won't be moved by words.

One night, she says, she was making love with her boyfriend, looking into his eyes. She felt secure in his embrace, cradled in the steady, loving constancy of his touch and his gaze. The shared rhythm of their bodies both comforted and aroused her in a delicate balance of pleasure. But as he rocked with her in his arms, she began to feel a giving-way, the heaviness moving, her hold on her feelings relaxing. All of a sudden, her heart seemed to crack open and, to her deep surprise, grief poured from her in a tide of tears. "My mother!" she cried, eyes locked with her lover's. "My mother is dying!" It was the very first time she had been completely present with that fact, understanding it, accepting it, *knowing* it.

Her boyfriend pulled her closer, holding her tight. "I love you, I love you, I love you," he said.

I don't guess they asked each other afterward, "Was it good for you, too?" Sometimes "good" just isn't adequate to describe an experience that has been referred to as the little death. Did you know that during orgasm, most of the brain shuts down? That with orgasm, raised levels of what are called the cuddle chemicals— oxytocin and vasopressin—lead to feelings of satisfaction and attachment? A study has found that women who regularly receive semen vaginally are less depressed than those who don't, says Helen Fisher, PhD, author of *Why We Love, The Nature and Chemistry of Romantic Love.* This could be because they really like their partners; it could also be because seminal fluid is awash not only with testosterone and estrogen but also with chemicals such as dopamine and norepinephrine, serotonin, and oxytocin, which can contribute to either elation or calm. Another recent study revealed the unsurprising result that the more often a person has sex, the happier he or she is. This could be because people who have sex often are more likely to be healthy and enjoying a good relationship. It could also be because sex exercises the muscles and the respiratory system; gets the circulatory system moving, which gives the skin a gorgeous glow; and according to Fisher's research, triggers the brain circuitry for romantic love and attachment. Why do we do it? Because it's fun. Because it can be the most powerful, concrete way to demonstrate love for ourselves and for someone else. Because sex helps us to remember. Because it helps us to forget. Because when we open ourselves to the experience completely, we become intimate with the world in a way that's otherwise inaccessible, and unique. Flooded with hormones that can release us from the moorings of self-consciousness and control, we can relax into a presence of mind that allows boundaries, momentarily, to dissolve. Sex can not only help us feel better—it can also help us to feel. ●

sexual energy:
feel the heat

Irresistibility isn't about perfect abs, blinding teeth, or aquamarine eyes. It's about warmth, desire, and willingness. At least that's step one, says **Amy Bloom.**

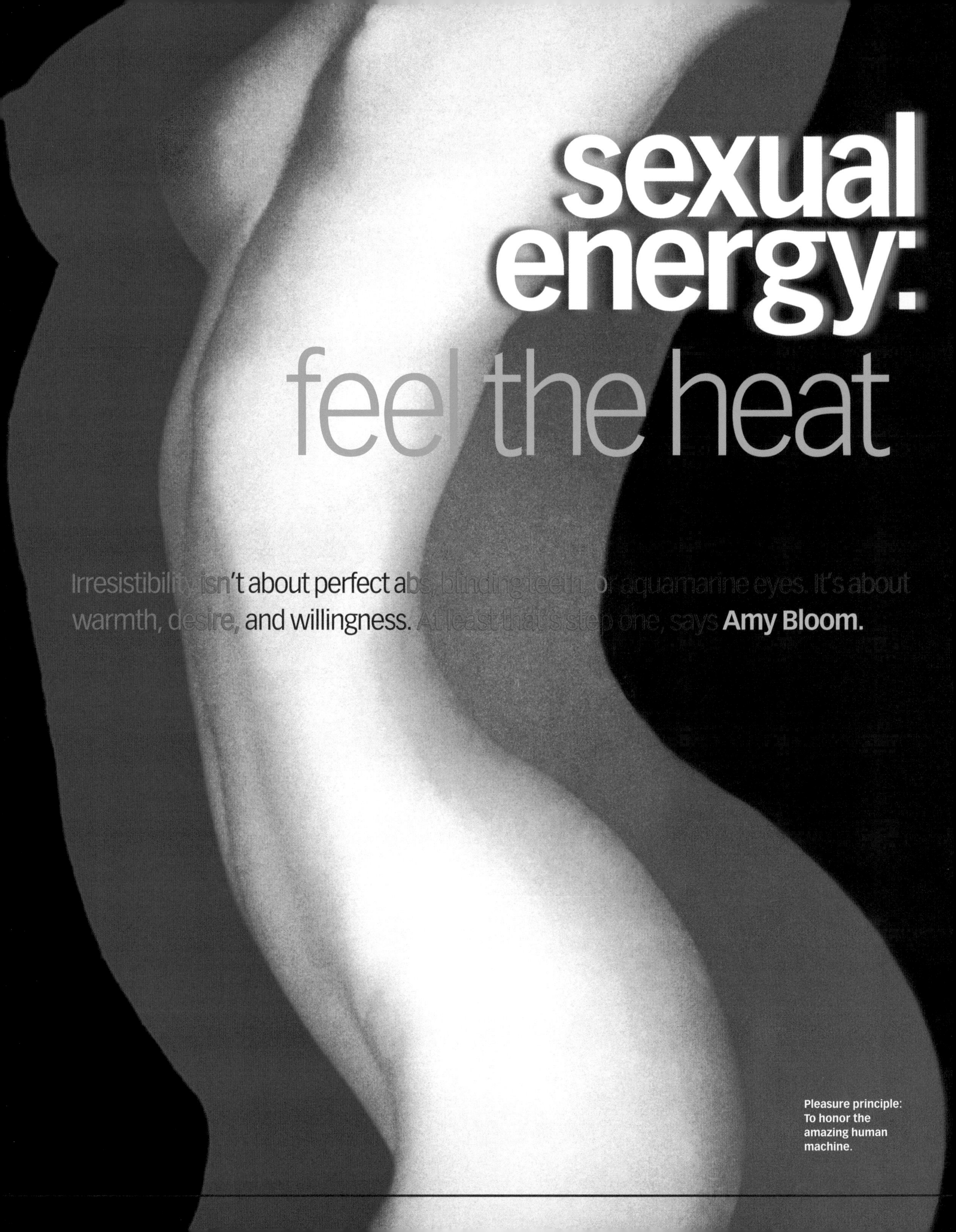

**Pleasure principle:
To honor the
amazing human
machine.**

Catherine Zeta-Jones's take-no-prisoners oomph. George Clooney's let's-do-it eyes. Hugh Grant's crooked smile. Halle Berry's everything. It's exhausting to think that we have to measure up to all that exceptional, multimagnified sex appeal. All of it so inaccessible, so expensive (what, no stylist? no trainer? no designer?), and so frankly impossible. Any sensible woman would conclude that you might as well pull up your faded comforter, grab some chocolate, and give up the idea of anybody ever finding you irresistible.

Please don't. Please consider that being irresistible is more a matter of interest and appetite than of anything else. You can forget about becoming everyone's physical ideal. Everyone has their preferences, their weaknesses, and even their hang-ups (even this author). There's nothing you can do about that. If he's mad for tall blondes and you're a short brunette, don't rush out for Clairol and three-inch heels. There's a better way. And forget about miniskirts (unless they look not only good but effortless on you). Forget about *Are You Hot?* and Lil' Kim and cleavage-to-there magazine covers; that stuff works only if you have all the equipment and not too much self-respect, and really, only if you have *all* the equipment. And if you do, you will of course wind up spending time with a guy who prefers the all-you-can-eat buffet to the great gourmet meal, and that might not be so much fun. But...irresistible is something else. It transcends the physical (not that the physical ever hurts—and your mother didn't lie; good posture is a plus), it plays fast and loose with the psychological, and it makes the world a bigger, more entertaining, more filled-with-possibilities place.

I have had two irresistible friends. One was a fat old man with plenty of minor illnesses, and despite qualities one and two, I can't count the number of times I had to push past attractive women of all ages to get to him. He wasn't rich, he wasn't powerful, but he had, to paraphrase Oscar Wilde, nothing to declare but his genius for making every woman feel she was a hidden treasure. He listened, he flirted, he responded openly; he made married women feel that he envied their husbands and that only magnificent self-restraint

kept him from throwing himself at their feet; he made single women feel that if he didn't so love his wife, he would make a fool of himself. Even when he was single, he managed to suggest, when flirting, that although there were some obvious, insurmountable impediments to true happiness for him and his current dinner partner/companion on the plane/ chance encounter in the bookstore, this moment, this hour or two, would always be one of the great pleasures of his life. He was unafraid to show interest, and even more, he was willing to show desire. He was willing to reveal that he was...willing. It was not a power struggle or a game or any kind of exploitation; it was a beautiful, charming dance, and it made his partners (whether for the evening or a long friendship) feel that they had been given a gift, however they chose to respond.

My other friend was only slightly more likely a player: a stocky, singularly unglamorous lesbian bartender. Like my older friend (and I'm sorry they didn't meet, but where would that have left me?), she understood that Venus, as Ovid wrote, favors the bold. She not only understood it, she had it made into a sampler hung above her enormously successful bar. And how did she come to own that bar? A devoted husband and wife, objects of her flirtatious affection and staunch friendship, bought it for her and, after spending $30,000, still felt they got the better end of the bargain because they had a great place to hang out and plenty of time to spend with her. She made men, gay and straight, feel that the only time she ever regretted being a lesbian was in their presence. She made old folks know she valued their wisdom and that it was a joy, at the end of a day, to move at a slower pace; she made young people feel they were the flowers of the world and she was delighted to admire them. And women—she made every woman she liked, gay and straight, feel that her presence was a joy, a brightening of the world. Her face lit up when she saw you, and that radiance made her beautiful. She never hesitated to say that she found someone irresistible; she never shied

away from attraction or the vulnerability that sometimes comes with it; she was never desperate or needy; she flirted from a happy abundance of love and lust, not a lack of either, and so she was our Lady Bountiful, our irresistible force, and at her funeral beautiful women, handsome men, famous poets—and her devoted companion—all wept as if their hearts would break.

And then there's appetite: The thing women are not supposed to have (except in music videos, and then it's so clearly on display for the benefit of the viewer that I don't get any idea what Madonna or Christina Aguilera or Eve really wants for herself). You can fake blonde. You can fake tan. You can even fake sexy—for a while. What you can't fake is the real and unmistakable scent and feel of someone who actually likes...sex. You can't fake that Bessie Smith growl, the easy warmth of someone who wants a little sugar in her bowl and who is prepared, under the right circumstances, to have and give a very good time. Who would you rather have dinner with: the flour-fearing vegan or the happy omnivore who looks on dessert as a special occasion, not a torment? So it is with sex. Shame, guilt, and aversion are not attractive to most people. Confidence and an adult appreciation of pleasure—and of the amazing human machine, which despite imperfections and wear and tear, can do such a glorious job of delivering it—is appealing. People who know that and show that they do are simply irresistible.

The heart of sexual energy is making others feel beautiful, wanted, clever, charming, making them see themselves in the warm, pink light of our unembarrassed attention and allowing some of the flattering light to fall on ourselves, our strong points, and our frank interest. It isn't the tenacious, almost hostile, approach of the lonely man or woman who is only a step away from turning on us if we disappoint. It isn't breaking up marriages or insulting one's spouse. It is embracing the world and the people in it; it is embracing desire and attraction as sources of pleasure rather than shame, and appreciating what we have to offer as well as what they, the lucky objects of our desire, do. ●

"How Do You Ask for the Sex Life You Want? Very Carefully"

If your partner isn't the same amorous stud muffin you fell in love with, **PHILLIP C. McGRAW, PhD,** has a three-point romance restoration plan.

I HEAR IT FROM SO MANY OF YOU— "My husband doesn't seem interested in sex," "I always have to initiate," and "I don't want to cheat, but my hormones are raging." The cliché of the frigid wife who doesn't want sex has been replaced by a new reality: Women who are married or in a committed relationship want to be having *more* sex. Sometimes the issue is simply about intercourse—they're not getting enough, or what they're getting just isn't that good. But in my experience, when women say they want more sex, often it goes beyond the physical aspects of a relationship to include a wish for more support, intimacy, tenderness, sensitivity, and acceptance. You want to know that your husband considers you a sexually desirable woman, and many of you just aren't feeling that.

Bringing the passion back into your relationship is not solely up to you. But since the only person you control is you, it's a good place to start. Is it fair for you to be the one doing the work? Probably not. Should you have to go to great lengths to make your husband want you? Probably not. Is figuring out what you can do differently the most efficient way to get what you're looking for? Absolutely. This process is not about a quick fix—five moves that will leave him begging for mercy tonight and every night thereafter. It's about taking an honest look at yourself, getting in stride with your partner, and together making a plan to break out of a rut and turn up the heat.

FIRST, DO A LITTLE THINKING

If you want to see your sex life improve, start by diagnosing the problem. Examine your life: Are you so busy that it's impossible for the two of you to be sexually intimate on a regular basis? Have you gotten out of the habit because sex is incompatible with all your other obligations? Days turn into weeks, and weeks turn into months, and before you know it you can't remember the last time you made love. Sex is a pattern, and unless it happens on an ongoing basis, other things will crowd it out. Use it or lose it.

Try to trace the pattern back in time and figure out how sex got moved down the priority list. Was it when you started having kids? One of the biggest mistakes that couples make is that they stop being friends and lovers because they've become moms and dads. It's a mental shift; all of a sudden, being a romantic partner is no longer important. It's like we decide, *Adolescence is over. I'm a mother or a father now, and I have to act like one.* Add to that the time and energy required in raising children, and sexually, the cards are stacked against you. But being a parent is just one of the roles we play, and neglecting the role of partner and lover is a huge error.

Now ask yourself, *What might I be doing—or not doing—to contribute to the situation? And what can I do to change things?* Back when there was passion in your relationship, were you taking more pride in the way you looked? For better or worse, men are responsive to visual stimulation. You can't be oblivious to that fact. You may need to make some small changes in your appearance, like getting rid of old sweatpants, cutting your hair, or losing the weight you've been complaining about for years. None of this is to say that *his* worn-out sweats and protruding gut are a turn-on. But it goes back to one of my life laws: You create your own experience—so get started. You may want affirmation from him—that you look beautiful, that your haircut is flattering, whatever it may be. I can't promise you that you're going to get it, which is why you have to decide within yourself that you are making the most of who you are and what you have to offer. Give yourself credit for that and find security in it, even if it's not externally validated.

And indeed, your self-image is crucial. Say to yourself, *I'm not just a mommy. I'm a hot number.* And then act like it. Talk yourself into it. Instead of waking up thinking about how many dirty diapers you're going to change that day, tell yourself, *I am going to seduce my husband today.* Try spending less time coming up with a plan to avoid traffic on your way to work and more time figuring out how you're going to inspire your lover. As a starting point, think back to when you and your partner were having sex more often and enjoying it. Remember what worked at that time in your life, and replicate those things. Have a conversation with yourself. Give yourself permission to get what you want. Claim your right, and give a voice to your needs. Being sexually

satisfied and feeling wanted by your partner are legitimate and healthy parts of a relationship.

NEXT, BRING HIM IN ON IT

Once you've thought about what's lacking, where the problem lies, and what role you play in it, you need to talk to him about it; he cannot read your mind. How do you tell someone you're not satisfied with the sex life you share? Very carefully. It's important to come at this straight. You need to sit down together and mutually recognize: "Our physical intimacy hasn't been there lately. We may have gotten distracted or

allowed too many other things to absorb all our energy." You are acknowledging, as a couple, that you've gotten out of the habit of focusing on each other romantically and that you want to make sex part of your lives again.

Now let's talk about timing. The time to raise the issue is not during a marital crisis. Your needs may be valid, but he'll resist you if you include it in a litany of complaints or bring it up in the middle of an argument. Getting defensive or figuring out who's to blame won't get you very far, either. If you'd rather argue about whose fault it is and try to convict your husband

Chemistry Notes

Judging from the mail I've been getting, a lot of you would like to know how hormones play into this I-want-it, he-doesn't situation. So I put some of your questions to Andrew Messamore, MD, an internist who focuses on hormone problems, from my old stomping ground of Plano, Texas.

Q: I think my husband has a low sex drive. He's warm and caring, but he never initiates sex. What can I do?

A: This is not at all uncommon. I have seen a lot of male patients with a low sex drive due to low testosterone levels. It may be genetic or related to his age—testosterone production decreases as men get older, and from ages 50 to 80 it can decrease to half its youthful level. If you suspect the problem is low testosterone, your husband should see a physician. He may be at risk for osteoporosis, loss of muscle mass, and heart problems. The doctor can give him a simple blood test and discuss therapy options like hormone supplements. If his testosterone levels are normal, psychotherapy might be in order.

Q: I just went off birth control, and I'm experiencing a hormonal surge that is driving me crazy! I am a devoted wife, but my mind and eyes are wandering constantly. What's happening to me?

A: Under normal circumstances, a woman's hormones don't change much until menopause, except for her regular

monthly fluctuations. But going off the Pill can cause a change in hormones, which can lead to a heightened libido. (The same thing happens when you've just had a baby or recently stopped nursing.) Your hormones can become hyperstimulated after a period of suppression, but your body will find its balance and go back to normal—probably within a few months.

Q: My partner comes home from work stressed and not at all in the mood. Does stress affect hormones? What can I do?

A: Yes, prolonged stress can cause overproduction and then depletion of hormones—so the levels rise, then fall off sharply. (Cortisol is a stress hormone, but all hormones are linked, so testosterone is also affected.) To make matters worse, this depletion is often accompanied by a lack of energy, and when we're drained, we don't want to have sex no matter what our hormones are doing. Still, in the vast majority of cases, sexual dysfunction is psychological. If your partner is overstressed, the cure may be as simple as helping him relax when he comes home. (That goes both ways, of course!)

for falling asleep with the remote in his hand night after night, then I ask you, Do you want to be right, or do you want to get some lovin'? I thought so.

I once met with a woman who was depressed that her husband wasn't interested in her sexually anymore. She told me that she did a striptease for him, and he just tried to look around her to catch a score on TV. Only later did she mention that it was the fourth quarter of a playoff game! Come on—you've got to pick (and time) your battles and set yourself up for success. Victims pout; players play. Stop complaining about what you're not getting, and start creating what you want.

What if he doesn't want to talk about it? Years of watching *Sex and the City* (not to mention my show!) may have helped you understand that your sexual needs are legitimate, and that talking with your partner about what you want is as reasonable as discussing where to go for dinner. But he may not want, or be able, to hear you. There may be underlying issues that are manifesting in the sexual domain—problems that have absolutely nothing to do with you. It's so easy to feel hurt or disappointed if he's not initiating sex, but don't take it personally. His struggle with intimacy may be a result of too much stress at the office. When the pressure is on, we tend to strip away what we actually need most: sleep, comfort, companionship—and sex. Is he depressed? Could medication be diminishing his sex drive? Also, men tend to measure their self-worth as a function of external circumstances. He may feel like less of a man if he doesn't have a job, for example, or even after something like heart surgery. Take a look at the situations that may be affecting him, and see how you can help. Would bringing a different passion (sports, a hobby) back into his life lead to more excitement in the bedroom? The two of you need to talk about what's going on. But if he's reluctant to be open about it, encourage him to at least look inside. Suggest that he ask himself what might be killing the deal for him. If you can find the source of the problems, you can tailor your intimacy to meet his needs, and yours. And if all else fails, try to convince him that one session of couples therapy is the key to getting your feelings out in the open and starting to make changes.

NOW, SHARE THE HEAVY LIFTING

You might wish your lovemaking would be Hollywood perfect with no effort on your part, but that's not how it happens. Anything worth having deserves some effort. Put your sex life on project status. Make a conscious decision to recommit to each other, to move sex higher up on the list, and to protect the time you make for it. You shower regularly, right? Something as important as the physical intimacy of a relationship deserves at least as much

> Anything worth having deserves some effort. Put your sex life on project status.

emphasis as a shower! Start by making small changes to put the odds in your favor. Resolve to get the kids into their beds at a reasonable time. Stop falling asleep on the couch, watching some stupid movie that you don't even want to see. Try getting into bed at the same time as your partner—otherwise you're knocking down one of your few opportunities to be together with no distractions.

Carve out time for lovemaking. Yes, it takes away spontaneity when you have to pencil in sex, but at least you'll be having it! After you do, you'll say, "Now I remember why this was so much fun. Now I get why we used to do it all the time." Then you'll build the momentum to keep it going more spontaneously. It's about behaving your way to success, and the first thing you need to do is get back in the saddle.

Experts agree that an important element of sexual arousal is fantasy. And yet we so easily get into a pattern where we're just not fanciful or intriguing sexually. Some people feel shame or fear when it comes to asking for what they want. Speaking candidly with your partner about your desires doesn't make you perverted or kinky. Create an environment of acceptance and openness by agreeing in advance that you can say anything. If you have a hard time verbalizing your desires, give yourself permission to explore each other's fantasies any way you can. Write your partner a letter, or simply envision what it is that you want as you're having sex. Don't be judgmental about this.

There's nothing wrong with spicing up your sex life with some variety. And by variety, I don't mean different people. Try a different place in the house, a different time, or a different position. Discover your partner's fantasy, and be willing to play the game. Be specific about what you want and careful about how you phrase your desires. Your conversation shouldn't start with "You don't do this" or "You aren't interested in that." What I would say instead is "I want this" and "I'm interested in that." If he's quick from penetration to orgasm—which all men are, physiologically, compared to women—you have to make sure there's plenty of foreplay taking place before the actual penetration. And you have to be able to talk about it. Educate your husband so you understand each other's needs.

Ultimately, you can't dance with someone who doesn't want to dance, and there's no question that many women want to be getting down more than their partners do. We all go through changes in our lives, and in that sense our sex drives are no different. Be patient and, most important, turn toward your partner. This is exactly what's not happening, if you consider all this talk of women cheating on their husbands. Look within yourself, talk to your partner, and come up with a plan. And start right now. ●

O

Talking & Listening

attack of the killer comment

It comes out of the blue—a catty remark, a veiled put-down, a blatant backstab. **Michelle Burford** on the best defense against wolves in sheep's clothing.

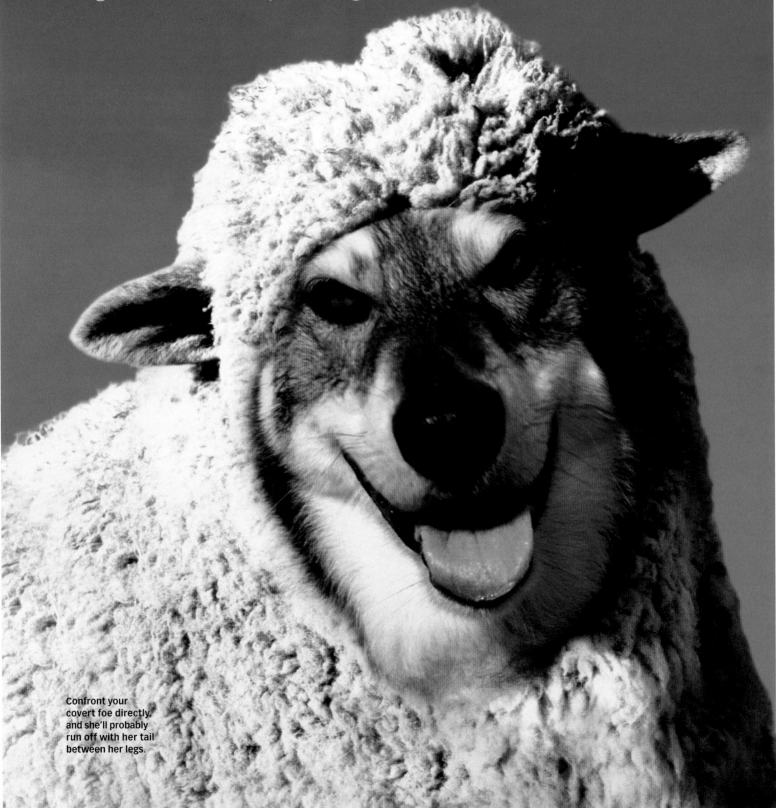

Confront your covert foe directly, and she'll probably run off with her tail between her legs.

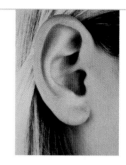

NEAR THE TOP OF MY LIST OF annoyances—right there under people who leave really long voice mails but don't give a callback number—is a mega-peeve: Engaging in catfights. I don't even like to *think* about them, so please allow me to boil my last near-rumble-in-the-ring down to short scenes. First: I find myself utterly bored, so I start a book club with friends. After three sessions of patchy participation, I throw out provocative questions just to crank up a debate. A week later, reports hit the girl-gossip chain that I'm a know-it-all who should be "dethroned." I realize whose campaign this is (she and I have history) and chuck it in the bin marked ignore this. Until the meeting when, as I'm exiting my living room to refill the bowl of stale popcorn, Suspect Number One says (she thinks out of earshot), "Yes, please go—we could use one less smart-ass in the world." I turn back and am greeted by silence and a row of red faces. Later—remember, I'll do anything to ward off a Thrilla in Manila—I corner the attacker with a kill-'em-with-kindness question: "Is my sense right that there's an issue between us?" After 23 seconds of squirming, she comes close to an apology. She never shows up in the club—or my life—again.

An attack by any other name would smell as putrid: a backstab, a dis, a verbal snipe, an outright attempt by an enemy to remove your head. Whatever its label, the aim is quick and dirty; you look down to discover a slow leak of blood forming a red pool at your feet. You may know the assailant well. You may not. She could be a longtime pal who is suddenly threatened by your recent weight loss, a colleague who is sure you've duped her out of a lucrative promotion, or a parent who is envious of how well your hubby communicates with you (who wouldn't be jealous of that?). The insults can be forthright or veiled: an eye roll when your head is turned, a "joke" that bites you in the butt, a word of humiliation in front of your boss. You know, you know:

Be wary of the person who fills you in on gossip that's circulating about you, supposedly as a favor.

It's not personal—it's the attacker's problem. But understanding that your foe never made therapy her priority doesn't mean you shouldn't draw up a plan of defense, and fast.

First, though, a peek under the hood: What drives this kind of hostility? And what makes it escalate? Aaron Beck, MD, a psychiatrist and the author of *Prisoners of Hate: The Cognitive Basis of Anger, Hostility, and Violence,* believes that people who are prone to attacking others—whether verbally or physically—regard life as a battle, often as a result of overcontrolling parents or other authority figures. They're continually mobilized to fight because of a pattern of perceiving belligerence in others' behavior, Beck writes. In essence, the antagonist concludes that everyone is seeking to oust or joust her—which is why she jumps for another's jugular before this "enemy" can take her down.

Jay Carter, the author of *Nasty People: How to Stop Being Hurt by Them Without Becoming One of Them,* calls such attacks invalidations—a term he uses to describe any attempt to injure. "The invalidator has to control you because she sees you as superior," Carter says. "If someone is invalidating you, she has probably been

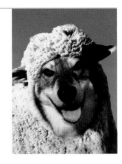

invalidated in the past." About 1 percent of invalidators are complete psychopaths who might eventually resort to a violent rampage, he says, but far more typical is the person who uses verbal attacks to score ego points.

Let's say you have a pal who has seen you through weddings and divorces, Berkinstocks and Manolo Blahniks. For years you've been trying to start a home business that finally jolts off the ground. She seems thrilled. Actually, she seems overly impressed: At every gathering, she feels compelled to announce you as "my friend, the brilliant entrepreneur" while slapping you on the back a tad too hard. You force a grin and thank her. A year later, as your venture continues to crank, you notice her daily phone calls drop to once a month—so you get in her face about it. "With your new business," she stammers, "I figure you're too busy to talk." You assure her you're not. You even hit the speed-dial more often yourself, but when you get her on the line, she seems brusque and offers subtle criticism of your business. You finally point this out, and she retorts, "Everyone knows you've always been so full of yourself." Splat.

Carter explains this shot in the forehead is your friend's way of leveling the power in the friendship. Never mind her own remarkable career; you now have something she's craved since the day she became a single mother—a flexible schedule and more face time with the kids. Her bullet of choice: an unfair judgment meant to knock you back down to size. In doing this, she attacks your self-esteem instead of addressing what's really bothering her—or going after what she wants.

Carter says put-downs also come in the form of cutting off communication (a

friend asks how you're doing but interrupts before you can say), manipulation (a colleague "forgets" to inform you of an important new policy), or rude comments that mask feelings the attacker is afraid to own ("After the meeting yesterday, everyone was saying how unprepared you sounded"). The smartest approach is to bring the conflict out into the open.

"A sniper can't snipe if there's nowhere to hide," says Rick Brinkman, the coauthor of *Dealing with People You Can't Stand.* "Since her limited power is derived from covert activity, once you've exposed her position, that position becomes useless." To do that, you have to cart out the big hammer that most women hope to leave in their toolbox: confrontation. Yet according to Brinkman, the head-to-head doesn't have to get nasty and can be accomplished with one of three approaches: (1) Stop, look, and backtrack ("Did you just call me stupid?"); (2) Ask "searchlight" questions ("When you say x, what are you really trying to say?"); or (3) Go on grievance patrol (by requesting a private meeting with anyone who might be harboring a grudge). "If the grievance is just," says Brinkman, "acknowledge its validity and admit to a mistake." Then say something like "If you ever have a problem with me again, I encourage you to come and talk."

Carter agrees that it's best to take the attacker to the side: "People who embarrass you in front of a group use the group for their power." When you go one-on-one, "the person learns to have respect for you because she knows you'll confront her." He suggests that after you corner the antagonist, you say "Do that to me again and I will have a little surprise for you." If she ignores your warning and tries it once more, greet her with: "There you go again trying to

embarrass me in front of everyone. Can't you think of a more professional way to handle yourself?"

A few more powerful moves from Carter: the stare-down (by looking directly at the attacker while she's in action, "you show her you know exactly what she's doing"); the question "Can you run that by me again?" ("Usually, the little coward won't repeat the insult"); and the mirror (when a friend says "I don't think you like me anymore," respond with "Do you like *me?*").

Be wary of the person who fills you in on gossip that's circulating about you, supposedly as a favor: "Sometimes informants are snipers in disguise," Brinkman says. He suggests saying to the bearer of bad news, "Does so-and-so know you're telling me this? Let's go talk to her." If you discover that the bullet might have been fired by someone you've trusted, Brinkman advises you to be straightforward: "Did you say this about me?" If she answers your question with "Who told you that?" say "That's not the question. Did you say it?" If the person denies it, just let it go and sweetly thank her for discussing it with you. You've done what you came to do: Put her on notice. Brinkman says creating this kind of discomfort is the goal. If you do it every time the assailant moves in for an attack, she'll have to keep adjusting her stance—and that means she'll likely lower her weapon and begin searching for less problematic prey.

Verbal assaults are so hurtful because they make you feel helpless. They're random. You can't always decode your attacker's hostility. Someone could hit you next Tuesday or next year—you can't know. What you can know is that at the first sign of warfare you'll be ready with your own bold plan of homeland defense. ●

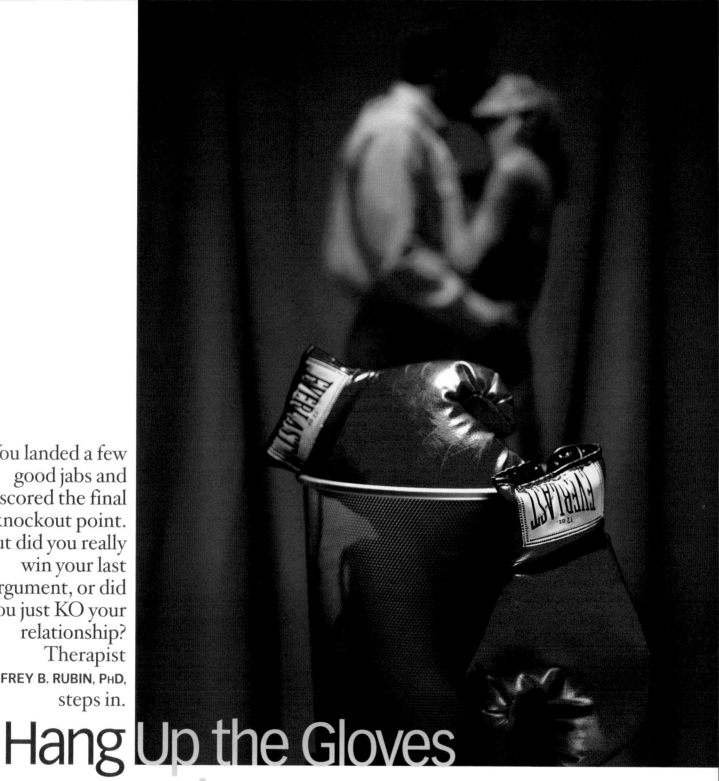

You landed a few good jabs and scored the final knockout point. But did you really win your last argument, or did you just KO your relationship? Therapist **JEFFREY B. RUBIN, PhD,** steps in.

Hang Up the Gloves

I HEARD THEM YELLING IN THE waiting room. By the time I emerged from my office to greet them several minutes later, the well-dressed couple in their early 40s were silently fuming. I introduced myself and ushered them inside. The wife, Cathy, sat on the sofa; the husband, Robert, chose a nearby chair. They glared at each other.

Stop fighting; start winning.

Without even waiting for me to ask why they'd come to see a therapist, Cathy exploded at Robert. "You're always working. You don't spend enough time at home. I feel like a work widow."

First Robert seethed, then he lit into Cathy. "Nothing is ever good enough for you," he said angrily. "I'm always working because you're always spending so much money."

She came right back at him. "At least I'm at home with the family, not married to my job. I might as well be single. In fact, I am."

"Yeah, but I'm not a critical bitch who's bankrupting the family."

It was time for me to intervene. "Throw me your wallets," I said. They looked at each other, then at me. "Hand them over."

They complied, intrigued enough to call a cease-fire. I took the wallets and put them on the ottoman at my feet. "Do you enjoy throwing your money away?" I asked.

They stared at me blankly.

"No," they both said.

"If you follow one principle—which I'll try my best to help you with—you'll save yourselves a lot of time, money, and tears," I said. "It's this: Be more interested in understanding your spouse than in winning. Otherwise, this process will take longer than it needs to, and you'll waste a lot of money trying to win. And you'll both lose. Guaranteed."

Now I had their attention.

In more than 24 years of practice, I've discovered that the biggest source of conflict for couples isn't money, sex, fidelity, child rearing, or in-laws. It's the urge to win. Wanting to win, to be right, is natural; it makes us feel strong and safe and grati-fied. It's also disastrous for a relationship. When the goal is winning instead of under-standing, partners are more likely to ig-nore, or trample, each other's feelings. That launches a spiral of escalating resent-ment and hostility leading to alienation—a troubling distance from each other that can become unbridgeable when communi-cation breaks down completely.

If the results are so dire, why do so many people continue to focus on defeat-ing their partners rather than on hearing and understanding them? For a variety of reasons. Some go for the win as a sort of preemptive strike—if they hit first, they believe on some barely conscious level that they can avoid being shamed, humiliated, or bullied. Others think that crushing their mate is the only course of action open to them—they're afraid that unless they're overpowering, they'll be overpowered; that unless they're hollering, or building an air-tight case against the other person, they won't be heard at all. They think the only available choices are conqueror or door-mat. Winning makes some people feel—for a moment—safe and triumphant, and these short-term gains fool them into thinking that they've chosen the right tac-tic. But, paradoxically, going for the win is the course of action least likely to get them what they really want.

You know you're getting stuck in this dead-end strategy when being right is more important to you than improving the rela-tionship, or when you constantly question or deny your partner's feelings and per-ceptions: One of you begins a sentence with "I feel..." and the other says, "No, you don't" or "You shouldn't." You know you're stuck when your conversations sound more like hostile debates than open-spirited col-laborations, when you regularly interrupt each other, or when, instead of listening, you mentally rehearse what you're going to say while your mate is speaking.

THE WAY TO BREAK THE cycle is by cultivating under-standing through compassion-ate listening. By that I mean hearing what your partner is really saying and feeling, instead of bracing for what you're sure he's going to say—and you're going to dismiss. In compassionate listening, also called empathetic or reflec-tive listening, you might not always agree with your partner, or enjoy hearing what he has to say, but you still strive to under-stand his logic and the deepest emotions beneath it. When each of you is committed to understanding the other's point of view, you begin to create an atmosphere of trust and safety that encourages working together to solve your problems and begins to extinguish the urge to fight.

Win-Win at Home

You can practice compassionate listening without a therapist. Remember, it takes patience; don't expect to master it immediately. Everyone values empathy, but in real life, being empathetic can seem like giving up territory. So each person waits for the other to go first, worrying, *If I empathize, you'll exploit me*. Having a set of guidelines can help end the impasse.

Set aside a block of uninterrupted time to talk on a regular basis, once or twice a week. Turn off the TV, and let the answering machine pick up calls. Lowering the lights can be helpful. Some people like to be physically close; others feel safer if they're not looking directly at each other. Speak in a heartfelt and gentle manner. Think about how to raise your concerns and needs without hurting your partner in areas where he or she is vulnerable. Instead of collecting evidence to build your case, listen deeply to what your partner is saying in an effort to find fresh solutions. If you start to feel uncontrollably angry or hurt, try shifting your attention to your breathing.

In that first session with Robert and Cathy, I explained the components of compassionate listening. I asked each of them to speak about one troubling issue, detailing their own feelings rather than attacking the other person. The listener's task would be to resist the urge to interrupt, criticize, or argue, and instead to repeat what the speaker said, including the deeper feelings beneath the content, until the speaker is satisfied that he or she has been heard. "When something your partner says triggers irritation or anger," I told them, "instead of getting emotionally hijacked by your reactions, you can do a quick exercise: Shift attention to the quality of your breathing, which may be shallow, constricted, or labored, especially if you're angry, and try elongating the exhalation." This relaxes the body and the mind just enough to short-circuit intense emotions and allow you to tune back in to what your partner is saying. Another trick for compassionate listeners who find themselves beginning to boil is to remind themselves, *I don't have to agree. I don't even have to solve this problem. All I have to do is understand what the other person is saying and feeling."* Looking into your partner's eyes can also quickly reconnect you.

Robert spoke first. He told Cathy that he was concerned about money.

"So am I," Cathy said, defensively.

"When Robert is finished, you can speak, Cathy."

"I'm scared," Robert said. "Everything feels like a house of cards."

Cathy's expression began to soften. Eager to heal the breach, obviously grasping the principle of compassionate listening and perhaps touched by the risk he just took, Cathy empathized with Robert. "You're really feeling pressure, aren't you?" she said.

"That's what I've been trying to tell you for years."

"I always felt you were attacking me," Cathy said.

"It's about me, not you," he said. "I feel fearful about money."

"I want to know what that pressure feels like for you," she said.

"I'm worried about our future," Robert said. "I feel we need to live on a smaller scale and have more of a safety net in case something happens to me. My father died at my age, you know."

Cathy was leaning toward Robert, listening intently. "I'd like to have more time with you and the kids," Robert said, "but in order to do that, I'd need to work less—and one way to make that possible is to lower our expenses."

"You're worried about our financial future. You feel great pressure, and you'd like us to spend less so you can have more time with the family," Cathy said. "Do you feel that I'm hearing you?"

"For once," Robert said.

I felt the sting of his accusation. Cathy looked as if she did, too.

"Understanding, not winning," I reminded him.

> When the goal is winning instead of **understanding,** partners are more likey to ignore, or trample, each other's feelings.

Robert took a deep breath. "Yes, I feel you heard me, Cathy. Thank you." Their small, tentative smiles gave me hope.

In the past, when Cathy and Robert argued about money, he felt she was mocking his fears. But she didn't hear fears—only attacks on her spending habits. So she'd strike back; he'd feel humiliated and he'd counterattack. Cathy, who came from a family in which her needs were often belittled or ignored, saw Robert's hostility as evidence that he didn't care about her feelings; she'd further retaliate by withdrawing or treating him with contempt, which made him feel even more humiliated, so that he said even meaner things to her.

But compassionate listening broke that cycle. Once Robert believed Cathy heard his concerns and would even help him to express his underlying anxiety, he felt more willing to acknowledge her frustrations. Cathy was able to tell Robert that she felt isolated and burdened, running the household and caring for their two children alone, unable to work more than part-time because of her responsibilities at home. As we neared the end of the session, Cathy said she felt for the first time that Robert was taking her seriously.

OVER SEVERAL SESSIONS, Cathy felt safe enough to tell Robert that she missed the self-esteem and sense of competence she'd gotten from her full-time job as a nursing administrator. And Robert was finally able to say that he feared turning out like his father, who hadn't been a great provider.

A spirit of mutual respect and cooperation replaced the bickering that had haunted their relationship. They worked hard to keep from attacking each other's tender spots when they discussed problems. And gradually, as their capacity to meet each other's needs increased, their problems shrank. When Cathy realized she was spending excessively in an attempt to make up for feeling deprived by Robert's absence, she decided, on her own, to economize. Robert realized that the family wasn't in as precarious a financial position as he'd believed. He began leaving the office earlier; he saw that he'd been working late not just because of his money worries but to avoid or punish Cathy. He moved beyond believing that it was his duty as a man to be the sole breadwinner and encouraged Cathy to go back to work. These were important subjects Robert and Cathy had stayed away from because they had no language for discussing them.

Robert and Cathy began spending more time together—walking several evenings a week after dinner and pursuing a mutual and long-neglected passion: dancing. Their practice of listening to each other brought them closer and made them stronger. Again and again, I've seen couples surmount seemingly intractable problems when they confront them cooperatively, with an urge to understand rather than defeat each other. When no one wins, both partners take the prize. ●

Dr. Phil's Six Rules of Talking and Listening

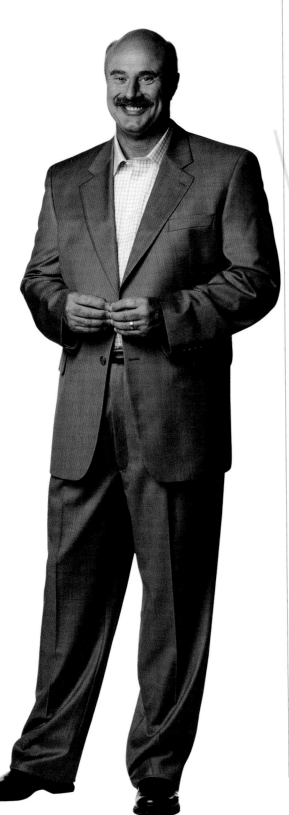

True or false: When you talk to other people, it's best to block your ears, dominate the conversation, and if they ask you what's wrong, chirp "Nothing." True!—if you want to live alone for the rest of your life. If not, **PHILLIP C. McGRAW, PhD,** has a conversation repair kit for you.

WHEN IT COMES TO RELATING TO each other, *communication* is perhaps the most overused term in our vocabulary. The problem is that most people don't really know what good communication is. But talking and listening are essential tools for learning about your partner's feelings, making your feelings known, and solving problems that arise within a relationship. As the saying goes, "It's better to light one candle than curse the darkness," so here's my attempt to shed some light on the subject and help you get better at the art of exchange.

RULE #1:
INSIST ON EMOTIONAL INTEGRITY

You gotta tell it like it is! You must insist that everything you say, imply, or insinuate is accurate, and if your partner challenges you on those messages, you must step up and own them. Mean what you say and say what you mean. You don't have to tell people everything you think or feel. But you do have to be accurate when you choose to disclose.

Suppose you're upset. When your partner senses that and asks, "Is something bothering you?" emotional integrity requires that you won't deny the message you're sending verbally or otherwise by saying, "Nothing is wrong; I'm fine." You may not be ready to discuss it, so the accurate answer might be, "I don't want to tell you right now; I'm just not ready to talk about it."

A lot of couples flagrantly violate this principle. Then they say, "We have trouble communicating." Of course they do—they both lie like dogs! And while we're on the subject: A material omission—leaving out something of crucial importance—is as much a lie as any actual misstatement.

RULE #2:
BE A TWO-WAY, NOT A ONE-WAY, COMMUNICATOR

A one-way communicator talks but never listens and pays no attention to whether the listener appears to be "getting it." You know what I mean. For her it's all about the telling, as in, "All right. What I want you to do is go out there, get this work done, give these people this message, put those kids to bed, and come back in here."

If that's how you communicate, all you know is what you've said, and you haven't got a clue about what the other person heard. Result: conflict.

But as soon as a one-way communicator asks for feedback, look what happens:

She: "Here's what I'd like you to do: A, B, C, and D. Does that sound okay to you?"

He: "Well, L, Q, R, and P don't make a whole lot of sense to me."

No wonder they're not getting along—they're not even talking about the same thing! When she checks to make sure that he has received the message, she uncovers a communication glitch. By soliciting feedback—by giving just as much weight to what is heard as to what is said—you put a spotlight on the issues the two of you, together, need to clarify.

RULE #3:
ESTABLISH A MOTIVE

Whether you're talking or listening, you need to be clear about why something's being said. Motive and message are important. If you've got a husband who says, "You're like the Spanish Inquisition. You're always asking me these questions and bugging me all the time," you need to look at what's behind those words. Is he trying to make you feel guilty because there's something he doesn't want you to see? Or are you trying to control too much of his life because you are insecure? In answering those questions, you'll figure out the motive and be able to move on from there.

RULE #4:
CHECK IN WITH EACH OTHER

You and your partner must agree to test each other's messages and respond honestly. No more b.s. Ask your partner, "Is what you're saying really the way you feel? Is that true?" Remember that when you ask the question, you have to be ready to hear the true answer. And you've got to be willing to take the same test yourself. If asked, "So you're really okay?" have the guts to say, "No, I'm not," when you're really not. Ask your partner the questions that will confirm his or her feelings.

RULE #5:
BE AN ACTIVE LISTENER

Most people are passive listeners. If you intend to become an active listener, you'll need to master two important tools. A famous psychologist named Carl Rogers called them Reflection of Content and Reflection of Feeling. I don't agree with a lot of what Rogers taught, but he hit the nail on the head with this one.

Reflecting a speaker's content means that you listen to the person; then you give him or her feedback that makes it clear you're receiving the factual message—but as you'll see, it ain't all about the facts. Here's an example of someone's getting the information but missing the message:

A: "Sorry I'm late. As I was leaving the house, my dog ran into the street and was hit by a car."

B (*reflecting the content*): "So your dog got hit by a car?"

A: "Right."

B: "Is he dead?"

A: "Uh-huh."

B: "So what did you do with the dog's body?"

Person B establishes that Person A has been heard, which addresses a fundamental need for A. But B has clearly missed the point. To be an active listener in an emotionally relevant situation, B has to do more than just reflect the factual information that A has conveyed. Reflection of feeling tells your partner not just that he's been heard but that you have "plugged into" his life and experienced it in some way, which is essential to his satisfaction. Reflection of feeling sounds like this:

A: "Sorry I'm late. As I was leaving the house, my dog ran into the street and got hit by a car."

B (*reflecting the feeling*): "Oh, my gosh—you must feel terrible."

A: "Well, I do. We'd had the dog for 12 years, and my kids really loved him."

B: "I'm sure they must be so upset; I'm sorry you're going through this."

Being able to reflect the feeling, not just the content, is essential to the success of your communication.

RULE #6:
EVALUATE YOUR FILTERS

When you and I engage in conversation, I can't control how well you communicate; I can only control how well I receive what you're telling me. I can go on the alert to things that may distort the messages you're sending me—I call them filters. To be a good listener, you've got to know what your filters are. Maybe you're coming into a given conversation with an agenda. Maybe you're judging the speaker and don't trust him at all. Maybe you're angry. Any one of these psychological filters can dramatically distort what you hear.

Filters cause you to decide things ahead of time. You may have prejudged your partner and decided that he's a hound dog, that he doesn't love you anymore. Result: No matter what he says to you, you're going to distort it to conform to what you're already thinking, feeling, and believing.

Take an inventory of your filters. If you're not aware of them, you can defeat the best communicator in the world because you'll distort the message, regardless of how well it was sent. ●

Talking Cures: A Crib Sheet

▶ **CHOOSE THE RIGHT COMMUNICATION ENVIRONMENT.** When the subject matter is weighty and emotionally charged, find a place where you won't be distracted and can devote yourself entirely to talking and listening.

▶ **PICK YOUR BATTLES.** People's willingness to listen goes down dramatically after the first criticism in a conversation. With each successive criticism, their defensiveness goes up and their receptivity goes down. By the third criticism, you might as well be talking to yourself. Don't wander into saying, "And it also really bothers me that…" If there's something you need to address, stick with that point and deal with other issues another time.

▶ **BEWARE OF UNDOING.** People will ratchet up their courage to say something extremely important, then sabotage their own communication by waffling. "You know, I think you're really mean and hurtful…and I know I probably bring that out in you." No; don't apologize for your real feelings. Deliver your message. Own it. Then stay with it.

▶ **MAKE USE OF "MINIMAL ENCOURAGERS" TO LET YOUR PARTNER KNOW HE IS BEING HEARD.** Minimal encouragers are the very least you must express to make sure the speaker knows you're listening to him. They are very simple: Make eye contact, nod your head, say things like, "Uh-huh; right; gotcha." What that says to the other person is "All right. I hear you. Keep going." Let him know that he's not speaking Greek to you.

▶ **DON'T DISGUISE YOUR FEELINGS IN A QUESTION.** "Are you going out with your buddies this Friday—*again?*" Really, what you're trying to say is that you want to spend more time with your partner. When your message is true, the response will be, too.

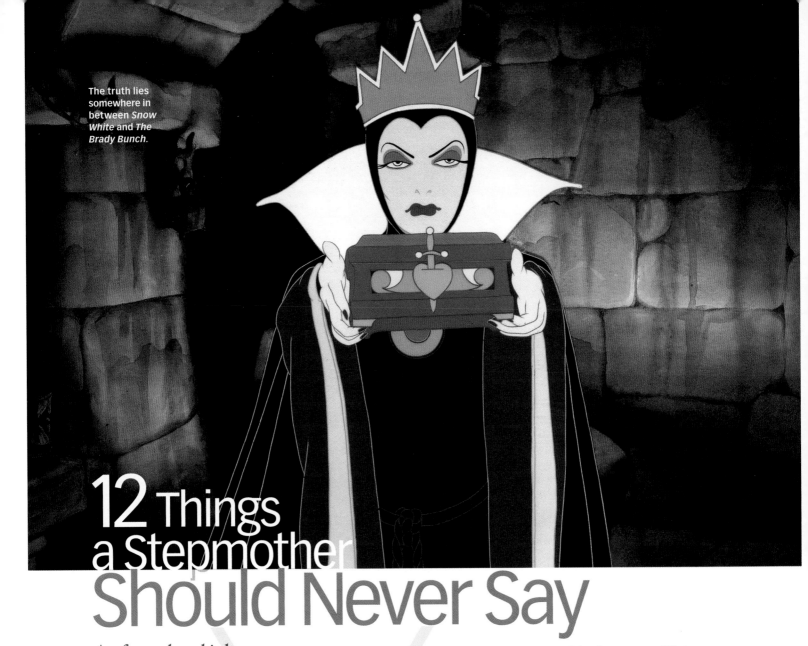

The truth lies somewhere in between *Snow White* and *The Brady Bunch*.

12 Things a Stepmother Should Never Say

As far as hard jobs go, it's up there with air-traffic controller and crane operator. Stepmothers preside over a minefield of hidden hurts, half-concealed traditions, and occasional tugs-of-war. Want the job? **ROSEMARY ROGERS** shows you around.

YOU SEE THEM AT THE MOVIES, visiting the zoo, and in restaurants. The stepmom is wearing a frozen, feeble smile and is a tad (sometimes a big tad) too young to be their mother, Dad is trying hard to please everyone, and the children are, well, distant. Actually, *hostile* is a better word. The stepmother hasn't felt this unpopular since her worst year of junior high: No mother-in-law—no prison matron, for that matter—could be as critical of her as other people's kids.

It's been said that parenting is the toughest job in the world. Wrong. It's the second toughest: Stepparenting wins hands down. Right now, approximately half of all Americans live in a stepfamily, which means that every day, millions of women are subject to the taunt—sometimes mournful, often angry—"*You're* not my mother!"

I've been a stepmother three times, starting at age 25, and now have two sets of stepgrandchildren. I know, from hard-won experience, that a great relationship with your stepkids is possible. Despite their occasional resemblance to feral little beasts, these are children who've been traumatized and had the bottom drop out of their lives. You didn't make them, didn't break them, and probably can't fix them—but they're kids you can grow to love and who will love you back. And if you avoid certain trapdoors like the 12 verboten phrases here, you'll not only get along but you'll never have to ask them to pick up their socks.

1. "Go ahead, call me Mom!" You're not their mother and you never will be. They're conflicted enough, and pushing them to use a mom-name will only confuse them more.
Corollary: "We're going to be one big, happy family!"

You might eventually become the happiest of stepfamilies, but it won't happen overnight. Studies show the new family dynamic takes at least three years to fall into place, and the first year is the toughest.

2. "Feel free! Do whatever you want." Almost as much as they need love, children need boundaries and are adrift without rules. Learn to say (not scream, please) the following phrase: "In this house, we..." so that time together will not be bogged down with endless negotiations.
Corollary: "Let's get down!"

No matter how close in age you are to your stepchildren, you're still a parent figure; try to be an example of mature living and not one of the gang. This is especially true if your stepkids belong to that group of psychotics euphemistically known as teenagers. Chances are they won't think you're cool for very long.

3. "I'll get it," "I'll drive," "I'll wash it," "Forget about me," etc. Don't let your stepkids (or their father) turn you into the creature everyone in the world resents: a martyr. Martyrs make people feel creepy and guilty, and when kids feel that way, they generally act out. You're better off being wicked.

4. "Why the long face?" Your stepchildren are allowed to be sad—they're in mourning. Let them grieve if and when they feel like it. Sorry, but they probably will grieve more around you, since you're the evidence that their parents are never getting back together. Don't call attention to their sorrow; remove yourself, and get Dad to be a mom at this point. Their depression will pass—they're kids.

5. "Your dad and I always..." Don't allude to the great times you have with their father when they're not around. They

already feel left out and probably imagine the two of you tossing your heads back laughing, spending wads of money, and throwing Ring Ding wrappers on the floor (not to mention the sexual fantasies going on in their fevered little brains). If you want to give them a positive image of a loving couple, just be a loving couple.

6. "Did your mother bring you up to do that?" Never bad-mouth the ex—and your husband (or partner) shouldn't either, even if the fur is still flying. Studies show that it's the ongoing conflict after divorce that hurts kids the most.
Corollary: "How could you have married such an idiot?"

Don't stand next to him when he's on the phone with his ex, making faces and sticking your finger down your throat. Don't write her letters or e-mails, and if she's a crank caller, get caller ID. Fighting about the ex—call it the ex hex—is the equivalent of having a stink bomb thrown into your marriage.

7. "Have you always done that?" Families have traditions that are meaningful to them. So if your husband and his children insist on watching *Hogan's Heroes* reruns, putting mayo on hot dogs, collecting rubber bands, or anything else you find distasteful, just keep your mouth shut.

8. "Your room is a pigsty!" Something's got to give, and neatness should be it. If the situation is desperate and the kids are growing subspecies in their space, get Dad to go in there and organize a cleanup. Life is messy, and it's even messier

> Your stepchildren are jealous of you. But admit it, you're jealous of them, too. If you make it a battlefield, **this is a battle you'll lose.**

when you choose a man with children. But remember: It's better to have a man with kids than one without kids who flosses his cat's teeth.

9. "Well, *my* kids and I..." If you have kids of your own who live with you and your husband, your stepkids may feel like they're getting the fuzzy end of the lollipop. Mentioning trips, restaurants, and the fun stuff you did the weekend they were with their mom feeds the illusion that your children are getting more. Be clear that there are no favorites and everything is even between both sets of kids.

10. "What's the matter, never heard of *thank you*?" Don't become a stepparent expecting gratitude. (Don't become a parent expecting it, either.) While you shouldn't tolerate rudeness, choose your battles carefully. Kids generally don't have the best manners; they get preoccupied and forgo social niceties. Don't be petulant; you're the grown-up.

11. "We're not made of money, you know." Their father's primary motivation is guilt. (Come to think of it, that's his secondary one as well.) Dad is guilty, the ex is angry, the battle is on, and money is the weapon. Stay out of the fight, work out a family budget, and don't discuss finances in front of the children.

12. "It's them or me." It will always have to be them. Your stepchildren are jealous of you. But admit it, you're jealous of them, too. If you make it a battlefield, this is a battle you'll lose.
Corollary: "Wake me when it's over."

Rather than enduring the time you spend with his kids, enjoy it. Tell knock-knock jokes, bake cookies, make dioramas—do anything other than withdraw and watch the clock until they leave. They're never really going to go away, even if you stay under the radar. Intimacy may be a long time coming, but, like so many other situations in life, you've just got to put in the time. Granted, it's a complicated dynamic, but the Beatles were right: *The love you make is equal to the love you take.* Or is it the other way around? ●

If the words *I'm sorry* ever stick in your throat, maybe you don't realize how good you're going to feel afterward—oh, yeah, and the other person, too.

MARTHA BECK

puts you on the road to contrition.

Always Apologize, Always Explain

"That's the dumbest thing I ever heard."

I WAS A MERE CHILD WHEN THE CLASSIC teargusher *Love Story* hit theaters in 1970, but I wept along with the adult audience as the dying Ali MacGraw told the darling Ryan O'Neal, "Love means never having to say you're sorry." Two years later, I saw another movie, *What's Up, Doc?,* in which Barbra Streisand's character repeated the very same line to the very same actor. This time, however, O'Neal had an answer. "That's the dumbest thing I ever heard," he said.

For me, that was a lightbulb moment. I'd been swept along by the romance of *Love Story,* but even as I'd watched it, I'd felt an uncomfortable tickle in my brain. Young as I was (practically fetal, I swear),

If only *Love Story*—starring Ryan O'Neal and Ali MacGraw— had been smarter.

something was telling me that real lovers say they're sorry quite often. Sincerely. Fervently, even. This is not because dismal feelings like shame and regret are necessary components of a relationship, but because without apology no relationship would be free of them. Everyone does things that bother or hurt others; a bit of inconvenient procrastination will do it, or a grumpy comment made in a stressful moment. When we lack the ability to say we're sorry, minor offenses eventually accumulate enough weight to sink any relationship. But the simple act of apologizing can reestablish goodwill even when our sins are much, much graver. Of course, it must be done right. A lame, badly constructed apology can do more damage than the original offense. Fortunately, the art of effective apology is simple, and mastering it can mean a lifetime of solid, resilient relationships.

WHEN TO APOLOGIZE

I've heard many clients discuss and anticipate the "perfect moment" for an apology, claiming that premature contrition would just be too darn hard on the person they've wronged. Here's what I think: The perfect moment to apologize is the moment you realize you've done something wrong.

This seems obvious when we're contemplating somebody else's sins, but in the harsh light of our own guilt, we often try to protect ourselves from shame or censure by waiting for the heat to blow over. We may try to postpone apologizing or avoid it altogether by lying, blaming others, making excuses, or justifying our actions. The impulse to go into such a stall is a big ol' signal. When you really don't want to say you're sorry, it's almost certainly time to do so.

On the other hand, you may be one of those people who apologize when they haven't done anything wrong. This is as false as failing to say you're sorry when cir-

Here's what I think: The perfect moment to apologize is the moment you realize you've done something wrong.

cumstances warrant it. If you frequently apologize for other people's bad moods, the limits of your own energy, Grandpa's political views, the existence of swine flu, and so on, it's time to stop. This kind of pseudo-apology may ease awkward conversations, but it's a form of crying wolf— it distracts attention from real issues and weakens meaningful apologies when the time for them arrives.

HOW TO APOLOGIZE

Apologizing is rarely comfortable or easy, so if you're going to do it at all, make it count. Aaron Lazare, MD, a psychiatrist and dean of the University of Massachusetts Medical School, has spent years studying acts of contrition in every context, from interpersonal to international. He has found that, to be effective, most apologies need to contain the following elements: (1) full acknowledgment of the offense, (2) an explanation, (3) genuine expression of remorse, and (4) reparations for damage. Here are some guidelines that may help you get the details right.

Acknowledge the offense.

Failing to fully acknowledge all aspects of an offense, says Lazare, is the most common mistake of ineffective penitents. If the time has come to eat crow, it won't work to nibble daintily on a drumstick; you have to eat the whole damn bird—claws, beak, and all.

Start by describing exactly what you did wrong, without avoiding the worst truths. Be blunt. Use accurate language. If you lied like a rug on your Match.com profile, your blind date won't be impressed when you admit to "fibbing." If you totaled a friend's car, saying you "dinged" it will just make things worse. Don't tell your Jenny Craig counselor you ate "some" cake if the truth is that you ate a whole cake.

Once the facts are out, acknowledge that your behavior violated a moral code, the unspoken social contract that allows human beings to trust one another. It doesn't matter whether you and the person you've hurt share the same ethics: If you've broken your own rules, you're in the wrong. Accept responsibility. Even if this can't put things right, it will stop them from being put wrong.

Effective acknowledgment:
"I did some tricky footwork in the stock market and ended up bankrupting some of the 'little people' who owned company stocks. I helped cause enormous suffering."

Ineffective acknowledgment:
"Okay, maybe I fudged a little financially."

SECOND:
Explain your actions.

Once you've confessed your errors, the person you've hurt will probably want to know why you committed them. A truthful explanation is your best shot at rebuilding a strong, peaceful relationship. At the very least, it will give your erstwhile victim some understanding and peace of mind. You may have to examine yourself closely to figure out the real explanation for your misdeeds. The core-deep explanation for your behavior is your key to changing for the better.

At this stage, beware crossing the line between explaining your actions and falling into a victim's whine. If you're blaming your parents or the manufacturers of Twinkies every time you swat at your parakeet, stop reading self-help books and memorize this instead: *Explanations good; excuses bad.* Explanations help you and your victim understand why you misbehaved and assure both of you that the offense won't recur. Excuses merely deflect responsibility. Leave them out of your apology.

Effective explanation:
"I mistreated prisoners because I'm basically angry and self-loathing, and I got high on having the power to control and humiliate someone who couldn't fight back."

Ineffective explanation:
"Everybody did it. I was just following orders."

THIRD:
Express remorse.

"If the victim does not perceive the party who is apologizing as remorseful," says Lazare, "the apology may have little meaning." Anyone who has been on the receiving end of the comment "I'm sorry you feel that way" knows the difference between sincere regret and an attempt to avoid responsibility for bad behavior. Few things are less likely to evoke forgiveness than apology without remorse.

For example, in 2003, MSNBC fired talk-show host Michael Savage for telling a gay caller, "You should only get AIDS and die, you pig." In his swan song apology, Savage said, "If my comments brought pain to anyone, I certainly did not intend for this to happen and apologize for any such reaction." Oh, I get it—Savage loves pigs, and meant "get AIDS and die" in a gentle, lov-

ing way. This little two-step ("I'm sorry for your reaction to my behavior") deftly removes blame from the guilty party and drapes it over the victim. For the apologizer, this feels much nicer than genuine remorse. Unfortunately, it leaves the offended party feeling more offended than ever—and rightly so.

Effective expression of remorse:
"I'm sorry I hurt you."

Ineffective expression of remorse:
"I'm sorry you felt hurt."

> An apology means real repair work: not just saying "I'm sorry" but rebuilding the neighbor's gazebo after that unfortunate experiment with the blowtorch.

FOURTH:
Make reparations.

"Okay, I said I'm sorry. What else do you want me to do?" This is often said by offenders who want their victims to move on, stop harping, get over it already! But if we want to tap the healing power of apology, we'll ask the familiar question in an unfamiliar way—as the first step toward reparation. An apology includes real repair work: not just saying "I'm sorry" but returning that pilfered sweater, going to

AA meetings, rebuilding the neighbor's gazebo after that unfortunate experiment with the blowtorch.

Often there will be nothing tangible to repair; hearts and relationships are broken more often than physical objects. In such cases, your efforts should focus on restoring the other person's dignity. The question "What else do you want me to do?" can start this process. If you ask it sincerely, really listen to the answer, and act on the other party's suggestions, you'll be honoring their feelings, perspective, and experience. The knowledge that one is heard and valued has incredible healing power; it can mend even seemingly irreparable wounds.

Effective reparation:
"What can I do to make things right between us? I'm completely committed to making it happen."

Ineffective reparation:
"Here's 50 bucks. Now shut up."

AFTER APOLOGIZING
When you really apologize, you should feel good about yourself. An effective apology is, as Lazare puts it, "an act of honesty, an act of humility, an act of commitment, an act of generosity, and an act of courage." But there's no guarantee that the other person involved will share your warm fuzzies. The final gallant act of apology is to release your former victim from any expectation of forgiveness. No matter how noble you have been, he will forgive—or refuse to forgive—on his own terms. That is his right.

Anne Lamott refers to forgiveness as "giving up all hope of having had a different past." The same words apply to apologizing. An apology is the end of our struggle with history, the act by which we untangle from our past by accepting what it actually was. From this truthful place we are free to move forward, whether or not we are forgiven. Apologizing doesn't make us perfect, but it shows our commitment to be honest about our imperfections and steadfast in our efforts to do better. It reminds us of what Ali MacGraw's *Love Story* character died too young to learn: that love means always being willing to say you're sorry. ●

O
Family

make your own mother

mother

You can custom-order bouquets of tiger lilies, the perfect pink paint, and every pizza under the sun. So why not the mother you've always wanted? Martha Beck on why—where the maternal is concerned—a mosaic of mothers is the way to go.

"WE ALL HAVE OUR LITTLE SORROWS," WROTE screenwriter Ronald Harwood, "and the littler you are, the larger the sorrow." Anyone who's ever felt like a motherless child—or an inadequately mothered adult— knows what he meant. It is when we are littlest that our needs are greatest, and consequently some of the greatest sorrows we'll ever experience come from our mothers. Unfortunately, motherhood is so difficult that virtually no one does it perfectly, and some parents are spectacular failures. Maybe your mother was flawless, but it's more likely she made mistakes. Perhaps she was occasionally impatient, unappreciative of the creativity you displayed by drawing that indelible Magic Marker mural on her kitchen cabinets. Maybe she was distracted by other concerns: finances, illness, alcoholism, frequent prison sentences. Whatever her errors, to the extent that your mother was not perfect, you inherited a legacy of sorrow. You may feel this as a subtle hankering, or as an emotional abyss that yawns within you like the death of hope. Either way, you can and should find a way to heal what psychologists call the mother wound. My favorite strategy for this is to stop focusing fruitless hope and blame on the woman who raised you, and make yourself another mother.

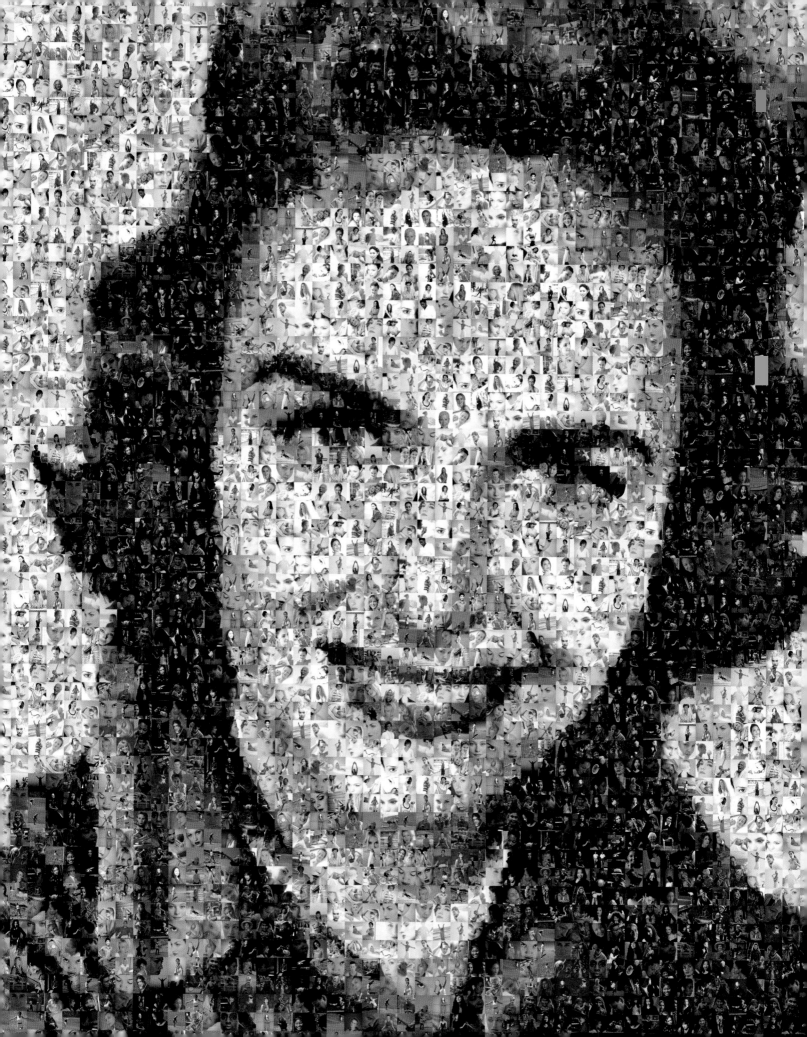

The way to go about this is to reconstruct your "maternal introject"; in other words, the image of "mother" you carry in your heart and mind. This internalized mother is based on your actual caretaker, and it continues to dominate your life even if your real parents are long gone. If your flesh-and-blood mother loved you unconditionally, your maternal introject will allow you to treat yourself compassionately forever. If your mother called you fathead and used you to extinguish cigarette butts, you're likely to keep hating and punishing yourself until you evict that shrewish mind-mother and replace her with a more sympathetic model. To do this, you must find real people who can model the behavior you wish you had found in your biological mom, then deliberately soak up the lessons they have to teach you. Here's the process my clients and I have used to make some of the most wonderful mind-mothers imaginable.

> If your image of mother is restricted to one mortal woman, it will inevitably prove insufficient to guide and comfort you through all of life's storms.

STEP ONE: THINK OF *MOTHER* AS A VERB

If your image of mother is restricted to one mortal woman, it will inevitably prove insufficient to guide and comfort you through all of life's storms. Thinking of the word *mother* not as a noun but as a verb ("to mother") helps change your internal definitions so that you stop looking to a human female for perfect parenting and begin to identify your mother as anyone who offers you maternal care. You're being mothered when anyone—I said *anyone*—offers you one or more of the following gifts:

Acceptance. This is not the anxious adoration of a mother who pins her hopes for happiness on her child's appearance or achievements. True mothering starts with unconditional love for another person, without demands or expectations.
Nourishment. Sustenance, comfort, and care, whether physical or emotional, are components of real motherhood. Anyone who nurtures you, in body, mind, or heart, is mothering you.
Instruction. Real mothers teach constantly, showing both by example and by explanation what their children must know in order to live well.
Empowerment. Real mothers are intent on working themselves out of a job, by building in those they mother the courage and confidence needed to become completely independent.

STEP TWO: MEET YOUR MOTHERLESS SELF

Once you've detached your concept of motherhood from a particular human being and learned to see mothering as a gift of love and strength, it's time to assess where you could use more mothering. Complete these sentences with whatever comes to mind:

I feel useless, unlovable, and disgusting when

_____ .

I feel empty and needy when

_____ .

I feel stupid and ignorant when

_____ .

I feel helpless and incapable when

_____ .

If none of these feelings are familiar to you, it's a sure sign that you've been very well mothered, by either your biological mom or an excellent substitute. But if the sentences above sparked clear associations ("I feel like a stupid, ignorant moron in board meetings," "I get incredibly needy around the holidays"), you owe it to yourself to find the kind of maternal love that can nurture your unmet needs. It's time to make yourself a patchwork mom.

STEP THREE: PATCH TOGETHER YOUR IDEAL MOTHER

After identifying the situations where you need more mothering, commit to finding people who can offer you acceptance, nourishment, instruction, and empowerment in those areas. If you think your biological mother is up to the task, great—go to her and ask for help and advice. But if your mom can't or won't provide it, open yourself to finding someone who can.

For example, because my mother never worked outside the home, she couldn't teach me much about combining child rearing with a career. That's okay, because as I embarked on this difficult process, I got a great deal on a rent-a-mom: a wonderful therapist who'd put herself through graduate school while raising five children. I grilled this poor woman endlessly about her methods of juggling personal life and professional life. Gradually, her answers made their way into the maternal introject I carry in my unconscious mind, and they remain there to this day.

I've helped scores of clients identify individuals who could mother them through various life dilemmas. If a client needs a verbose but committed cheerleader, I'm happy to become that part of her patchwork mom. But many people require mothering I can't give: someone to help them raise an autistic child, endure chemotherapy, cook kick-ass chili, or master infinite other challenges. Amazingly, once a client identifies a mother-need, someone always seems to show up to fill it. Within weeks—or at most a couple of months—each client encounters a person whose gifts of love and teaching can be sewn into the blank space that once marred the patchwork of the internalized mother.

I know this process works because of my own experience, as well as by observation. Whenever I feel uncertain, inept, or desperate, I begin looking for a mother to teach and encourage me. So far, every search has paid off. Sometimes I learn a few key lessons from a person who then leaves my life, but many of the people who contributed to my patchwork mother are continuing presences. Each one gives me something unique: Karen is so giving she'd do virtually anything to facilitate my happiness, and so accepting she'd be sincerely proud of me if I robbed a bank. Annette coaches my writing and spoils my kids like an indulgent grandma. Brilliant, kind Betsy shows me all sorts of professional and personal ropes. Lisa is the creative genius who gives me permission to have wild ideas. Every one of these women is my mother.

Once you begin to think this way, you'll find that mothers show up in forms you might never have expected. Some of my best mothering has come from men, like John, who would protect me to his last breath, or Roger, the massage therapist who cares for my body when it aches from a sleepless night or a hard workout. And then there are my "paper mothers," books that read like love letters written specifically to me, even though I will never meet the authors. Or, when words won't do and simple physical contact is all I need, there's my pathologically cuddly beagle, who has no line items on his to-do list other than snuggling, breathing, and loving.

When I look over my list, when I consider the phenomenal collection of beings who abide in the part of my heart labeled MOTHER, I can't imagine anyone in the world will ever be as well mothered as I am—that is, unless you want to try making your own patchwork maternal introject. The perfect mother is available to all of us if we're willing to let go of expectations that will never be filled, and to see what is being offered to us here and now. Though all mothers are limited, the force of motherhood is not. It surrounds us every day, in all sorts of guises, some predictable and ordinary, some startling and extraordinary. If you allow yourself to embrace it, I guarantee you'll find it waiting to embrace you. And that, to me, is the mother of all comforts. ●

how not to turn into your mother

Grant us the serenity to avoid using checks with seagulls on them, the courage to bypass poodle-shaped oven mitts, and the wisdom to know the difference between our mothers and ourselves. Suzanne Finnamore points the way.

As far back as I can remember, my parents and teachers told me that when I grew up, I could be anything I wanted to be. It was the 1960s; small girls were told this, amid a paradoxical sea of pink plastic kitchenettes and Barbie lunchboxes. What I was not told is the inevitable second half of that statement, which is: And then you will become your mother.

There are certainly far worse fates than becoming my mother. To begin with, she is that most capable and noble of all beings: a good mother, something I aspire to be. I have always adored her, except for a fleeting five-year period following my adolescence that hardly bears mentioning. She raised my brother and me single-handedly after my father left; she never faltered, even managing a kind of cheerfulness. She had only one rule: The first half hour after she came home from work, no one was to ask her for anything. Easing her shoes off as she walked in the door from her secretarial job at Heald business college, she would light up a Salem (again, the '60s) and drink one Harvey Wallbanger on the rocks—made with vodka, orange juice, and Galliano—in a chilled beer stein. She is droll, my mother. All the men in my life have kept in touch with her, as they would a particularly lovely ex-wife.

That said, I do not have an overwhelming desire to become my mother, in the same way that although I admire Cher, I do not wish to actually be Cher. I especially object to the insidious and almost supernatural way this daughter-to-mother evolution happens.

It begins slowly. Traveling with tiny sewing kits. Carrying extra hosiery "just in case." Rearranging furniture at 11:30 at night. Using your mother's catchphrases with your own children, in the exact tone your mother used and that once threw chills down your spine.

I remember the moment I knew it had finally come for me. It was last year, December 26, and I was shopping for Christmas ornaments, 75 percent off. I looked at the shopper next to me, a woman roughly my age. "This is it," I said. "I've become my mother."

Precautions may be in vain, yet I feel we must strive to resist this metamorphosis, in the same way we must spend two hours in line at airport security checkpoints, even though we are told explicitly that this will not ensure security of any kind.

Some simple strategies:
1. Never send a very helpful newspaper article to anyone.
2. Never avoid freeways because *you know a way.*
3. Never place your toilet paper in anything that could be construed as a "toilet paper holder." If it is crocheted or shaped like a poodle, you may as well surrender; it is too late for you.
4. Never block a sweater.
5. Never carry an umbrella in the car.
6. Never look back and describe a liaison with an extremely dashing man as the One Who Got Away. (All mothers have one; see that you don't.)
7. Never break in new shoes.
8. Never pack sensibly for a trip.
9. Never collect plastic bags.
10. Never have more than four refrigerator magnets. Those that double as picture frames or are cunningly shaped like frying pans with teensy eggs are lethal. Look at your mother's refrigerator. Now compare it to your own. Take time to grieve.

It's a slippery slope, my friend. Be vigilant. It may help to remember that no matter how nonchalant she appears, your mother is waiting for you to become her. She deserves flowers once a year, but she does not deserve this final victory. Not yet, not today. I'm going to the beach now, without a sweater, a hat, or a towel; I may even hitchhike. I suggest you do the same.

ask your mother to tell you a **story**

Sometimes our mothers have histories and inner lives that we can't even begin to imagine. With one quiet reminiscence, M.J. Rose's mother untangled all her daughter's confusion.

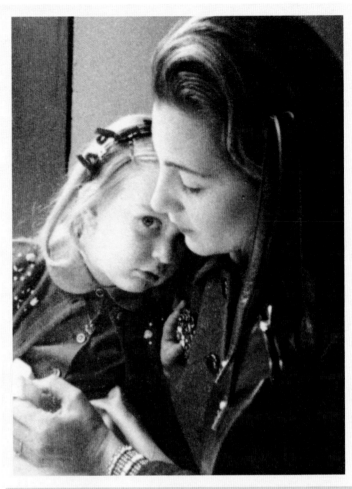

MY MOTHER'S VOICE LULLS ME, AS IT ALWAYS HAS WHEN SHE tells me a story. Her fingertips play with a lock of my hair. I close my eyes, and the familiar scent of her Shalimar comforts me. I might be six years old, lying in bed, waiting to hear how the tale is going to end, but I'm not. I'm 41 and she is 67.

This is a story she's never told me before. And hearing it now will change my life.

We're traveling from New York to Washington by train to see the

Vermeer show at the National Gallery. Somewhere just past Philadelphia, we lapse into reminiscing about the long train trips we took to Miami when I was much younger. "At night, I'd stare out the window and watch the lights streak by and be so happy listening to you tell me bedtime stories," I say.

Then, without knowing why, I ask her to tell me a story again: "There must be one you wanted to tell me but I wasn't old enough to hear."

So while the scenery whizzes by, my mother begins to talk about her childhood.

Her parents divorced in 1929, when she was a toddler. Three generations of her father's family lived in a big house in Brooklyn, and that was where she went to live.

Even today, for a father to get custody of a 2-year-old girl is unusual. In 1929 it was almost unheard of. "They told me it was because of the Depression. Since both my parents had to work, there would be more family to take care of me in my grandparents' house," she says.

I already know this—the amicable divorce is part of the family history, as is the fact of my mother's being raised by aunts and uncles, grandparents and cousins. But until now, I've never heard the rest: "Every Saturday my mother was supposed to come get me so we could spend the weekend together," she says. "I'd get up early and be dressed and ready hours before it was time."

My mother looks out the window so I can't see her face, but her voice is breaking. "Then I'd wait for your grandmother. But she hardly ever came. Those awful Saturdays would end with one of my aunts coming outside to sit with me on the steps, trying to distract me with cookies or the promise of a movie later on," she says. "I never really believed my mother wasn't coming until I'd see my dress-up skirt and blouse hanging in my closet again. There was nothing to do but start counting the days till the next weekend when, I was sure, she'd come."

I picture the 5-year-old, 6-year-old, 8-year-old, waiting.

"Did you cry?" I ask.

"No."

I am crying.

My mother might be in her late 60s, but her laugh is a young woman's. "Obviously, I got over it," she says, trying to make me feel better.

Yes, she did get over it, in a way. She grew up, went to college, worked, married, and had two daughters. And, at least from the outside looking in, she managed to establish a fine adult relationship with the mother who had all but abandoned her as a child. But underneath the facade are cracks that never have been filled.

Suddenly, all the excessive gifts my grandmother and her second husband shower on my mother, my sister, and me

My mother craved a connection that eluded her for her entire childhood. That experience shaped her—and me.

every Christmas make sense. And something else begins to make sense, too. My whole life, I've struggled with a fear of abandonment that I've never understood. As a child, if my parents were even five minutes late picking me up from a friend's house, I panicked. When I went off to summer camp, I needed to call my parents more often than the other kids did, and if my folks weren't home when I phoned, I worried incessantly. My need to touch base continued through college and beyond. I was more than capable of having a life of my own—but I was tethered to my parents in a way that few of my friends were, and that felt excessive.

The fear of losing those I loved sent me searching for a therapist, but I was never able to shake my abandonment anxiety.

Until, on the train, listening to my mother tell me about her own mother abandoning her, something clicks.

My mother craved a connection that had eluded her for her entire childhood. That experience shaped her—and me. In her overzealousness to be the mother she'd never had, she transferred her anxiety and I absorbed it. Being abandoned had been so traumatic for my mother that she over-compensated, and it backfired. She was always there, and that made me fear her leaving. She loved me too much.

After our trip, back in therapy for a short time, I finally understand what I've always thought of as an irrational fear. At last I can start to overcome it.

Our mothers hide many facets of their lives from us. We don't get to know them as children, girlfriends, lovers, or wives. They try to protect us, especially from themselves. But we still absorb their attitudes about relationships, femininity, and their bodies without knowing it. We can— as other daughters have told me—inherit propensities for adultery, substance abuse, and stubborn neuroses that we can manage better once we see their origins.

Understanding that our mothers have far more complex inner lives and histories than we imagined as children can help us understand our own inner lives. As adult daughters, we need to invite our mothers to share the stories that felt too intimate to reveal before.

In the context of "What haven't you ever told me?" my mother introduced me to a sad little girl named Jackye who held the missing piece of my emotional puzzle. I also learned something important about the person who became my mother.

And for me, that's a happy ending. ●

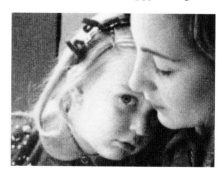

Thought this might interest you?!

Your mother sends you articles about local bear sightings and premature quintuplets. Your father mails bulletins on faulty toaster ovens and the cost of home heating. **JULIE KLAM** and **JANCEE DUNN** examine the dear, perplexing phenomenon of the family clipping service.

IT USUALLY STARTS WHEN YOUR PARENTS retire. The clippings arrive in the mail—articles about 401(k)s, the dangers of Botox, the energy rating of your air conditioner. These well-meaning bulletins, carefully cut from newspapers and magazines, often have a note from your mother or father scrawled across the top, saying "Just in case" or "Worth a look." The further you find yourself removed from your parents' care—both chronologically and geographically—the faster the notes pour in, and what starts as a trickle becomes a flood when you reach your 30s. By then, of course, you actually are interested in clutter-busting hints and how to prevent bone loss. All of our friends have a story: One receives clippings from her in-laws culled from *The New York Times*—the very paper where she works as a senior editor. Adam, a screenwriter, gets dispatches from his father on health issues with comments written on the top: "If you don't take potassium supplements," his dad jotted on one, "you are only fooling yourself."

In our informal survey, the clippings break down into just a few categories:

MEDICAL FEARMONGERING These articles feature an unlikely but potentially fatal risk, like "Gum Disease: The Silent Killer," "The Perils of Throw Rugs," or "What You Don't Know About Pâté." Lisa, a pharmaceutical salesperson, was puzzled when she received a note in the mail titled "Hepatitis: The Insidious Spread of a Killer Virus." "In case you're thinking about getting a tattoo," wrote her mother on the top. (Lisa hadn't ever contemplated any form of body art.) Our friend Erica, a nurse from Chicago, remembers, "One time my mother sent my husband a clipping about tea tree oil healing toe fungus. Let's just say he was a little embarrassed that I'd told my mother about this."

YOUR INEVITABLE FINANCIAL RUIN These are the flashing red lights of parental clippings—usually sent by our fathers, dealing with tax shelters, investments, and retirement planning. The tone of the notes are doomsday-slash–smiley face. Jancee recently received an article about a Roth IRA, with a Post-it that read "I know you don't want to die old and broke! Love, Dad." Julie's father sent along a cautionary tale from his local paper about a man who filed his own tax return rather than entrust it to a professional and went on to owe the IRS $1.5 million. (Her father tucked his accountant's phone number in the envelope.)

POTENTIAL HAZARDS From our parents' perspective, ordinary life is one vast minefield, and they are ever vigilant. We'd never leave our house if we took seriously every bulletin our parents sent: ads for carbon monoxide tests, tips on fire prevention safety, the dangers of standing in front of the microwave. (Actually, after reading these clippings, we wouldn't feel safe *in* our homes without a hazmat suit.)

But when our parents really mobilize is in times of crisis. And for many parents, your being single—no matter how happy you are—qualifies as a hazard. Jennifer, who's unattached in a big city, says that her all-time favorite parental clipping is about unmarried women: "Single, Successful & Dateless!" "What's most disturbing is that

it's from a Dallas newspaper," she says. "And my parents are in Oklahoma City." To this day, she doesn't know how they found it.

Some parents feel that their missives are too urgent for ordinary mail. Tracy, a recently divorced mother of three from Connecticut, received a fax machine from her parents so their clippings could arrive at lightning speed. "I never imagined that my personal travails would turn into a hobby for my parents," she says. "As my marriage started to sour, they barraged me with articles ranging from how to detect a

cheating spouse to how to protect your assets. They even sent me articles on the divorce of former GE chairman Jack Welch." On top of that fax, Tracy's mother suggested that she contact Mrs. Welch's attorney, presumably to keep her off skid row.

"FUNNY!" We especially like bulletins from the hometown paper—usually human interest stories of a goat befriending a rooster, or about the local chapter of the Polar Bear swim club—with "Funny!" invariably scribbled on top. Two weeks after September 11, Julie's mother sent the cover story of the Glens Falls, New York, paper, an article on a local man who helped popularize disco. She thought it'd be a comfort to Julie to know that in some part of the world life was beginning to go on. Jancee's father recently passed along a review of Cranford, New Jersey's new sushi restaurant. "Good

as NY but no parking fees!" he wrote. And then there are the cartoons: Three of our friends received the same *New Yorker* cartoon of a dog telling his canine pal that "On the Internet, nobody knows you're a dog." "The Family Circus," "Cathy," and "Baby Blues" all seem to speak to parents. ("Who does this remind you of?" is usually the standard commentary written on the top.)

BUYING A NEW WHATEVER Although their appliances are from the Cold War era, our parents somehow know the foam capacity factor of the latest cappuccino maker. Nothing gives Jancee's father more pleasure than her mentioning she's in the market for a new dishwasher or a vacuum cleaner. He races to his stack of *Consumer Reports,* which he's archived back to the early nineties, highlights the specs—efficiency, cost, user ratings—and mails them off as fast as he can. Fathers have a horror of potentially faulty appliances. "I told my dad I needed a new toaster oven," says Heather, a Boston chef. "I immediately got reviews for several, and written in red pen next to the one that I'd planned to buy was the warning 'This toaster has been known to burn the tops of corn muffins.'"

HIDDEN AMONG THE TIPS FOR LOW-cost moisturizers (Crisco! Olive oil!) and "101 Uses for Grass Clippings" is one unmistakable message, and it's that our parents want us to know they're thinking about us. And they're on the case. Even with the small stuff. For mothers, especially, these notes are about connecting, the equivalent of a daily phone call. It's a way of saying "I, unlike your friends, remember that in 1992 you mentioned that you liked cats, so please enjoy these feline-related clippings." For our fathers, the goal seems to be preparedness. Jancee once asked her dad, "Why the onslaught of clips from the Kiplinger financial newsletter?" He said, "We don't want you to make the same mistakes that we did." Faraway dads can't inspect your tires or make sure your fire alarm is up to code, but even from a distance, they can put some things in order.

When your folks live elsewhere, your day-to-day lives don't overlap. And you know what? Crisco works pretty well, and it's cheaper than Crème de la Mer. •

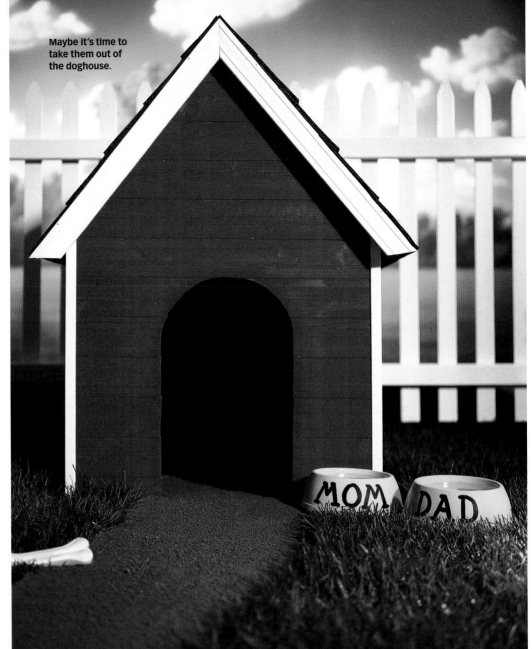

Maybe it's time to take them out of the doghouse.

MOM DAD

They're the twosome it's hardest to see clearly. And easiest to blame. But letting them off the hook, psychologist **ROBERT KAREN**, PhD, says, is the first step toward happiness, self-acceptance, and maturity.

Forgiving Your Parents

AN OLD FRIEND TELLS ME THAT she can never forgive her now dead parents and that she shouldn't have to, given how awful they were. And they *were* awful, treating her as the black sheep, relentlessly belittling her for being bookish, homely, and odd. At one point, this friend, a fellow writer, was giving me feedback on a book I was writing on forgiveness. She particularly loved one passage: "Even if the grievousness of the wrong is never acknowledged or atoned for, we may want to feel our way back to a caring place. It's the place we'd rather live."

And yet when it came to her parents, she had not thought to apply it.

I had an encounter involving forgiveness with another old friend. He made it clear that he believed so strongly in its importance that he could barely understand why anyone would withhold it. He marveled at how the people in the Balkans kept their tribal feuds going for decades. "What's that all about?" he asked. "I can't understand it!"

I said, "But you should understand it. You haven't spoken to your father in 15 years." He stiffened. "That's different,

Bob," he said, without a trace of irony. "He's a monster."

THE SINS OF PARENTS ARE among the most difficult to forgive. We expect the world of them, and we do not wish to lower our expectations. Decade after decade we hold out the hope, often unconscious, that they will finally do right by us. We want them to own up to all their misdeeds, to apologize, to make heartfelt pleas for our forgiveness. We want them to give us the love we've always craved. And this desire for love has very specific wishes attached: Why don't you give me better birthday gifts? Why don't you remember what I tell you about my life? When will you start being more generous with money? We want our parents to embrace us, to tell us they know we were good children, to undo the favoritism they've shown to a brother or sister, to take back their hurtful criticisms, to give us their praise.

There's nothing wrong with wanting this. It is a natural want. No one is perfectly mature, and we may hunger for our parents to repair whatever damage they've done long after we've become adults. We get into trouble, though, when we let this hunger rule our lives.

Nursing resentments toward a parent does more than keep that parent in the doghouse. We get stuck there, too, forever the child, the victim, the have-not in the realm of love. My writer friend feels her parents do not deserve her forgiveness. Even after their deaths, she doesn't want to give them that satisfaction. But as a result, she still lives with them psychologically, still has the horrible opinions of herself that they fostered. Strange as it may seem, a grudge is a kind of clinging, a way of not separating, and when we hold a grudge against a parent, we are clinging not just to the parent but more specifically to the bad part of the parent. It's as if we don't want to live our lives until we have this resolved and feel the security of their unconditional love. We do so for good reasons psychologically. But the result is just the opposite: We stay locked into the badness and we don't grow up.

I had a patient who, even as a grown man in his 30s, was still waiting for his father to be the father he should have been and was destroying his own life in the process. A part of him had remained a small child, riveted to a father who was often unavailable and insensitive. My patient couldn't move on with his life, he couldn't really *have* a life—not a job, not a girlfriend—because to do so would mean moving away, separating from his dad in some way. As long as he remained a misfit, a patient no therapist could fix, he could stay

> Strange as it may seem, a grudge is a kind of clinging, and when we **hold a grudge** against a parent, we are clinging not simply to the parent but to the bad part of the parent.

emotionally entwined with his father and still dream of the perfect paternal rescue.

Blaming his dad for his failures freed my patient from having to face himself. I once said to him, "When you're lying in the gutter with a bottle in your hand, dying at 48, you'd rather say, 'Dad was such a bastard!' than 'Boy, did I fuck up my life.'"

The sad thing about clinging to a parent in this unforgiving, infantile way is that we foreclose the possibility of getting the love we need from others. And it is this love—available love—that could heal us. I have two women in my practice, one in her 30s, one in her 60s, who know their husbands love them and yet are unable to experience that love. It feels empty, unimportant. It never quite reaches them. They hide this fact from their husbands and feel ashamed of it, as if it's proof they are misfits when it comes to love. As kids, they were deeply wounded by their rejecting mothers and now they can't get unglued. They're like small children who lose their

mother in a big store and nothing will soothe them but getting her back. They don't want their husband's love. Only Mom's will do.

The failure to come to terms with the ways our parents have failed us does not always lead to such drastic consequences. But we do end up in an uncomfortable relationship with them: distant, dutiful, rageful, clinging, false.

Before we're able to locate our forgiving self, we have to process our hurts and anger from the past. A woman tells me she doesn't want to dredge up bad experiences from her childhood. "I don't want to feel angry at my mother. I don't want to hate her. I don't want to lose her." She believes she has a good relationship with her mother. The irony is that she doesn't. It's all pretense. This woman would never think to be less than a good daughter. But the unfelt anger is keeping her from feeling any real warmth.

Forgiving our parents is a core task of adulthood and one of the most crucial kinds of forgiveness because it reverberates throughout our psychic lives. We see our parents in our mates, in our friends, in our bosses, even in our children. When we've felt rejected by a parent and have remained in that state, we will inevitably feel rejected by these important others as well.

We've all had this experience, which we might describe as being "overly sensitive" or "paranoid," or as "having our buttons pushed." A lover doesn't call back soon enough and we begin to feel unwanted, cast aside, small, unattractive, depressed, and then out for vengeance. Our child acts pouty, angry, unwilling to make up with us, and we cease to perceive him as a child. He is our tormentor, our rejecter, turning our life to misery. This is part of what is at stake in our failure to let our parents off the hook. We re-create with the people we love our worst experiences with our parents.

Most parents love their children, with surprisingly few exceptions, even among those who beat their kids or molest them. But no parent is perfect—which means that everyone has childhood wounds. If we're lucky, our parents were good enough for us to be able to hold on to the knowledge of their love for us and our love for them even in the face of the things they did that hurt us. The real tragedy of the parent-child relationship occurs when the bad side of the parent is so bad that it overwhelms the child's capacity to hold on to the good. That's when we harbor feelings of being unloved, unlovable, unloving. And that's when we cling to the bad parent and our childhood wishes that can't be fulfilled.

There is a joke in which one psychoanalyst tells another, "You know, I made the most extraordinary Freudian slip the other day. We were at my mother's for dinner and I meant to say, 'Would you please pass the salt?' But what came out was, 'Boy, did you mess up my life, you hideous old bag!'"

It is, of course, delightful to think that analysts are as ensnared in the aftereffects of childhood misery as the next person. Yet it is not so much the past that haunts the analyst in the joke as the way he holds on to it. If a man repeatedly sticks the knife of rage into his mother for what she did to him when he was little, it's not the past that's killing him but the knifings themselves. His chronic hatred is part of being glued to her.

Being glued to a hated parent inevitably means that the worst aspects of that parent live on in one's head as a debilitating presence—judging, blaming, finding fault. The analyst's gross verbal slip (the impossible grossness of it is more than half the laugh) reveals not just what he feels about his mother but that he is still living with her and controlled by her—indeed, is still *enthralled* with her in some way.

WHAT, THEN, IS THIS place we'd rather live, this place of forgiveness? Let me say first what it's not. To forgive is not to condone the bad things our parents have done. It's not to deny their selfishness, their rejections, their meanness, their brutality, or any of the other misdeeds, character flaws, or limitations that may attach to them. To forgive them is, rather, to do two important things: First, to separate from them—which is to stop seeing ourselves as children who depend on them for our emotional well-being, to stop being their victims, to recognize that we are adults with some capacity to shape our own lives and the responsibility to do

so. And second, to let them back into our hearts. When we do that, we can begin to understand the circumstances and limitations they labored under, recognize the goodness in them that our pain has pushed aside, feel some compassion perhaps, not only for the hard journey they had but also for the pain we have caused them.

Jonathan, a fellow psychologist, had a father who was a violent alcoholic. He left home and abandoned Jonathan when he was 6 and allowed Jonathan's stepfather to adopt him. Jonathan saw his father periodically, treasured his times with him, even worshiped him in some ways, but was bitterly hurt by his father's relentless insensitivity and selfishness. Finally, when Jonathan was in his 20s, they had a falling-out that was not repaired until his father was on his deathbed decades later.

We re-create with the people we love our worst experiences with our parents.

"He had a stroke," Jonathan told me, "and was entirely incapacitated. All he could do was make a desperate guttural sound, 'Auch! Auch! Auch!' like a wounded animal. And I could see that at this end point of his life, when all his faculties had been taken from him, he was trying to say something very loving. And I think at that point I was able to let go of the anger. I just let it go. I felt a great sense of relief and a sense of forgiveness and a sense of compassion."

Jonathan was also able to see that he had contributed to their long and painful estrangement: "All my life I felt a lot of love for him, and that's where my anger was coming from, because I felt rejected. And I also felt he loved me a lot. It was something that got badly out of whack, probably because of my ego and because of his ego."

Others come to a similar place by different means. Sometimes we get insight into our parents and are able to understand

and forgive them when we become parents and see how hard it is to get the job right. Sometimes we see that our grudges have been horribly unfair, that we've made one parent the scapegoat, the other the god, or been unjust in some other way. Some of us achieve forgiveness by taking a vital inner journey to deal with our hurts.

Perhaps the most crucial aspect of that journey is allowing ourselves to feel the longings that have been pushed aside and made unconscious—to feel that part of us that is still a child, desperately in love and horribly hurt and hoping against hope that the parent will be good again and make everything right. When we can feel these childhood longings, understand them, talk about them, cry perhaps, a subtle change takes place within us. We are able to care about our own hurt. Not in a self-pitying way. It is as if the adult part of us, the secure part of us, is able to embrace and soothe the child. This is the beginning of a process that can lead us out of our bitterness, away from our entwinement with the bad part of the parent, reintroduce us to the good part that we may have forgotten, and pave the way toward forgiveness.

To forgive our parents is a gift not just to them but to ourselves, because it brings us back to the good part of the relationship with them, where we experience ourselves as loving and lovable people. It strengthens our own sense of self because, like it or not, we are always identified with our parents. And, finally, it gives us the opportunity to better enjoy the time we have left with them and to get from them what they may now be able and even longing to give.

But as valuable as forgiveness is and as important as it is to strive for, no one can forgive deeply felt wrongs in an instant. Getting to a forgiving place, finding the forgiving self inside us, is a long and complicated journey. We have to be ready to forgive. We have to want to forgive. The deeper the wound, the more difficult the process—which makes forgiving parents especially hard. Along the way, we may have to express our protest, we may have to be angry and resentful, we may even have to punish our parents by holding a grudge. But when we get there, the forgiveness we achieve will be a forgiveness worth having. ●

the well-trained mother

In 42 years, Lisa Kogan and her mother, Rosestelle, have forgiven, forgotten, let it go, sucked it up, driven each other nuts, and made each other laugh. Is history bound to repeat itself?

"Gwynff," I say.

"Gwynff?" my mother repeats.

"That's right, I'm going to name your one and only granddaughter Gwynff."

Silence. "Is that an actual word?" she asks calmly.

"Yes, I believe it's Welsh for 'We're not telling people the name we've chosen,'" I answer with equal calm.

"Middle name?" attempting nonchalance.

"Nosferatu," attempting to preserve privacy of middle-name decision.

"Ava is a nice name," she says, floating a trial balloon.

"Yes, you've mentioned that," I say, bursting it.

"I mean, not that you have to go with Ava or anything.... Lauren, Emma, Rachel, they all work."

"Gwynff," I say.

My mother and I

go back more than 42 years. It took a lot of time, but I've trained her well. She no longer tells me my paintings hang too high or my hemlines hang too low. She doesn't suggest I get my head out of the clouds or the hair out of my eyes. In exchange for which I refrain from complaining bitterly that she served broiled chicken with a side of Birds Eye frozen green beans virtually every night from 1974 to the bicentennial. She doesn't throw my inability to parallel park at me, and I've quit addressing letters home to "the woman who forced me to wear a coat over my Halloween costume." We've managed to forgive each other's frailties, to accept that she's neurotic and I'm, well, even more neurotic. We understand that I will never wear anything that involves appliqué and she will never eat anything that involves calories. It's a complicated truce, but it generally works for us, and when it doesn't, we moan to our respective shrinks and live to love another day. Others are less fortunate.

My friend Robin insists that the next time her mother decides to slip her phone number to a divorced orthodontist from Great Neck, she fully intends to fake her own death. I applaud Robin's creative problem solving and hereby volunteer to show up at her phony memorial service and repeatedly sob, "Oh, dear God, I guess all that blind dating finally did her in."

They say good

fences make good neighbors, but I look at the mothers and daughters I know and find myself wondering if the fence must be electrified to keep one's mother from straying into dangerous territory. Will this little person who's currently occupying space in my uterus have to one day line the borders of her heart with razor wire to stop me from chipping away at her choice of laundry detergent and footwear? How do we keep from becoming trespassers in each other's lives?

I ask my mother

about this, but all she says is that everything will be fine. She insists I'll know what I'm doing, and that if I don't, little Gwynff Nosferatu will train me. Her vague response annoys me to no end. I'm looking for some hard-core mothering here, for a Campbell's commercial in which we're wearing chunky hand-knit sweaters and sharing deep truths over piping hot bowls of tomato rice soup. I want her to brush my hair and call me Cupcake and say the kind of things you read in Hallmark cards—but that's just not my mother's style, nor was it her mother's, and for better or for worse, I'm pretty sure it won't be mine, either. Instead I'll leave my daughter irritating phone messages suggesting she switch laundry detergents and invest in better shoes. And because I'm a writer, I'll probably write her all the things that my mother has said to me over the years—if not in word, then in deed:

Always try. Always

care. Always believe in what you're doing. Always respect yourself. Always know that you are loved. And always remember how happy you've made me just by showing up for the big dance. ●

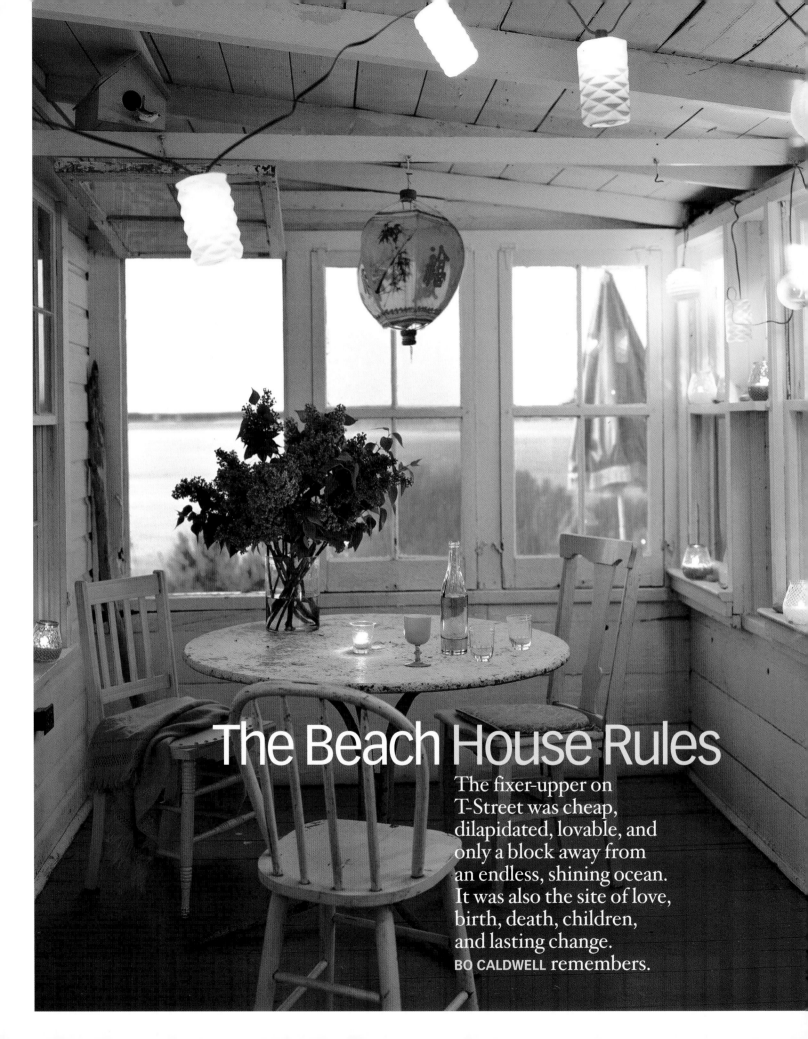

The Beach House Rules

The fixer-upper on
T-Street was cheap,
dilapidated, lovable, and
only a block away from
an endless, shining ocean.
It was also the site of love,
birth, death, children,
and lasting change.
BO CALDWELL remembers.

IN FEBRUARY 1967, MY PARENTS bought a beach house. They were driving around with a real estate agent, when white writing on one of the ocean-facing windows of the house caught my mother's eye: for sale $35,000. "You don't want to see that one," the agent said. "It's a mess." That only made her want to see it more: She and my father had already bought and sold a few fixer-uppers, and the fact that the house was a mess was more bait than deterrent.

The agent wasn't lying—the house was a mess. To start, it was filthy; you could scrape grease off the living room's wood-paneled walls with your fingernails. The five bedrooms were painted bright 1960s colors—neon blue, purple, green, yellow—and that wood paneling in the living room was a garish 1950s rumpus room orange. The floor throughout the house was linoleum. An ironing board stood in the living room; the kitchen was shoddy and outdated.

My parents were instantly serious. They saw through the mess, and by the end of the afternoon, they were signing papers.

I was thrilled. I was in sixth grade, and I knew that a beach house could give me some much-needed junior high clout, a kind of implied leverage: *If you're nice to me, I might invite you to my beach house.* And even then, I loved the beach. I loved it early in the morning when no one was there and the sand was all smooth from the beach cleaner. I loved it in the middle of the day, when you could lie there and listen to the radio or to the people around you talking and the sun's heat was so strong it felt personal. I loved it in late afternoon when people started packing up and walking to their cars, and if you were lucky enough to be staying with someone with a beach house, you didn't have to go yet. And I loved it at night, when you could come down late and walk on sand that was so cold it felt much finer than in daytime, like some other substance altogether, and you could swing on the swings over a dark black sea, and maybe see the grunion run.

The house on T-Street became my mother's career that spring. We lived a little more than an hour away, in San Marino, and if she left home at 6, she'd be at the beach house by 7:30 or so. With help from friends and people she hired, she cleaned the place from top to bottom and painted the bedrooms and kitchen and hallways and baths. A friend stripped the living room walls and stained the wood a lighter driftwood shade. My mother would get home at 9 o'clock at night, and on the weekends it was the same, only my father was with her.

When the house was finally in good shape, there were carpet and furniture to think about. My parents found a secondhand-furniture store in town and

> At sunset we'd straggle into the kitchen to find pans of lasagna and my mother saying everyone could stay, as long as they called their parents.

bought as much as they could from the owner. Over the next 30 years, they would take back what wasn't working and trade it in for something else. There were linens to buy, no small thing for a five-bedroom, two-bath house. My mother found a place that sold towels by the pound; she bought sheets as though she owned a hotel. When my brother came home from college in June, he and a friend spent their summer painting the house's light blue exterior a dark beige.

Since then, I've spent part of every summer at T-Street—when I was growing up it was with as many friends as my parents would say yes to. We'd lie on the beach slathered in baby oil or cocoa butter, working on our tans, listening to Three Dog Night and Chicago and Cat Stevens on

transistor radios, and for lunch we'd get tortilla strips and hamburgers and Diet Coke floats from the snack stand. I'd invite a dozen kids home for dinner, and at sunset we'd straggle into the kitchen to find pans of lasagna and my mother saying that everyone could stay, as long as they called their parents. (It's only now, as the parent of teenagers, that I am appropriately awed by this ability of hers to make dinner for a dozen at a moment's notice.)

Over time certain traditions established themselves. The Fourth of July, for example, was always an occasion—Hyannis Port West, my dad called it. At night we sat outside and ate barbecued chicken and corn on the cob that someone had bought at a stand that afternoon. Friends brought fresh strawberry and peach pies for dessert, and after dinner we'd watch the fireworks launched by the city from the end of the pier, a quarter mile north. The quality of the fireworks varied, but nobody minded.

The middle room of the house—my brother's when we were growing up—is now the boys' room, shared by my nephew and my son. The tiny bedroom that was mine is the girls' dorm, shared among my nieces and my daughter; with a double bed and a trundle bed, the room can be turned into wall-to-wall beds. In high school when friends stayed over, the boys were given the bedroom farthest from mine, at the exact opposite end of the house, as far as East is from West. At 11 o'clock, the hour my father decided was the appropriate time for everyone to retire to their quarters, he would ring a brass ship's bell that he'd mounted in the living room, probably with that express purpose in mind, and we would disperse. My friends were soon calling the house Camp Caldwell.

Dad's notes, still taped up around the house, remind us of things like not turning off certain lights (they're on timers), and not fooling with the sprinkler system (no one knows why), and putting the garbage out on Sunday nights (because if we didn't, he would need to haul the garbage home in the trunk of his Oldsmobile—my mom knew a woman who froze her garbage, then took it home to throw it out). I knew I was truly an adult the first time I stayed at the house alone and no one from my family called to remind me to put the trash out. I think I was 38. My father's role was Master Craftsman, and there is evidence of his handiwork everywhere: a huge bolt here, a funny latch there, a cupboard inexplicably nailed shut, the tools in the garage hung on the wall with Dad-made twisted wire loops. He was also Chief Exterminator, constantly waging Wile E. Coyote battles against the gophers in the backyard (they always won), and Chief Gardener, working again and again to rid the back corner of the yard of an industrial-strength banana tree and, more recently, fooling with the automatic sprinkler system, which always seems to be out of whack.

Because it falls in summer—August 21—we've always celebrated my mother's birthday at the beach house. Last year everyone was there: my brother and his family, my family, Mom and Dad—the whole gang. We sat around the kitchen table eating too many chips, then ate rotisserie chicken for dinner, and afterward Mom opened her presents. The day was similar to many others before it, but there was apprehension in the air: Four days later, my father was scheduled to undergo surgery to repair an abdominal aortic aneurysm, and although we had all talked about what a relief it would be to have it over with, Dad was quiet that afternoon and evening, and his somberness worried us.

That night was our last celebration as that whole, intact family. Five days later, following the surgery, a stroke robbed my father of speech. Ten days after that, a second stroke robbed him of mobility, and a month and a half later, a third stroke stole his consciousness. He died two months and six days after my mother's birthday.

I THINK OF THAT NIGHT OFTEN this summer. We decided not to celebrate Mom's birthday at the beach house this year; there would be too many reminders of Dad. I want to hold on to that night the way I often want to hold on to things here: the way the ocean looks, the smudged colors of the sky at dusk, the wink of phosphorous in the waves at night. I look outside dozens of times a day, and I always want to capture what I'm seeing.

But I'm trying something new this year: I'm telling myself to let go. I think how great my mother's birthday was and how we were as a family, and I tell myself that I don't have to hold on to it to make it last. It's my lesson and my homework this summer: not holding on so tightly to what is, and trying to make room for what will be. I have my work cut out for me; I'm not good at letting go, whether it's of memories or relationships or habits. Or kids. My veterinarian told me that his rabbi says that if you don't let go of your kids, they have to let go of you, and I gritted my teeth when he said this. When my kids were younger—from the time they were toddlers all the

> Because
> the beach house
> has been
> such a constant,
> it is here that
> I practice letting go.

way through elementary school—I cried the night before each birthday. *She's 7,* I'd think, or *He's 5,* trying to get used to the idea of my kids growing up.

My son will turn 16 in the fall, and in a few weeks my daughter will start her senior year in high school. She looks at schools thousands of miles away, and I sometimes wake in the night with a feeling approaching panic: *A year from now, she'll be gone—what will I do without her?* I imagine packing and goodbyes, absence and empty rooms, things I hate. I try to come up with ways to fill my time once she's gone, and I picture myself as the world's oldest candy-striper. The image is not comforting.

There are other changes. It has been a year in which Mom has lived alone. She has done great, and everyone, including me, marvels at her. Lately, she has mentioned moving from the house she's lived in for 40 years. And even though I know that selling may someday be the right thing for her, the idea of her not living there is foreign.

The beach house without Dad was also foreign at first. Everything was. Since his death I have dreamed of him often, and in the dreams he is always silent. I have come to think that his silence has something to do with my holding on to him too tightly. But letting go of him is easier said than done.

There are so many reminders at the beach house: his conspicuous repairs—and all those notes, which, for some reason, he took to signing with my brother's name in recent years. And there is a new reminder of him this year: the ocean itself. On the first Sunday in January, my brother drove the hour from his house to T-Street. When he got to the beach, he put on a wet suit and paddled out on the surfboard he'd borrowed from his teenage son. He wore a backpack. When he'd gotten past where the waves break, he just sat for a while. And then he took a canister from the backpack and scattered our father's ashes into the ocean, in sight of the same kitchen window that our mother had spotted from the street so many years ago.

I know that a phase of my life is ending, one where the kids are at home and Mom and Dad live in the house I grew up in. The rhythm of my days and our holidays and our family is changing. I also know that these are very minor worries in the scheme of things and that I am fortunate to have these as my main concerns. But they still make me sad.

All of this is a little easier to accept at the beach house, though, because over the years it has been such a constant. And so it is here that I practice letting go. I bite my tongue when I feel myself about to give my son or daughter unwanted advice, and I tell myself that even when they're grown up, I'll still be their mom. I think of my own mother, and I remind myself that home has more to do with the people you love than with the place you live. And when I think of my father, I try not to tell him how much I miss him but rather to be thankful for who he was.

As I look out at an ocean that is my friend, I try to let these things sink in. And I try not just to ready myself for the next part of the journey but to welcome it, and to move forward with a little bit of grace, and with thanks for what is past. ●

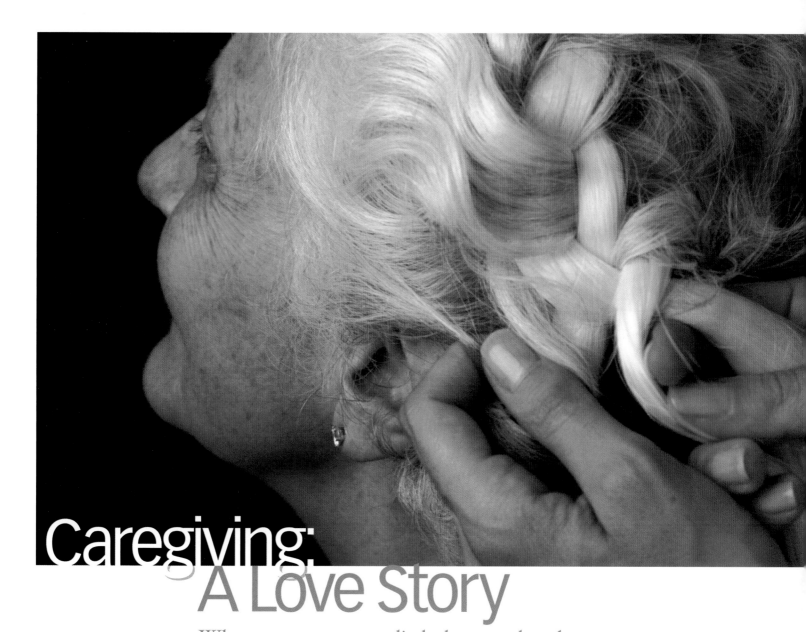

Caregiving:
A Love Story

When **ANN PATCHETT** was little, her grandmother drew her baths. Now grown-up, she feels privileged to return the favor. A granddaughter muses about age, youth, reversals of body and mind—and love's long haul.

WHEN I WAS A LITTLE GIRL, MY grandmother lived in Paradise, California, and based on the summer vacations my sister and I spent at her house, the name of the town was fitting. She taught us to knit and sew and make our own doughnuts. Beneath her sink was a box con-taining turpentine, brushes, and three dozen tiny bottles of enamel paint, and we spent afternoons making pictures of frogs and quail on the smooth rocks we brought home from Lake Shasta.

Life could not have devised a better grandmother. She owned a dog and was not interested in

> "I shampoo, braid, and pin," says Patchett. "We have a routine."

television. She let me fill up books of S&H Green Stamps and spend them any way I pleased. At night I stood on a stool in front of her kitchen sink and she rinsed my hair with lemon water.

Over the years, we have changed our roles: She drove me places, now I drive her places. We used to talk about the books we read, then she was reading the books I wrote, then her eyesight failed and I was reading books to her. For years I had lunch with her every day and we'd watch her soap opera, but then she couldn't remember who was who and the whole thing became an irritation to her. That was during the 16 years she lived with my mother. Her friends had died and her eight siblings had died and her husband had died and she was biding her time. When the process seemed to be going too slowly to suit her, she went on a hunger strike that was worthy of the IRA. When she got to 103 pounds, two years ago, we put her in assisted living. She was 92.

The world is divided like this: One day my mother goes to visit, the next day it's me. I take my grandmother to my house, bend her over the sink, and wash her hair. We have a routine. Once it was painting rocks and baking molasses cookies; later it was shopping, or just trips to the grocery store. Now it's grooming. I have become one of those little Egyptian birds that stands on the back of a crocodile, digging its beak in between the scales. I shampoo, condition, blow-dry, braid, and pin. I put her in the perfect light of my kitchen window and tweeze the invisible hairs from her chin, and then she runs her fingers across her chin to check me. "Missed one," she says, tapping. I file her fingernails and paint them if she's in the mood. I fill my blue Le Creuset soup pot with warm water and apple cider vinegar and soak her feet. Then I sit on my kitchen floor and do her toes.

A NOTE ABOUT THE BIBLICAL significance of foot washing: There is real humility in the act. When people tell me I have a very glamorous life, I smile and think, *You know nothing about the feet.* My grandmother has been known to squeal and say, "Ow! That was too close!" before I

ever touch clipper to nail. Fancy pedicures are available at the assisted living home. I took her once, thrilled to have found such a meaningful way to spend my money. I sat with her through the whole thing, and while it seemed to go very well, she told me at the end that it wouldn't happen again. She did not like placing her feet in the hands of a stranger. "If you won't cut them, I'll do it myself," she said. But my grandmother's feet are as far away from her as China, and so I returned to my job.

Back in the days when my grandmother had a wallet with money in it and knew what she wanted to buy, I would count out the change for her in checkout lines. "Where would I be without her?" she would say to the disinterested teenager receiving the money. Then she would turn to me and say, "What's going to happen when you're my age? Who will take care of you? You'll be all alone."

And it's true. I have no children, and I never will. There will be no one who loves me, who will pluck out my chin hairs or run a Q-tip around in my ears, but I've never thought that the hope of free custodial care was reason enough to reproduce. At 39 I have to wonder what the chances are that I'll see 94 anyway. Life is, after all, a long obstacle course filled with car crashes and cancer. Certainly something will knock me off along the way.

"I'm saving my money," I tell her. "And when I'm your age, I'm going to rent myself the nicest granddaughter in the world. I'm going to rent one who's much better than I am. And when I die, I'm going to leave her everything." It's true, actually. That is my backup plan in case I live too long.

"You're smart," my grandmother says, squeezing my wrist. "You shouldn't have

a baby." What she means is that she is my baby, and she would rather not share me.

AFTER SHE WENT INTO AS-sisted living, my grandmother made friends with food again and ate her way up to a record-breaking 180 pounds in a year and a half. When I took her to the doctor for her physical, she was mortified. "One eighty?" she said to me. "They must have weighed me with my sweater on."

"A 75-pound sweater?" I asked.

She handed it to me. "It's wool."

The doctor is pleased about the weight. Aside from her slipping mind and bad eyesight, my grandmother appears to be in glorious physical health, very possibly good for another ten years.

I want to believe I will be good for another ten myself. I remember my grand-

I remember my grandmother
sitting on the edge of the tub, scrubbing my back when I was a child. Now she is in my tub and I am washing hers.

mother sitting on the edge of the bathtub, scrubbing my back when I was a child. Now she is in my tub and I am washing hers. They give good showers at the assisted living place, but there is nothing like a bath. Her skin, so recently stretched out, is pink and flawless. Her breasts are full. I wash every inch of her. She is mine, my body.

There was a time I thought that love was kissing, sweaty palms, desire. Now I know that love is this: sticking it out, the long haul. I pull her out of the tub, my chest and arms soaking, and stand her on a towel to dry.

"What is that stuff?" she asks. When I tell her it's lotion, she says that she's never heard of such a thing before. "But I like it," she says. "It's good."

I believe that liking lotion is a clear sign of life. I slather it on. ●

On Being a Parent

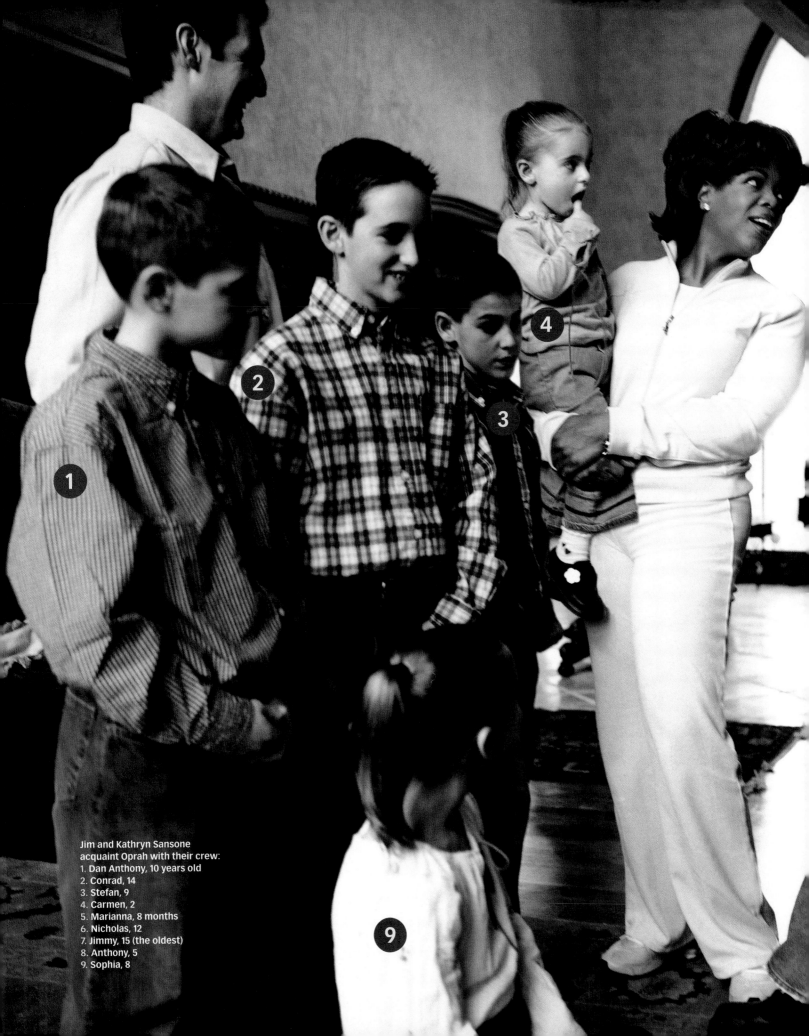

Jim and Kathryn Sansone
acquaint Oprah with their crew:
1. Dan Anthony, 10 years old
2. Conrad, 14
3. Stefan, 9
4. Carmen, 2
5. Marianna, 8 months
6. Nicholas, 12
7. Jimmy, 15 (the oldest)
8. Anthony, 5
9. Sophia, 8

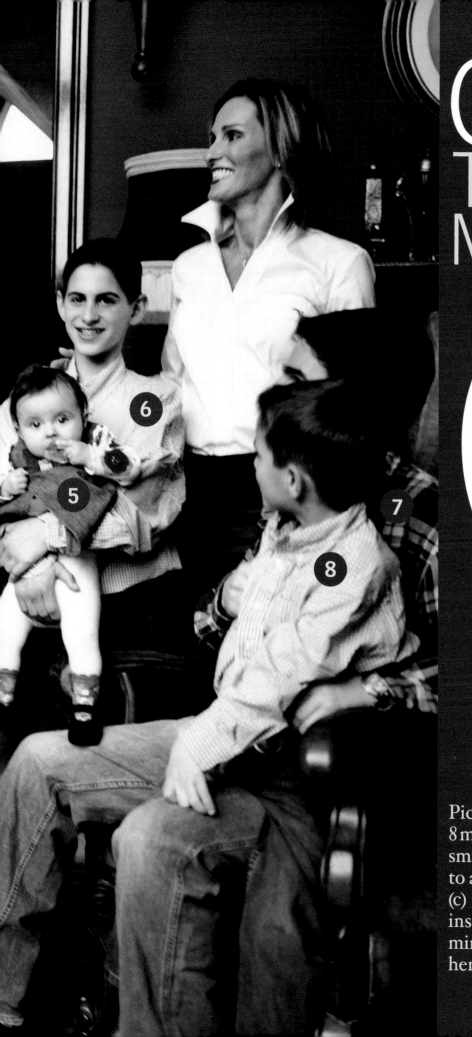

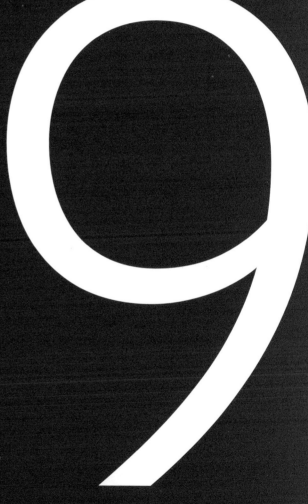

OPRAH
TALKS TO A MOTHER OF
9

Picture having 9 kids ranging in age from 8 months to 15 years. Do you (a) start your own small country, (b) have yourself committed to a home for the terminally exhausted, or (c) think about having more? Oprah gets inside Kathryn Sansone's very organized mind and house to find out how she keeps her sanity…to say nothing of her shape.

A AFTER FIVE MINUTES IN THE St. Louis home of Kathryn and Jim Sansone, I know this family is a clan unto itself: nine kids, each exuding the kind of spirit and confidence that doesn't happen by chance. I first met Kathryn in May 2002 when she was in the audience of my show. Then six months pregnant with her ninth child, she stood to explain how working out with weights had transformed her body. One year and 700 guests a day later, I sit across from a woman I find unforgettable: a mother whose greatest joy comes from raising respectful and responsible children.

The Sansone family, by the numbers: six boys and three girls, ages 15, 14, 12, 10, 9, 8, 5, 2, and 8 months; four in braces, two in preschool, one in high school, four taking piano lessons. One Saint Bernard dog. One swing set behind their house on three and a half acres. One homemade ice-skating rink in the backyard. One Texas-size table big enough for everyone to sit around. And two parents who call each one of their children a gift: Jim, a 42-year-old lawyer who co-owns a real estate development business, and Kathryn, whose passion is to do what I believe is the most important spiritual work on earth—mothering. The three of us sat beside a fireplace and talked.

OPRAH: *Growing up, how many children were in your family?*

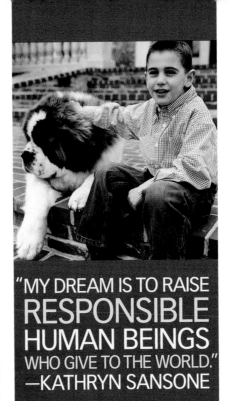

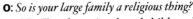

"MY DREAM IS TO RAISE **RESPONSIBLE HUMAN BEINGS** WHO GIVE TO THE WORLD." —KATHRYN SANSONE

KATHRYN SANSONE: I'm one of three girls, and my husband is from a family of eight. We knew we wanted children—we just never talked about having nine. After our oldest child, Jimmy, was born, we wanted him to have a sibling. With every child we were blessed with after that, we just adjusted and were thankful.

O: *Are you Catholic?*

KS: Yes, I converted from Greek Orthodox when I married.

O: *So is your large family a religious thing?*

KS: No. I've always just loved children. Before I got pregnant the first time, I was an elementary school teacher. I got pregnant on my honeymoon.

O: *Did you leave teaching after your first baby?*

KS: Yes, I left after I had Jimmy. As a teacher I always wanted to bring out the self-esteem in a child, and that's what I want as a mother, too.

O: *I felt that the moment I met your kids. Each one has such a strong sense of self.*

KS: Thank you—that's such a huge compliment.

O: *One child is as well behaved as the next. To raise children like this is one of the hardest jobs on earth.*

KS: We're still working hard at it, especially now that we're getting into the teen years, with all the crap that's going on out there. We've put parental controls on our computer, and we took off the instant messaging. Otherwise I might not know who my children were talking with.

O: *What's your dream for your children?*

KS: My dream is to raise self-confident, respectful, responsible human beings who can give a lot to the world. After I drop off the kids at school every morning, I go to a monastery and sit in front of the Blessed Sacrament and give everything over to Our Lady and to Jesus. My prayer is always the same: "Use me." I get a lot of strength that way. I want to do the best for the kids, and since I've got so many, my mind is always in a million places.

O: *How do you keep everything organized?*

KS: I'm an organizational fanatic. I created a locker room that the children pass through when they come in the house. Each child has a personal locker, and every day when they arrive home from school, they dump their stuff there—backpacks, shoes, soccer uniforms. I organize them by season: In summer I put their swimsuits in the locker room, and during winter the hats and gloves go there. As for keeping their clothes organized, thank goodness for school uniforms! I lay out their clothes on their dressers the night before, and until last September, I made all their lunches. I also try to get any school papers and tests signed and ready to go back in the morning.

O: *How many bedrooms in this house?*

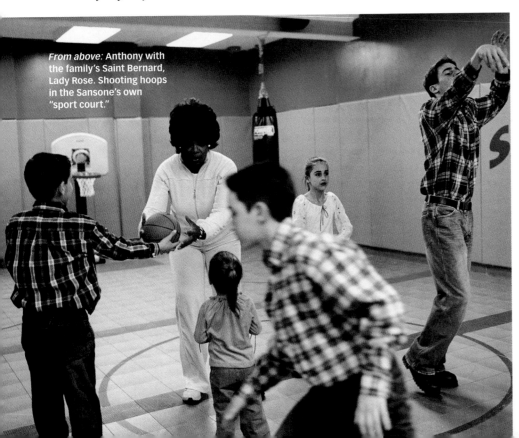

From above: Anthony with the family's Saint Bernard, Lady Rose. Shooting hoops in the Sansone's own "sport court."

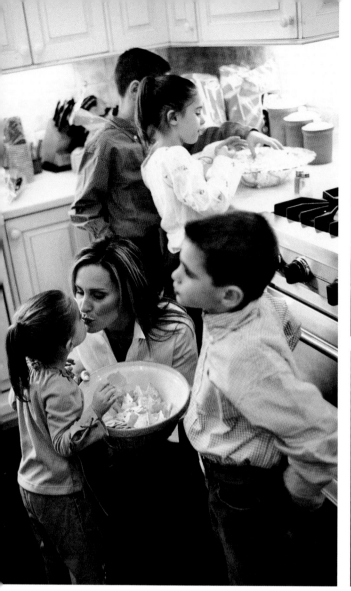

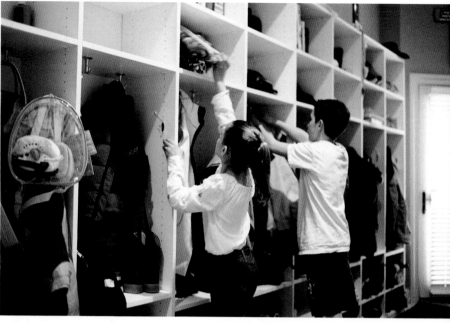

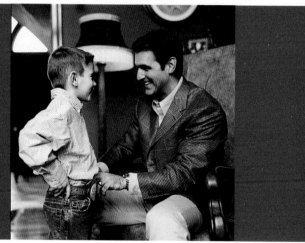

KS: One for us, four for the kids. They're all doubling up—two boys, two boys, two boys, and three girls. But they only use two of the four bedrooms because they all end up sleeping in one another's beds.

O: *What are mornings like around here?*

KS: Very smooth. The key is the big shower we had designed for the kids. It has four showerheads, so we just throw the boys in there together.

O: *Hold on a sec—I think Anthony needs something.* [Five-year-old Anthony opens the door.] *Anthony, what do you need?*

ANTHONY: I need my dad.

O: *Goodbye, Jim. Okay, Kathryn—what were you saying about the shower?*

KS: After the shower, they drop all their clothes down a chute to the laundry room. Then they dress, and we all have breakfast.

O: *What kind of breakfast do you prepare?*

KS: I'll make eggs and French toast, bagels with cheese, and I'll throw some bacon on the George Foreman grill. That thing is a huge hit.

O: *You cook like that every morning?*

KS: On school mornings. I usually don't make a big breakfast on weekends. Sometimes Jim cooks.

O: *Do you take all the children to school?*

KS: My husband drops off our high schooler, and I take the other five in our SUV at around 7:30. By that time, a caretaker comes in to watch the three youngest children.

O: *What do you do when you're back home?*

KS: I spend 30 to 45 minutes alone every day—that was my New Year's resolution. It's outstanding.

O: *Has that made a difference in the rest of your day?*

KS: Huge. My kids have even noticed. They say, "You seem calmer, in a better mood."

I've always been into getting my workout, but I still felt unbalanced because the spiritual part wasn't all there.

O: *How long are your workouts?*

KS: Thirty minutes of cardio, another half hour for weights. After quiet time and a workout, I take two of the children to preschool.

O: *What do you do with the rest of your day?*

KS: Depends on the day—but I can tell you that I never sit down. I check to see that all the beds are made, I clean the bathrooms, I straighten the house. Some days I go up to the children's schools and help with hot lunches there. Other days I make lists of groceries and keep track of what the children need. When you've got eight kids in school, somebody always needs a pen, a backpack, shoelaces, or a folder. I tell the children to write down what they need and put it on my desk. A few weeks ago, my sixth-grade son left me this note: "Mom, could you please xerox the *World Book of Greece?*" I thought, *This can't be right.* When I called the teacher, she clarified the assignment: My son needed a copy of just the section *on Greece* in the *World Book.*

Keeping up with all their appointments is a challenge. We've got four in braces, and the orthodontist wants to see each every four weeks—and they're all on different schedules. They also have appointments with the eye doctor and the dermatologist, and then there are regular checkups. And of course, the baby always needs to go to the pediatrician for shots.

O: *Do you have any cleaning help?*

KS: I have a housecleaner come in every other week.

O: *Other than your quiet time and workout, is there any other part of your day just for you?*

KS: I find time between 7:30 and 3:00, when most of the kids are at school. When I pick them up, I want to be ready for them. Three o'clock is hell hour around here—that's when the homework and all the "Can so-and-so come over?" start. Some of the kids have four or five hours of homework, which they start before dinner. And after school, I coach my son's basketball team.

O: *Would you define yourself as a supermom? If this ain't super, I don't know what is.*

KS: I don't define myself as a supermom. I define my husband and me as superparents. We do this together. I could never handle this alone.

O: *What hours does your husband work?*

KS: He leaves early when he drops off our son, and he's home by 6:30.

O: *Do you all sit down for dinner together?*

KS: Yes. We just bought a big round table. The children help: One gets the pitcher of water, another sets the places. I've taught a couple of them to barbecue.

O: *What's for dinner—chicken nuggets and fries?*

KS: I usually do a salad, maybe something from the grill, and I cook a lot of pasta. I make vegetables of some sort—and, of course, there's hot bread.

O: *Please don't tell me you make the bread.*

KS: No. It's Pillsbury all the way. At the table, we all tell what our day was like—my husband and I want to get our kids used to public speaking. Then if we have time and everybody's in the mood, we play *American Idol.* Three of us will be the judges, and the others will put on outfits and sing for us.

O: *You do all this during dinner?*

KS: After dinner. That's our time to just relax and hang out. Then they hit their studies again or we've got sports practices.

O: *Do you ever feel overwhelmed?*

KS: At times I can be overwhelmed with the hustle and bustle of everything.

O: *Are you a yeller?*

KS: Oh, yes—I yell.

O: *But you don't feel like you're going crazy most of the time?*

KS: No.

O: *And you don't feel like you've lost yourself to your kids?*

KS: Not at all. Jim and I go out alone during the week, and our kids watch one another. We go for coffee on Saturday and Sunday mornings. We tell them, "We're going out, and don't call us on our cell phones." They know that's our time.

O: *All that and you still look great. Are you all made up when you're preparing breakfast every morning?*

KS: Gosh, no. I literally just brush my teeth. And unless I'm meeting someone for lunch, I often stay in my workout clothes and sneakers all day.

O: *Do you put on a little makeup before Jim comes home?*

KS: I make myself look presentable. Maybe I'll throw on some lipstick. I'm always clean. I don't make up my face and go to the malls all day—I'm too busy for that.

O: *Friends with two kids say it's difficult to make each one feel important. How do you make nine feel validated?*

KS: On vacations my husband and I set aside special days for each of them—one may go to breakfast with us, for instance. And every day, I find one-on-one time while we're riding in the car. I'll say things like "I'm proud of you" or "You're awesome." There are always opportunities to give each child attention: One can help me cook, another can be my special laundry-person, and someone can drive with me to the grocery store.

O: *Kathryn, we have another visitor—hi, Jimmy.* [Fifteen-year-old Jimmy passes through the room.]

KS: Jimmy, say goodbye to Oprah.

O: *Where are you going?*

JIMMY: I'm going to my brother's game. Bye, Oprah.

O: *Nice to meet you. Good luck through adolescence—may it treat you well.*

JIMMY: Thank you.

O: *All the kids seem to like one another so much.*

KS: They love one another. And in a sense, they've raised one another.

O: *How do you feel about your role as a mother?*

KS: I feel like I'm being used for a higher purpose. I've been blessed with a lot of strength. When I pray for guidance, I feel like I get it—and I try to filter it to them.

O: *Do you think you could do this without a spiritual foundation?*

KS: Never. Maybe I could do it for a bit, but not for the duration. And raising the children is really a partnership. Jim and I have known each other since we were 16 and 17, and we both come from strong families. We're lucky to be blessed with so much support from our extended families.

O: *Do you want more children?*

KS: I'm 40, and I'm not getting any younger. But I never want to just say never. [*Laughs.*] I probably won't say no even when I'm 55 or 60.

O: *Do you take precautions not to get pregnant?*

KS: Yes—we watch it. I know my body really well. With the baby being just a few months old...

O: *You don't want another one right away.*

KS: Correct.

O: *What do you say to moms who feel overwhelmed with just two or three children?*

KS: Do more for yourself—it's okay. It's not selfish. Exercise. Spend quiet time. It will empower you to do the work you're supposed to do. I see a lot of parents who do so much for their children that they just spin out of control. But to take care of others, you really do have to care for yourself first.

O: *What is your wish for yourself this Mother's Day?*

KS: To be thankful for all the blessings I've been given—truly.

O: *I bet Mother's Day is big in this house.*

KS: It's a fun day. The kids go out and shop for flowers; they bring me breakfast in bed—and every year, I just cry over their cards. They tear me up. One year one of the boys gave me a card that said "I thank God every night for putting me on this earth with a mother like you. You're the best mom a kid could ask for. I love you, Mom." For me, that is the greatest gift. That's all I could ever want. •

The Truth About Mommy Time

New mother **LISA KOGAN** had a choice—she could write this article, or she could wash her hair.... Does anybody have a hat?

ONE YEAR AGO THIS MONTH, I TOOK a second job. And though it doesn't offer a dental plan, sick leave, vacation pay, profit sharing, a Christmas bonus, an expense account, a 401(k), or even a company softball team, it does provide plenty of job security: I will be a mother every day for the rest of my natural life.

Raising a child—alone or with a partner—may be a labor of love, but, as anyone who's ever sung "The Wheels on the Bus" 11 times in a row can tell you, it's still labor. So imagine my weariness when I picked up a magazine in the pediatrician's waiting room touting the virtues of a little something called mommy time. Apparently the concept involves making it a priority to get out there and enjoy a manicure, a movie, a long lunch with an old friend—it's all about taking time for yourself on a regular basis. But here's the thing: I took 42 years for myself; now I'm taking time for a Cheerio-encrusted 21 pounder with three teeth, mashed banana in her eyebrows, and a tendency to wake up at 5 a.m. for breast milk and *Blue's Clues.*

Who are these manicured mommies analyzing the latest indie flick over salad niçoise? Are they the same women who bake from scratch, do Pilates, run multimillion-dollar corporations, volunteer at nursing homes, and campaign for clean air while having soul-shredding sex with their adoring husbands 4.7 nights a week and twice on Sundays? Because I don't know any mommies like that. Maybe they hang out at a special playground located in old Doris Day movies—they sure don't live in my neighborhood. The women I know feel victorious when they actually manage to pick up their dry cleaning. We're a motley crew all in serious need of a haircut and a shot of caffeine. Like the Marines, we do more before 9 a.m. than most people do in a day. We've seen things in diapers that would send plenty of members of polite society shrieking into the night. There is no surface in our homes that doesn't feel sticky, no blouse in our closets that hasn't been irrevocably stained. There is no part of our physical beings that hasn't been gummed, sucked, gnawed, or spit up on. We live mostly on teething biscuits, rice cereal, and the edge...and that, for better or for worse, till preschool do us part, is mommy time. God may have rested on the seventh day, but let's be honest here, that's only because he sent his son to live with another family. In the words of the late, great Warren Zevon, "I'll sleep when I'm dead." ●

**Got milk?
The author's
daughter, Julia
Claire Labusch,
at 6 months.**

THE STRONGEST LINK

From cooing baby to whiz kid, her son has been her light, love, and learning curve. Now that they've grown up together, what happens to that primal bond? **Valerie Monroe** reports.

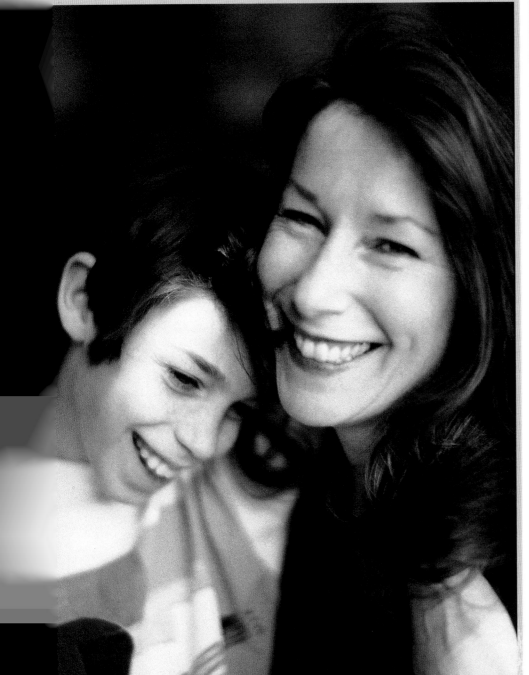

I SO LOVED BEING PREGNANT that I wished I could carry my son forever. The bigger I got, the more luxuriously contented I felt. And not just contented: commanding, sorcerous. Who needed to pull *this* bunny out of the hat? In the end, the doctors had to tie me down and remove my son surgically. My obstetrician, who performed the Cesarean section, would say that my cervix had incompletely dilated. That's what *he* thinks. I simply refused to give my baby up.

One evening when my son was about 8 months old and I had not yet weaned him, my husband and I left him with a sitter so that we could take in a ballet. By the end of the performance, my throbbing breasts were signaling that I'd been away from the baby long enough. When we walked into our living room, the cheerful young sitter was holding him by the hands as he stood, his fat legs wobbly, on her lap. In the moment before he saw me, his expression was one of careful determination, as if he knew he'd had one too many, but that he could stand on this lap without falling over, dammit, if he just tried hard enough. When his eyes met mine, though, he burst into a brilliant, drooly grin, leaning toward me and bouncing crazily in his excitement. I picked him up. He clutched my neck and started snuffling around in my blouse. As I settled on the couch to nurse him, I felt absolutely whole and complete, the way I'd felt during my pregnancy. It is this powerful, primitive, empathetic connection, this merging, this heady blend of joy, satisfaction, and easy competence that is also the deep grief of motherhood. Because to raise a child successfully, you have to let him go.

As a new parent, I was ambushed by the intensity of the attachment; I had no idea how my feelings would evolve over the course of my son's childhood, from his early loud and stubborn stirrings for independence to his current status as a 20-year-old college student and world traveler. The first time a sitter took him out in the stroller, I stood at the window, my face pressed to the glass, waiting for her to round the corner on their return. The idea of my son's ever crossing a busy city street alone? You might as well have said that he'd be walking on the moon. Tentatively, I shared a confession with one of my mother-friends: "I know I'm not supposed to," I said, "but I love my baby more than I love my husband." "What can you do?" she said. "Me, too."

YET DAY BY DAY, AS MY son grew, our connection somehow became elastic enough to accommodate his need to establish himself as separate from me: At 3, he suggested a playdate at his best friend Nicolette's house. Really? He wanted me to leave him there alone? "Yep," he said, "pick me up later." At 6, he wanted to join an after-school program; at 9, to go to sleepaway camp; at 12, to spend the weekend at a friend's in the country; at 17, to go to school in Minnesota; at 19, to study in Japan.

The summer before he left, I couldn't get enough of him; I took every opportunity to be home when he was. One day I asked him if he agreed that the closer a child is to his parents, the farther away he has to go to become independent of them. "I don't know," he said, "maybe." Is that why he chose to go to Japan? "Oh no," he

> It is this powerful, primitive, empathetic connection, this merging, this heady blend of joy, satisfaction, and easy competence that is also the deep grief of **motherhood.**

said. Then: "Maybe." The day he left for Kyoto, I felt as queasy as the first time he walked to school alone. Only he was no longer a small, slender shoot, bearing the heavy fruit of his backpack, overripe with books—he was tall and strapping, firmly supporting the weight of his decision to leave everything familiar for eight months of the unknown. "We're doing this quickly, like taking off a Band-Aid," he said at the airport when it was time to say goodbye. He hugged me and my husband tightly, turned around, and walked to the plane. I waited till we got to the parking lot and then cried—I cried in short bursts for weeks. I kept thinking, *The sweetest part of my life is over. How can I stand it? What will take its place?*

About halfway through his stay, we visited him. He met us at the airport. He was easy to spot, a couple of heads taller than everyone else in the crowd. "Just follow me," he said, as he led us through the maze of people, passageways, and ticket booths to our train. "Follow me," he said, as he bought our tickets, as he helped us find our room at the hotel.

When he was on his own, he rode around Kyoto like the Japanese, on a bicycle. The bike was a little small for him—as was almost everything else—which made him seem bigger than when he'd left home. Or maybe he was bigger; I wasn't sure. His host family obviously adored him. Though I couldn't understand their conversations, the mutual kindness and respect they shared with my son needed no translation.

For two weeks, my husband and I followed him like baby ducklings. And by the time he put us on the train to Osaka for our flight home, I understood that the sweetest part of my life was not over but that it was expanding, the way the connection between my child and me has always been expanding, to include experience and satisfaction and joy I could never have imagined. I wish I could love everyone in my life the way I love my son: cleanly, without jealousy or neediness; wanting for him happiness, success, strength, and many more people who love him as I do. ●

It took 30
years and one
transatlantic
phone call for
the actress
to understand
what her
mother was
talking about.

Christine Baranski's Aha! Moment

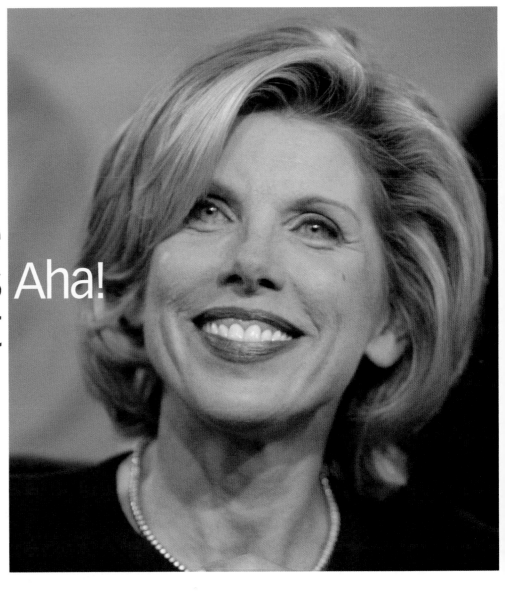

WHEN I WAS 19 I RECEIVED A $1,000 scholarship from Juilliard awarded to a girl or a boy who was hardworking, promising, and needed money. And when they gave it to me the administrator said, "Now you make sure you use this money to live on next year." Well, the next day I went and got my passport to go to Europe. And I called my mother. She was absolutely appalled and said, "You can't do that! You can't travel alone! What if something happens?" The poor woman, right? I said that she didn't understand, this was an opportunity, blah, blah, blah.... I was so high-spirited, so determined. There was no discussion, and I was gone. I traveled in Europe by myself for six weeks.

And I remember my mother showing up at the airport when I got back. She was so happy to see me, so grateful that nothing had happened. *Then* she said, "I'm so proud of you."

Fast-forward to a few years ago. My 16-year-old daughter spends a school year in France living with a family—something called School Year Abroad. She's like me: headstrong, adventurous. She tells me she's

going with another girl to Rome. By themselves. So this is not with the family, this is alone. I tell her, "I don't know if I want you to do this. You'd better be careful, blah, blah, blah.... And hold on to your money. The trains there are very dangerous—I've heard a lot of stories about theft."

So she goes to Rome. And I think to myself, Well *I* did it—I have to let her do it.

But then we got a call very early one morning. "Mom," I heard this quiet voice saying, "we had our money stolen on the way to Rome. Can you wire us some more?" And of course I said, "I told you! What did I say!" Oh, the anxiety we felt, and the anger, and the oh-my-God-my-daughter's-in-Rome-by-

"Now I can see how strong my mother was to let me go," says Christine Baranski.

herself panic. And then it hit me. This is what my mother experienced raising a high-spirited, independent girl like me. Because my daughter is just like me. And I thought, *This is really hard. Things can go wrong! How did my mother do it?* Now I can see how difficult it was and how strong she was to let me go. I understood the depth of her feeling, her love, and her fear that something would happen. I felt such an appreciation for that, so many years later.

When my mother died, I found myself standing in the midst of her things, filled with all this emotion, this longing and missing. I realized once again how much she gave me, and all I want to do is give my children the same: the strength to love someone profoundly, and in the end let them be who they are. ●

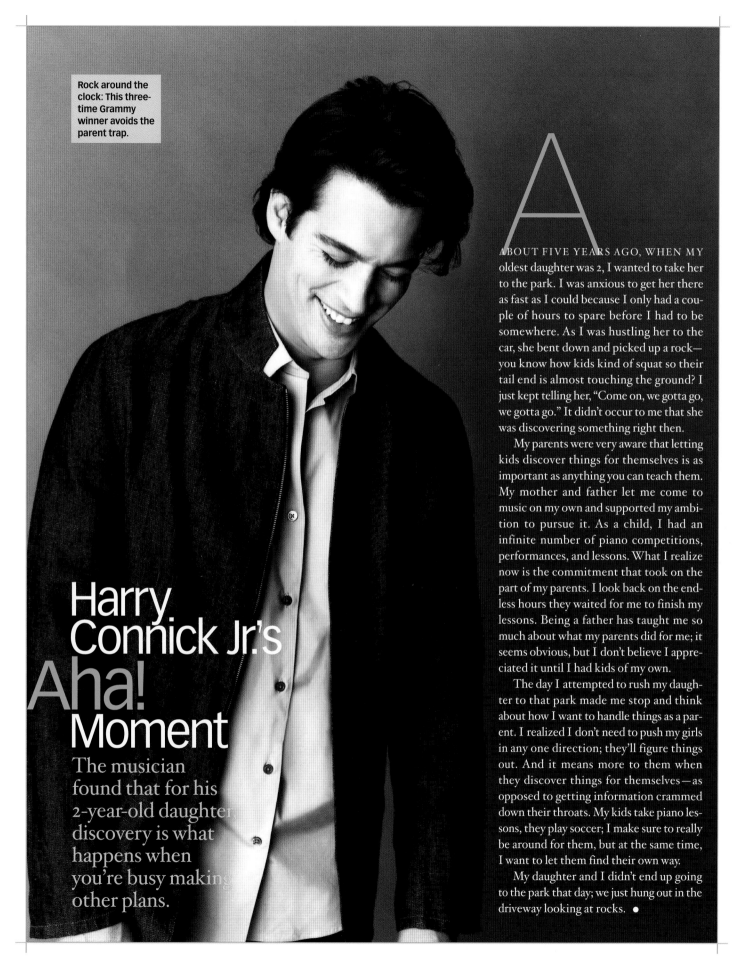

Harry Connick Jr.'s
Aha! Moment

The musician found that for his 2-year-old daughter, discovery is what happens when you're busy making other plans.

A

ABOUT FIVE YEARS AGO, WHEN MY oldest daughter was 2, I wanted to take her to the park. I was anxious to get her there as fast as I could because I only had a couple of hours to spare before I had to be somewhere. As I was hustling her to the car, she bent down and picked up a rock—you know how kids kind of squat so their tail end is almost touching the ground? I just kept telling her, "Come on, we gotta go, we gotta go." It didn't occur to me that she was discovering something right then.

My parents were very aware that letting kids discover things for themselves is as important as anything you can teach them. My mother and father let me come to music on my own and supported my ambition to pursue it. As a child, I had an infinite number of piano competitions, performances, and lessons. What I realize now is the commitment that took on the part of my parents. I look back on the endless hours they waited for me to finish my lessons. Being a father has taught me so much about what my parents did for me; it seems obvious, but I don't believe I appreciated it until I had kids of my own.

The day I attempted to rush my daughter to that park made me stop and think about how I want to handle things as a parent. I realized I don't need to push my girls in any one direction; they'll figure things out. And it means more to them when they discover things for themselves—as opposed to getting information crammed down their throats. My kids take piano lessons, they play soccer; I make sure to really be around for them, but at the same time, I want to let them find their own way.

My daughter and I didn't end up going to the park that day; we just hung out in the driveway looking at rocks. •

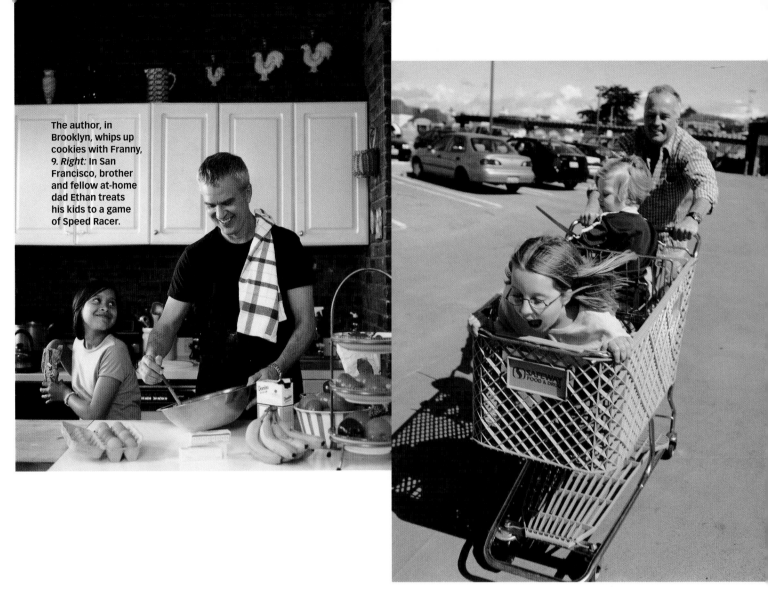

The author, in Brooklyn, whips up cookies with Franny, 9. *Right:* In San Francisco, brother and fellow at-home dad Ethan treats his kids to a game of Speed Racer.

The Stay-at-Home Dad

Coincidentally, their wives both have high-octane jobs. Coincidentally, he and his brother cook, clean, schlepp kids to school, and question the foundation of their lives. SEAN ELDER reports on the ups, downs, grievances, little joys, and nagging ambivalence of house-husbandry.

MY WIFE OFFERED TO BUY ME A STOVE for my birthday. We were having dinner at a neighborhood restaurant when she made the suggestion—just a suggestion, she assured me, a joke, if I wanted to look at it that way. But the joke was on her. I just blinked and said, "The 30-inch Wolf range?"

I've always been the cook in our house, and not just a weekend warrior, either. My mother was such a bad cook that when I was a boy I would pretend I was a prisoner of war being forced to eat her creative offerings—macaroni and cheese studded with sliced hot dogs, say. My younger brother, Ethan, and I learned to fend for ourselves in the kitchen, and after our parents divorced we took turns cleaning, along with my younger sister, while our mother was out earning a paycheck. What used to be called women's work has always been second nature to us.

But I never thought of it as my calling. Whatever satisfaction I derived from cooking or schlepping laundry or changing diapers came in part from the knowledge that I would soon be doing something else. My job—writing and editing—often allowed me to work at home. I mocked weekend dads as gentlemen fathers, as cut off from the real toil of parenthood as gentlemen farmers were from plowing the fields, but the truth was that I no more wanted to be Mr. Mom, a full-time househusband, than I wanted to get behind the mule.

Well, hee-haw. Two years ago, I was laid off from my last full-time job, and it turned out I was ahead of the curve. People who had been calling me with job offers were suddenly calling me for leads, and the only reason I haven't seen them selling pencils on the sidewalks of New York is that we all use computers now. My wife, Peggy, meantime, is making a salary more than three times what I pulled down last year.

My brother was laid off late in 2001 from the high-tech parts company he sold for in Silicon Valley; almost immediately afterward, his wife, Leah, took a lucrative position with a nationally known cookware retailer. Suddenly, we were both home taking care of the kids—he has two (a son, Finnegan, who's 3, and a daughter, Ali, 8) as do I (Franny, 9, and Adam, 18)—plus the house and all that implies.

I know we're not alone. In the markets and at the matinees I see them: Millennium Men dragging their children on errands or being dragged themselves to Nickelodeon movies, all the time wondering where their work went.

In the past year, Ethan and I have compared notes, via e-mail and cell phone, on grocery shopping and the fortunes of the Giants. Sometimes I send him recipes; sometimes he sends me porn.

Are we not men?

Some are married to women who can make more money. Others do it because they want to. HANNAH WALLACE reports on

MEN BEHAVING DADLY

When Peter Baylies founded the At-Home Dad Network in 1994, there were few resources for a full-time father like him. One day while his son John was napping, Baylies decided to start a newsletter.

He began a conversation with 20 at-home dads over the Internet and asked them for submissions. "I was flooded with articles," he says. The result is a national organization for stay-at-home dads (SAHDs) with more than 50 local groups, each with 50 to 100 members, and an annual convention—held on weekends so the men can get away while their wives watch the kids.

Today, thanks to organizations like Baylies's (athomedad.com) and slowlane.com (a URL whose irony is not lost on anyone who's ever stepped off the fast track to run after young kids), a househusband who would have felt isolated in his own neighborhood ten years ago is no longer alone. Baylies estimates that there are 2 million men at home raising children. One small sign that SAHD ranks are expanding: At restaurants and rest stops around the country, the men's room is just as likely as the ladies' room to have a Koala diaper-changing table. According to Koala's vice president Brendan Cherry, the number of new businesses ordering two tables, as opposed to one, has grown exponentially over the past five years.

Libby Gill, author of *Stay-at-Home Dads: The Essential Guide to Creating the New Family*, attributes the increase of SAHDs in part to economics. "Two out of five women outearn their husbands," she says. If one parent is going to care for the kids, the choice has less to do with gender than with who has the bigger paycheck and the most job security.

Men still struggle with their new role, however. "In the beginning, I had this macho thing about 'a guy's gotta work,'" says Todd Vossler, a primary caretaker of two, whose wife makes a good salary as a certified public accountant.

Vossler founded a chapter of DC Metro Dads, a network for Washington-area stay-at-home fathers, which organizes lunches and play groups. "You need that adult conversation," he says.

Tom Smith, also raising two children, remembers a party he went to after moving to Brockport, New York. "An older gentleman walked up and said, 'So you must be the new professor.' I said, 'No, that'd be my wife.' 'What do you do?' he asked me. When I told him I was a stay-at-home dad, he looked at me, turned around, and walked away."

Despite stories like this—and every dad has at least one—Libby Gill thinks the stigma of being a SAHD is gradually disappearing. "There's been a shift over the last generation. It's gone from 'Jeez, I'm the weirdest guy on the planet' to 'I'm really proud of the contribution I can make to my family and to my children,'" she says. "It's becoming normalized now."

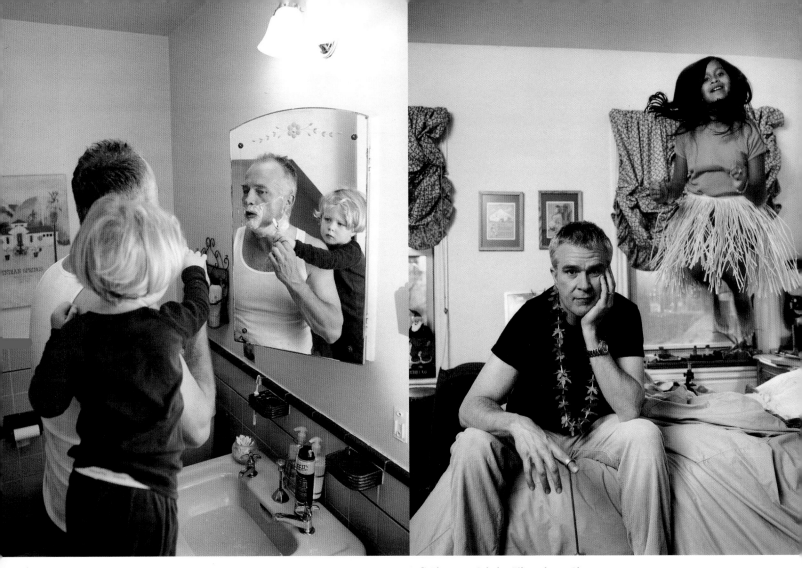

Left: Finnegan, 3, helps Ethan shave. *Above:*
Sean and Franny play dress-up.

Despite the time difference between San Francisco and Brooklyn, Ethan and I are on pretty much the same schedule. The toddler gets up at about 6:15, so Ethan tries to beat him by 15 minutes for what might laughably be called "me time," which for him consists of reading yesterday's front page before today's paper arrives.

He e-mails me on the first day of Finn's swimming lessons at the Y: "I'd pictured a helpful teenage girl taking Finn and showing him how to kick, breathe, etc. No, not the case. Boom box blasting 'The Wheels on the Bus' and parents in the pool singing and bobbing with kids. I envision our childless friends standing on the side saying, 'See, that's why!' Finn starts to have fun, and so do I. After a half hour, my arm starts to hurt. This is what my doctor refers to as two-year-old arm. I take her advice: I switch arms."

I recall the days of two-year-old arm rather fondly myself. Franny lets me hold her now with the resigned air of a hostage, though that aloof 9-year-old routine seems like a pose, a rude T-shirt she's trying on. Some parents have told me that 9 is the adolescence of elementary school. For girls, maybe. When Adam was 9, he acted like a 9-year-old boy, i.e., Bart Simpson. Maybe aloof is better.

MY KIDS ARE IN SCHOOL, which opens up my day considerably. Or would. We have an old house, and we tapped ourselves out buying it five years ago. Now the floors are buckling because water is getting in from somewhere into the subfloor, warping the wood. Before I can get the floors fixed, I've got to find someone who can figure out where the leaks are. Before someone can figure out where the leaks are, he has to come look at the rear walls. In New York, getting somebody to come do anything, even haul away furniture you're donating, is a full-time job. I'm on the phone to the floor guy and the waterproofing guy trying to coordinate their visits, when my son calls. He's left his homework on his desk. Could I fax it to his school?

ETHAN CALLS WHILE I'M grocery shopping that afternoon; he's doing the same thing in San Francisco with Finn in the cart and Ali in tow. Over the phone I can hear Ali yelling. They are already in the Safeway parking lot, and I'm still at the Key Food deli counter, waiting. "Speed Racer!" she cries, audible a continent away. This, my brother later explains, is when he runs through the parking lot pushing the cart with Finn in the child seat and Ali hanging on the front, imperiling all of them and innocent bystanders to boot. Like to see Mom do *that*.

ONE DAY I DECIDE TO make chocolate chip cookies with Franny. Although it's a reward—she has finished her homework, practiced piano, and washed her hair—I have an ulterior motive: I really like chocolate chip cookies. But where our last experiment in cookie baking was a raging success, this time nothing goes right. The dough's lumpy. There's not enough sugar. And then, for reasons I can't fathom, the oven won't get hot enough to bake them. They just sit there, sweating in little warm lumps in this ancient Tappan oven that was new when I was still listening to the Sex Pistols. My daughter loses interest, and I put some water on for pasta (at least the range still works). Peggy said she'd be home about 8.

Thinking about the Sex Pistols must have reminded me of college, because soon I'm brooding about my wasted English B.A. as I dice vegetables and try to drown out my regrets with *All Things Considered*. I had wanted to be a real writer, the kind whose photo you find on the back of books, and instead I'm questioning Marcella Hazan's predilection for butter. I am reminded of a John Cheever story in which a housewife hangs her college degree over the sink until the joke gets old and she puts it away. I think I'm becoming a feminist.

DON'T KNOW IF IT'S CABIN fever, but some days I feel trapped," Ethan tells me in an e-mail. "Most days I can't even seem to squeeze in a workout. Any of my other forms of relief are none too healthy for body or marriage."

Then he tells me that a job he's been courting is on and he should be back to work by January. I feel like a South Vietnamese soldier in Saigon watching the last U.S. helicopter leaving. He's got tickets to tonight's World Series game, too, he says. "Watch for me on TV—I'll be the guy in the Giants cap with a beer."

The Giants win that night but lose the series, four to three. The waterproofing estimate comes in at $4,500. The floor work is estimated at a relatively modest $1,400. Meanwhile, our mother seems to be losing her marbles, and Ethan has started looking at retirement homes in the Bay Area. He took her on a tour of one; afterward she said it was okay but she didn't like a lot of old people.

He e-mails me the next day: "I took Finn to a Montessori school for a visit this morning and watched them gently test him. I had to fight myself not to yell the answers and move the blocks myself. This is how I feel with Mom. I wish I could

In the markets and at the matinees I see them: **Millennium Men** wondering where their work went.

turn back time and bring her mind back into sync. Every day I realize more that this will never happen."

I'd love to fly out there and provide support to my brother, but I can't afford to leave. Franny's piano teacher tells me that her timing is off. I say mine isn't so good, either.

PEGGY AND I GET INTO A huge fight coming back from the Home Depot Expo one Sunday. Turns out the Wolf range I had my eye on needs six inches on either side because they run so hot, which would mean replacing the kitchen counter and cabinets. Ours are tragically prefab anyway and falling apart, and when they go, so goes the dishwasher, the sink, and the leaky faucet. The floors, as I mentioned, are pretty well shot, and while we're at it, those pantry shelves should go, too, along with the refrigerator. We've gone from a $4,000 range to a $50,000 kitchen remodeling in the course of a few hours, and the conversation that follows—touching on money, responsibility, opportunity, and all the places we've never been—is as sudden and ugly as a dust devil. Funny how you

can go from window-shopping together to visions of joint custody. Afterward, we take turns saying we're sorry, uncertain of what we're apologizing for.

I call Ethan the next day, and of course I don't talk about the fight with my wife. Instead we speculate about where Giants manager Dusty Baker will end up next season. Ethan just signed the papers on his new job. "Now that it's the end of my stay-at-home stage, I'm already missing it," he tells me, and I find myself filled with resentment. *Short-timer,* I think. It's a lot easier to wipe up one more spill when you're not thinking of doing the same thing tomorrow and tomorrow and tomorrow. My pettiness depresses me.

FOR $130, A BALD RUSSIAN comes and replaces something called the bake igniter in my oven, and soon Franny and I are making cookies again. The sweet smell fills the house and makes me forget my bitterness. As much as I chafe at my life and its boundaries, there are times when I think I could spend eternity baking with my daughter.

I decide to give my son a shaving kit I'd been saving for Christmas. My father was not around for me when I was a teenager, so I probably attach more significance to the gesture than Adam does: I feel like I'm offering him a leg up into the adult world, the world of shaving and travel and unfettered possibility. "Cool," is all he says, and turns up the stereo.

AN E-MAIL FROM ETHAN: "Shaving in the bathroom. Finn walks in, 'Wha' are you doing?' 'Shaving.' 'Can I shave?' 'No, sweet boy, you have to be big to shave.' Leaves, comes back with two sticks, one big, one small. Holds the big one upright and uses the little one to play it like a cello while humming. I ask, 'What are you doing?' He says, 'Singing.' I tell him he looks like he's playing the cello. He says, 'I play jello.' I ask, 'Can I play jello?' He says, 'No, you have to be little.'"

As much as I made of giving Adam a shaving kit, I am reminded of the appeal of no responsibility and the music only little children can hear. Make us all little again. ●

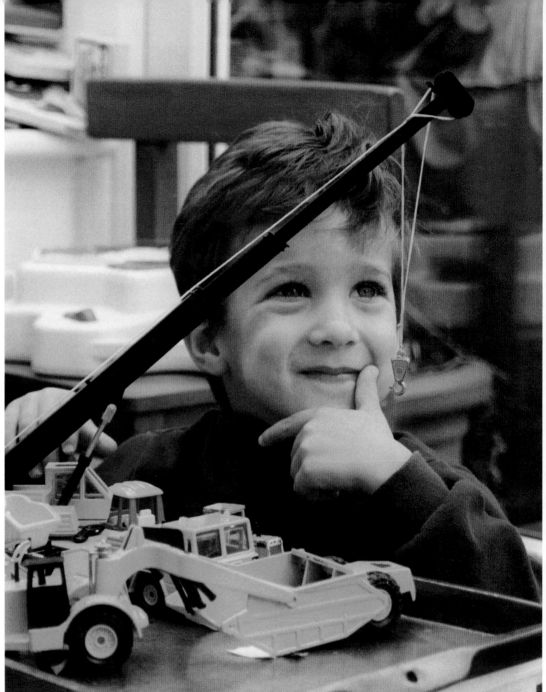

Nico, with the machines that flattened his mother's opinion of men.

The Road Warriors

They don't want to play with dolls or read about charming French orphans. They want to dig, blast, shovel, detonate, and steamroll! No one told LISA WOLFE that having sons would put her on a collision course with her own feminist expectations.

"CAN WE BUILD A ROAD?"

"Can we build a *rooooad*?"

"Can *we* build a road?"

A 3-year-old will try anything. My son Nico is changing the intonation of the question so I might forget I heard it ten minutes ago, and ten minutes before that. So I might forget that I did build a road with him many of the times he asked—today, yesterday, and the day before. Can he be serious? All we *do* is build roads! All we *do* is gather every toy digger, dumper, steamroller from every corner of the house and zoom the vehicles around the floor making noises like "*Brrrrrmmm!*" "*Nee-naw-nee-naw!*" and "*Eeewwweeewww!*"

It's not that building roads can't be fun. It can be a lot of fun. If I crash one of my vehicles into one of his, the kid gets so excited you could melt. But every 90 roads or so, I think it might be nice to do something else.

"Why don't we read a book?" I gently suggest.

"No."

"Why don't we make a *picture?*" I learn from him and change the intonation of my question.

"No." He learns from me and won't be fooled by toddler tricks.

"I know!" I say. "Why don't we play with your fantastic *doll?*"

"Because I want to build a road," Nico says.

WHEN HIS 1-YEAR-OLD-brother, Aidan, wakes up from his nap, I have another idea. We'll go outside. There's something both sexes can enjoy together—the great outdoors. The boys are delighted. It's a chance to be in the dirt.

They have been playing for more than an hour, running fingers, sticks, rocks, and anything else they can find through the muck, when Christina, the 5-year-old who lives in the house attached to ours, prances out the door all dressed in white. She is wearing a wedding gown her mother made her for Halloween and a shiny tinfoil crown.

"Christina!" I cry, getting all excited. "You look beautiful!"

"I'm getting married," she beams.

"Who are you marrying?"

"My daddy!"

"Boys," I say. "Look at Christina! She is dressed as something we call a bride...."

The boys don't look up from the dirt.

Christina's mother walks out, sees her daughter in white and my boys in the dirt, and says with a smile I can't say I appreciate: "So much for 'It's all in the upbringing.'"

I don't smile back. Instead I tuck one filthy boy under each arm and march them indoors for a bath. Then I feed them din-ner, put his brother to bed, and tell Nico he is allowed to watch one videotape before it's his turn to go to sleep.

"*The tractor tape!!*" he cries.

"Nico," I say in my best loving voice. "You watched the tractor tape last night. And the night before that. What about something else tonight, like *Mary Poppins?*"

"No."

"But you love the chimney sweeps! Remember how dirty they get?"

"I love *the tractor tape!!*"

I have no one to blame but myself. I am the one who bought *the tractor tape!!*—a video whose official title is, I believe, *Road Construction Ahead,* which came packaged with a small yellow excavator. The thrill I felt as I carried the thing to the cashier is nothing if not a testament to how much I love my son.

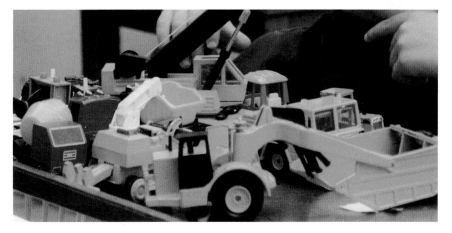

I pop the tape into the VCR. Nico holds his breath. I press play. Diggers start digging, dumpers start dumping, drum-intensive music pumps the room. "*The trac-tor tape!!*" Nico cries, jumping up and down and punching the air like a guy whose team has just won the Super Bowl. "*The tractor tape!!*"

"Hi," says a man in blue jeans and a red hard hat, who is plowing some dirt. "My name is George, and I'm usin' this bull-dozer to put in a new road."

Nico shrieks. More diggers dig. More dumpers dump. George points to a gray mountain of rock. "When there's solid rock like this where a road has to be built," he says, "then it has to be moved."

Nico knows (as he ought to, having viewed this tape about a third of the days he has lived) that his favorite part is coming up, the part where they blast the mountain of rock. Dynamite is tied, holes are dug, my son starts whirling like a dervish. He pivots on one foot, then another, chanting, "Yes...yes...yes...yes...." By the time the dynamite is buried, the love of my life is frothing at the mouth. There is a loud bang. Rocks shoot through the air. Nico has never looked so thrilled in his life. No amount of singing or cuddling or

storytelling, no visit to any playground or petting zoo or farm has ever managed to elicit from him such an ecstatic response.

I appreciate that what I am watching is one of the most gorgeous things I'll ever see: the exuberance of a happy, healthy child. On the other hand, my child is so happy it's making me sad. *Who* is *he?* I wonder. Who is this person, high as my thigh, realization of my deepest desires, who is so

Who is this person, high as my thigh,

transfixed by the sight of rocks

and gravel flying through the air?

transfixed by the sight of rocks and dust and gravel flying through the air?

I don't know. That's the thing. I don't know how anyone can get so excited about rocks and dust and gravel flying through the air. I don't know how anyone as female as I could have produced a child as male as this, or his brother.

At first, like so many women I know, I tried to feminize my boys. I bought them their infamous doll. But we could never find her; the poor thing was invariably lying at the bottom of a pileup. Nico says her legs make "really good road bumps."

woman for which secretary. At college, some of my feminist professors made my mother and grandmother seem pictures of female contentment. And as a young single woman in New York, I would spend hours on the phone with my friends whenever one or another of us had her heart broken, reciting the litany: Men are not as emotionally sophisticated as we are. Or as articulate. Their brains are simpler. They are driven by baser instincts. Boys are harder to raise than girls, with all that wild boy energy. Then once you finally raise them, they shoot out the door. (My

way the firemen could get in!"), I can't help thinking he wouldn't do this if he were a girl. But at least I'm trying. Trying for once not to see my sons or other men through my condescending female lens. Just because their responses to things might be different from mine does not make them bad.

I look over at Nico, who is leaning against the sofa, spent. The hair I combed so neatly after his bath has been flung in every which direction. His airplane pajamas are hiked up to his chest, exposing a big round milk belly. Such a little person

I realized I had spent a good chunk of my life denigrating the penis people. I didn't do it maliciously; I did it more for sport.

Then there was the Madeline book. I loved nothing more as a kid than my Madeline book. My mother, hearing that I was pregnant, confessed she had been saving it for me all these years. We hugged in tearful anticipation of my reading the book to my own children. There is just one problem. My children won't listen. Only one page holds their interest, the one that reads "To the tiger in the zoo Madeline just said pooh, pooh!" They love it. "She said pooh pooh! She said pooh pooh!" Nico runs joyously through the house shouting. "Pooh pooh! Pooh pooh!" his brother follows him, chanting.

Slowly the message began to penetrate the layers of tulle in my head: These boys weren't going to change. Change was up to me. And it wasn't going to be easy. Though my father, brothers, and husband are among the kindest souls I know, I had spent a good chunk of my life denigrating the penis people. I didn't do it maliciously; I did it more for sport. Most women I knew were playing. When I was a little girl, I listened to my mother and grandmother go on about which man had left which

grandmother—whose dying words to me were, helpfully, "Promise me you'll keep going until you have a girl"—never tired of repeating: "A daughter is a daughter for all her life, a son is a son till he gets himself a wife.")

I probably would have kept this up if I'd had daughters. But I had sons. And so I had to confront my prejudices—a process I initiated shortly after the pooh parade. I was forced to realize not only how wide-ranging my assumptions about men were, and how I had come to accept them over the years as absolute truth, but how hypocritical I was. For all my ranting, in college and after, about how unfairly men had stereotyped women, I was doing the same thing to them. In fact, if you replaced the words *boy* or *man* with *girl* or *woman* or *African-American,* it would be illegal to say the things I was saying. I was a sexist pig!

I'd like to be able to tell you that as soon as I realized this, I packed up my prejudices and put them away. But you already know this isn't true. When Nico salivates over *the tractor tape!!* I still get pangs. When he asks for a dollhouse, and we get him one, and the first thing he does is smash all the windows ("But there was a fire! It was the only

to have such big issues about. And, of course, it isn't only me. If prefeminist society favored boy children, postfeminist society seems to favor girl ones. I get numerous phone calls from panicked pregnant women who find out they're having a boy. "What will I *do* with a boy?" they ask, with fear so palpable you can feel it over the receiver. "Love him more than you imagined possible," I always say.

walk over to my son and scoop him up in my lap. He smells like a mixture of baby shampoo and himself. Like a dog, I bring my nose to the back of his neck and start sniffing around. I can't describe what I am looking for, but I will know when I find it. It turns out to be a spot behind his left ear, under a curl. I plant my nose there and inhale as deeply as my lungs will allow, hoping to stash the smell in a place where I might, please God, never forget it.

Some sort of large machine (Nico could probably tell me what it's called, but I'm not interested enough to ask) is spraying a bold yellow line down the freshly paved highway. "The new road is finished," says George, "and ready for traffic." ●

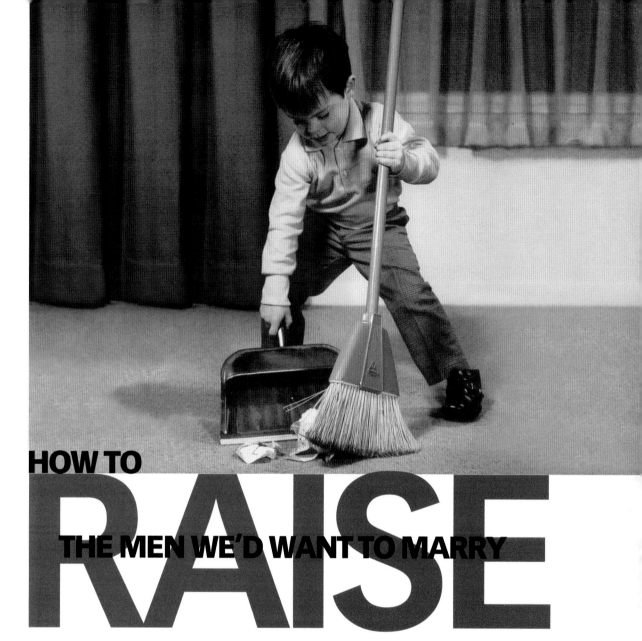

HOW TO RAISE
THE MEN WE'D WANT TO MARRY

I WAS DESCRIBING IN PRODIGIOUS, enthusiastic detail the trip to Japan from which I'd just returned with my then 15-year-old son. "And he's so much fun to travel with," I went on to my patient friend. "His observations were really interesting, and when we met new people, he was such a good listener, and he seemed willing to try almost anything," I said.

"Well, of course he's a fine companion," my friend said. "You raised him to be."

I felt a sharp urge to deny that, as if she'd accused me of something selfish. But I *have* raised a boy who's smart and observant, sensitive and kind, who listens well and is remarkably honest and articulate about the way he feels.

Attention mothers of sons: Women of the future are counting on you. Valerie Monroe tells how to bring up a good, kind, happy, mindful, nongrunting husband-to-be.

Lest you think I'm bragging—oh, never mind, I *am* bragging—there are many more mothers like me who've broken what William Pollack, PhD, calls the boy code, the persistent, largely unspoken but pervasive belief that we should bring up boys to be stoic, to hide their feelings, to become quickly independent of their parents (their mothers especially). In short, not to be like girls. Pollack, assistant clinical professor of psychology at Harvard Medical School, and author of *Real Boys,* believes that for boys to be happy and healthy, they must be allowed to have feelings, to show empathy, to be able to express the range of emotions encouraged in girls. Until I had a son, I thought, well, naturally you want to raise your child—boy or girl—to have a full emotional life. Then I tried to. And I discovered that there's a big difference between believing a boy should show his feelings freely and actually having a boy who does.

WHEN MY BEST FRIEND'S older son and my son were both around 3, her boy delighted in swathing himself in glittery tulle and prancing around with a fairy wand. My friend took it in stride, providing generous amounts of fabric and making aesthetic improvements—more sparkles, a bigger star on the wand, etc.—to her son's great and often delirious satisfaction. On the face of it, I supported her and her boy, but I confess I was also relieved that my son didn't express quite the same level of interest. It was such a small thing: A boy, barely out of babyhood, innocently enraptured by clouds of tulle—why was it even the slightest bit threatening to me? For the same reason that when my mother (an adoring grandmother in every way) saw my son weepy with hurt feelings when he was 10, she asked me reprovingly, "Do you think it's good for him to be so sensitive?" Or that when a friend who noticed him at 14 snuggling with me on the couch later asked, "Is he interested in girls yet?" A sensitive, affectionate boy risks being perceived as a "mama's boy, tied to her apron strings." Isn't it interesting that we have no such phrases to describe a girl who is attached to her mother? And that "daddy's girl" completely lacks the pejorative connotation?

My mother's and friend's questions scared me because they suggested that the closeness between me and my son was in some way inhibiting his path to a healthy manhood. Should I have sent him signals that I expected him to reject the intimate bond established between us? There are many reasons mothers might feel the need to withdraw from their sons, says Olga Silverstein, family therapist and author of *The Courage to Raise Good Men.* We're afraid that we'll contaminate our boys with "female"

qualities. We believe that boys must grow away from their families, and so we want to protect ourselves and our sons from the inevitable pain of separation. We think we're incapable of modeling qualities important to becoming a man, or that our closeness will make him homosexual. Or we believe that because he is male, he is unknowable to us, or that our affection and bond will be construed as seductive.

"It's absolutely necessary to shift the way we think of those qualities we call feminine," says Silverstein. "As a culture, we perceive empathy, nurturance, talent for friendship and relationship as belonging only to women and less valuable than independence and other kinds of strengths traditionally associated with men," she says. "Women have to believe that feminine strengths are valuable not just in women but in humans. Then we won't worry about feminizing boys." This isn't to say that we shouldn't respect the differences between boys and girls, whatever we perceive them to be. But the idea of defining male and female as opposites (as we do in this culture) is misguided and leads us into trouble, Silverstein says, because it implies that boys must not only separate from their mothers but reject the qualities associated with them. Does this sound unfair? Even misogynistic?

We know what we get when a boy is raised with the code, says Pollack: a mask of masculinity, false bravado, the need to be aggressive and to win, and to ignore or repress feelings of vulnerability. These are the men who seem strong but who are, ironically, weakest in many ways because they're hiding or are unaware of their neediness and are poorly equipped to engage in any kind of honest relationship. But those boys who get affection, love, respect, and compassion, grow up whole, not unconsciously seeking what they needed from their parents. I see these boys everywhere among my son's friends. They have pals who are girls. They are friendly with their mothers. They *like* their mothers.

One afternoon when my son was a senior in high school, a group of his friends gathered in our living room to play video

games. From the kitchen, I was aware of a sea of voices, deep and loud. Exclamations of playful frustration and surprise rose and fell in waves, over a steady undercurrent of exchange about schoolwork and teachers. After a while, I waded into their midst. They all glanced over at me.

"Hi, Reid's mom," one of them said.

I had a question for them, I said, related to a story I was writing: "You guys are 18, right?" I said. "Do you still tell your mothers that you love them?"

There was an earsplitting commotion as the game players wiped out the enemy. The playing stopped and silence swept the room. I stood there uncomfortably.

"Well, sure," one of the boys said finally.

"Of course," said another.

"Why not?" said a third.

A fourth boy, whose mother is a doctor, stretched his legs and leaned back in his chair. "My mother raised me and my brother and sister pretty much by herself," he said. "My mother is a goddess." No one snickered. It was a statement of fact.

HOW DID OUR BOYS TURN out like this? Silverstein suggests some important ways to ensure that our sons grow into whole human beings. We must continue to talk to them about our feelings and their own and not let them get away with putting us off. We should not be afraid to demonstrate our affection or anger or disapproval. We need to be honest about what we like and don't like about the way they act, supporting empathy, self-knowledge, and respect for feminine qualities. We can help them understand that both men and women can model how to raise a good person.

A child who is fully and deeply loved, who learns to acknowledge his feelings and is well equipped to express them, and who learns to take responsibility for his actions, to value compassion and live it daily—this is the boy who will grow into a man who'll make a loving companion. That's good for the woman he marries. Even better for the man he becomes. ●

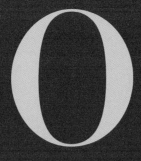

O

Friends

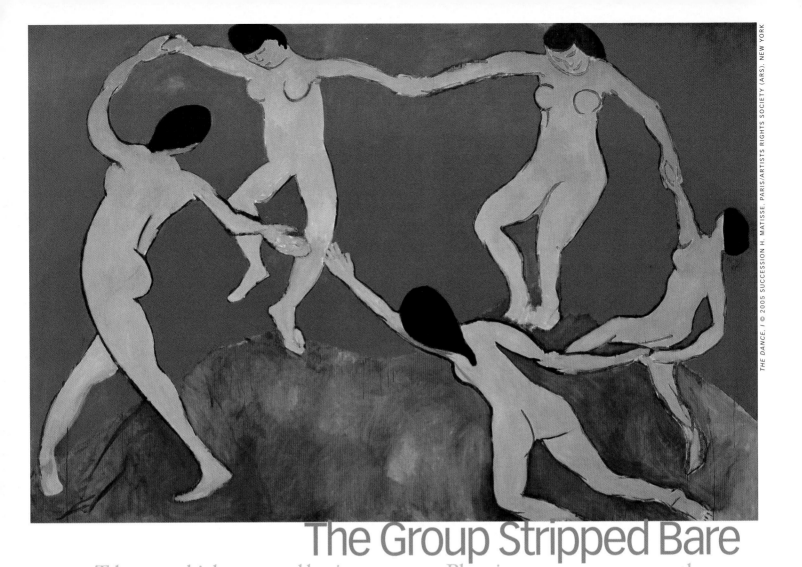

The Group Stripped Bare

Take some high-powered businesswomen. Place in a room, once a month, for 17 years. Stir in one therapist...and watch what happens. **BY JONI EVANS**

WE CAME TOGETHER BY ACCIDENT: nine women, all part of a national women's organization, to plan a panel discussion on aging. We ranged from our late 30s to our early 60s, and we got so involved in talking about the topic that I can't remember if we ever put on the panel. We decided to meet once a month to discuss, encourage, exchange, sympathize, network, scold, forgive, confess everything that was happening in our lives. We've hardly missed a month in 17 years.

We could have been the cast of a sitcom: one CEO of a law firm, one founder of a company, the owner of a hosiery company, president of a monthly publication, publisher of a book company, partner in a search firm, venture capitalist, officer of an investment real estate firm, and vice pres-

ident of an advertising agency. In total privacy and total trust (we never talked out of school), we shared life's most shocking jolts: deaths (two of our members lost to breast cancer), birth (one baby girl born to an overworked mother), divorces (three: two heavily contested, one marriage that died a natural death), new jobs, firings, IRS audits, retirements, facelifts—you name it, we lived it. We exchanged lawyers, tax shelters, birthday presents, psychiatrists, computer technicians, jewelry, gum surgeons, dreams, sex toys, Frédéric Fekkai appointments—you name it, we shared it.

But by around 1999, it was clear something was off. Our attendance was erratic, we'd come late, we'd argue, we'd be too polite. We were reluctant to

Henri Matisse's *The Dance, I,* 1909.

tell the whole truth. We were too timid to challenge each other, or too angry not to wound. We were hurtling toward a dead end.

We decided to do something about it. We invited in a psychoanalyst with the hope that he could get us unstuck. Jeffrey Rubin, PhD, was in private practice in New York City. He was not only an author (*Psychotherapy and Buddhism* and *A Psychoanalysis for Our Time*) but a practitioner of meditation and yoga. He seemed to have no ego. He was more interested in hearing what we had to say than imposing his own agenda. Every other month, paper and pencil in hand, he sat on our living room couches and listened. (We would come to understand that Listening Is an Art.)

THE GOAL, JEFFREY SAID, was to create an atmosphere of trust so that we could communicate more authentically. (He started each session with a meditation period that lasted five or ten minutes. For me it lasted a lifetime. I hate meditation. But after a while, I learned to appreciate the quiet transition between the tension of the day and the shelter an evening with my friends provided.) Jeffrey pointed out that many groups fall into bad habits, especially a group as long-lived as ours. He suspected that we had slipped into fixed roles, making honest communication almost impossible. Before that first session was over, we were able to identify those roles:

The Judge: the silent critic.

The Victim: feels inadequate ("Oh, woe is me"); hides her competence.

The Supercompetent: always in control, ferociously independent, has trouble asking for what she needs (me!).

The Conflict Avoider: jumps in to get rid of tension and bail out anyone struggling ("Oh, don't be silly, you're perfect").

The Maverick: really doesn't participate or receive.

Jeffrey encouraged us to slow down, hold a mirror up to ourselves, and give and get what he called compassionate feedback. (We would come to understand that Feedback Is an Art.) For example, if we were addressing the Victim: "When you say, 'Woe is me' each month, I feel that you don't take in the advice we give you. I feel that you're stuck. Is there anything I can do to help?" Each member would give feedback, then Jeffrey would ask the Victim, "How did what you just heard make you feel?" Here we each had to consider our initial reaction and examine why we'd said what we did. Then we had to express how it would feel to have it said to us. By slowing the communication and miscommunication, teasing out underlying feelings, and finding a constructive and compassionate way to rephrase what we'd said, we went deeper.

Over the next months, we learned to listen *to* our fellow members, not listen *for* the old stuff we thought we were going to hear. (We would come to learn that listening *to* is very different from listening *for*.)

A general theme for one member was the bitterness she felt toward her bosses: how they'd failed to recognize her excellence, how office politics were holding her back. Before Jeffrey, we would have categorized that as "Oh, there she goes again." Now we broke out of the old assumptions and really listened. How long had this been true? Was her unhappiness spilling into her home life? Was it possible the holdup in promotion wasn't office politics at all? Maybe she wasn't as good a leader as she thought? In the end, by asking questions and giving her feedback, we helped her see for herself that it was not her management skills but her creativity that made her unique, and she moved to a different job.

> Our choice was
> intimacy,
> no matter how scary
> it became.

But just around this point, things got rough. Uncovering the truth for this member had been difficult. We began to realize in the process of revisiting some old hurts, old arguments, that not all of us were comfortable on this path. It was amazing to find out that something said in 1996 was still a hot button in 2003. You had to have the stomach for these sessions. Having never been in therapy, I wondered if this is what it felt like: lump-in-the-stomach time, tears spilling over, even fear.

For example, many years before, I had blurted out to one member that I was uncomfortable with her parade of boyfriends (too many of them, why didn't she value herself? too much sex talk, why was she showing off? etc.). At the time she had yelled at me, and I immediately backed down and said I was sorry. (But I wasn't! I was sure I was the only one in the group brave enough to speak the truth.) Now so many years later, she told me what she'd felt when I'd criticized her, how it had humiliated her and, worse, kept her from express-

ing herself honestly from then on. How having these men as concurrent boyfriends was her choice and sex was her joy (no, she wasn't showing off).

I'd like to say that all seven of us survived this process. But that wasn't the case. Two members grew profoundly uncomfortable with our new direction. Maybe it was too personal. Too threatening. "Too mean," one of them said. We lost them both. And we all lost something—that kind of history cannot be duplicated. It felt like a divorce: hurt feelings, guilt, and blame. But still we stuck to the path, believing strongly in what we were trying to do. Eventually, we invited someone else to join us, and we are now a dynamite half-dozen chicks.

Recently, we've been exploring the effect of our work lives on our close relationships. As Jeffrey explained it, the very qualities we've needed to succeed—self-sufficiency and the ability to hide weakness—have made it difficult to be open and vulnerable with friends and loved ones. So lately we've been talking about what we appreciate about each other—and what we need from each other. We feel safe enough now to be able to admit: "I'm lonely." Or "I'm afraid to love him. What if it turns out the way it was with my first husband?" Or to ask: "Could you all call me on Friday nights?" Or "How can I deal with this new management when I don't trust them?"

After four years, each of us is finding a fresh excitement, a deeper caring we had no idea we could achieve. This has not been an easy journey. It takes courage. Our choice was intimacy, no matter how scary or uncomfortable it became.

We've created an environment of tolerance and openness. We see possibilities, we listen with new ears, we hear each other better. Now we have to handle our new closeness. This is a family of our own choosing. What a privilege.

In that first meeting with Jeffrey, we asked him, "How long do you see us doing this with you?"

"A good consultant should eventually put himself out of business," Jeffrey said. "The goal is to help you be able to do this on your own."

It's time to see how we do. •

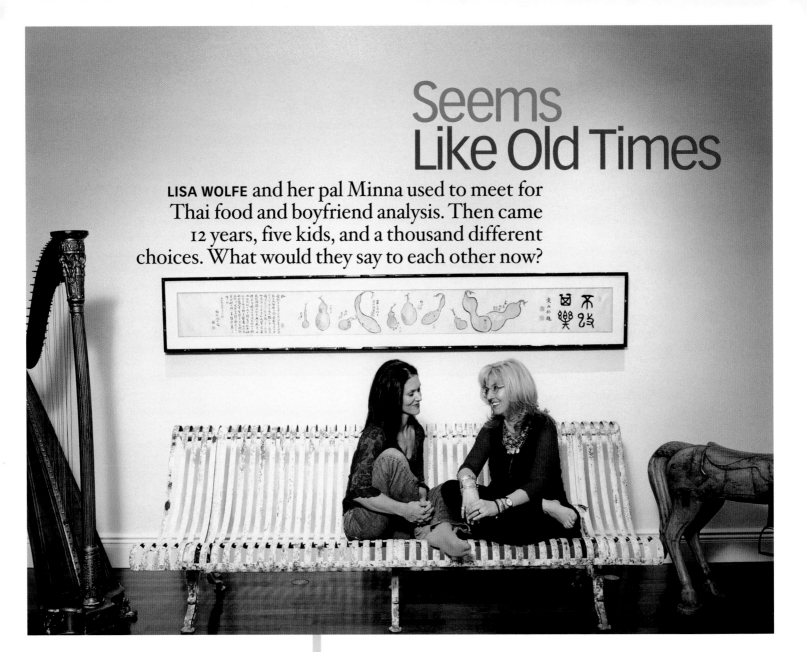

Seems Like Old Times

LISA WOLFE and her pal Minna used to meet for Thai food and boyfriend analysis. Then came 12 years, five kids, and a thousand different choices. What would they say to each other now?

Friends for life? The author (*left*) and Minna Towbin Pinger reconnect.

I AM STANDING ON THE CORNER of 79th Street and Columbus, waiting for my friend and feeling nervous. I shouldn't be feeling nervous. I know that. I repeat it to myself like a mantra. Minna is my *friend,* for God's sake. My best friend. At least she used to be. I don't know what she is now. Or what it will feel like to spend time together.

We've been trying to arrange this date for 13 months, since I moved back to New York. But it hasn't been easy. A lot has sprung up in our lives since the days we used to meet for Thai food or a movie at the drop of a hat. (Namely, between us: five kids, seven moves to different cities, two determinations to relaunch careers—she as a jewelry designer, me as a writer—and two husbands who, though thankfully rel-

atively liberated, are still entitled to sometimes expect old-fashioned things like attention and food on the table.) Once her son had an ear infection; once my son had strep. Once she had to check out a new pediatrician; once I had to look at a new school. We saw it as a sign of our closeness that we could say to each other, as she said to me one day, "I'm so inspired to work, I can't not take advantage." Or, as I once said to her, "I'm just too tired to move."

But if I'm honest, which I don't always like to be, I think there was something else, too. I think the fact of having lived so far apart for the previous dozen years had created a distance between us. We swore it wouldn't happen, and I will never forget helping her dress for the wedding to the man who would move her to Los Angeles—me zipping, she fluffing, and both of us promising we would write, call, visit as often as needed to make sure we didn't grow apart. To be fair, we tried very hard. We phoned each other regularly (until I got married and moved to London, creating an eight-hour time difference), and then we wrote lots of letters (those things people used to stamp and put in the mail). We were the last two people I know to surrender to e-mail, and I'm glad about that, because now I have a boxful of her letters that I can hold and read when I'm a little old lady.

A few years apart wouldn't have changed us very much, but 12 is a whole other story. Especially since we spent them in such different places. Always a hugely individualistic artist, Minna let loose even further in L.A., wearing things like sarongs

Minna has two boys the ages of mine, 8 and 6, and this daughter, Zyla, who's nearly 2. I knew she'd be bringing her along today. But still it shocks me to see the stroller. I'd forgotten about strollers. There was a time when I didn't know what it felt like to walk down a street and *not* push a stroller, but that suddenly seems like a different lifetime. Minna looks, how shall I put it—because I really hate to put it the way that it strikes me—*old* to be pushing a stroller. She's adorable, and has long blonde hair and legs that come up to my armpits, but in the merciless glare of this mid-August sun, there is no pretending to miss the lines that traverse her face like our flight paths of recent years, the baby croissants of puff beneath her eyes, the gray roots sprouting not just at her temples but everywhere, because who has time to color

pered, upon reaching the in-box of the foreign editor, "You should see this guy; he is *intense*."

Minna was so cool and creative and had such a happening circle of friends, I couldn't quite get over it when she wanted me to be part of it, too. I was so boring compared to her. After our nights out together, I would invariably go home to read, and she would invariably go downtown to stage a drug intervention. She was always staging drug interventions. She wore clothes that were ugly and didn't match long before it was fashionable. She danced with her eyes closed. She was the only person I would allow to meet certain sexy sexist boyfriends, and she never got high-minded about any of them.

"She wants to show you her boots."

"What?"

If you want a poignant lesson in the passage of time, get together with a friend you haven't really seen since the two of you were in your 20s.

with pink bras and red sneakers; using expressions like "What up?"; sending her kids to a school where they spent a good chunk of time painting the walls and she spent a good chunk of time tape-recording what they had to say about it. Ever in touch with my inner Canadian, I, on the other hand, became more formal in London, shunning running shoes except when I exercised, writing thank-you notes to people to thank them for writing me thank-you notes, sending my children to a Montessori nursery where they were required to wear uniforms and forbidden to run or raise their voices. The couple of times Minna and I got together on summer vacations over the years, the initial rush of seeing each other was followed by mutual, if benevolent, bafflement: How do you let/force your children to act that way? How do you let/force *yourself*? I love you, you know that, but what is the deal with your life?

"HEY!" A VOICE CALLS FROM the left. I turn to look. And I see her rushing toward me, pushing a stroller, hair and necklaces and earrings flapping in the wind. "I'm so sorry I'm late!"

your hair as regularly as you have to now? Plus there's a royal blue splint from her left forefinger up to her elbow.

"What happened?" I ask.

"Oh, nothing," Minna says, with a grin I know to mean it's no big deal at all to be dragging a 2-year-old and her stroller, diaper bag, and bottles around Manhattan with just one hand.

"But why do you need it?"

"Oh, it's stupid. I was picking her up one day and something snapped. But please, it's boring. How are you?"

"I'm..." I'm wondering whether I look as old to her as she looks to me. "Fine, thanks," I manage to say.

Neither of us is that old, just 40. But if you want a poignant lesson in the passage of time, get together (preferably outside on a sunny summer day) with a friend you haven't really seen since the two of you were in your 20s. Minna and I met the first day of my first job after college, at the *New York Times,* a place so cold and scary I nearly ran away that first morning rather than have to walk through the door. Imagine my relief when the copy kid assigned to show me where to put which piece of copy was wearing earrings to her shoulders and a smile the size of the metro desk, and whis-

"She wants to show you her boots."

So that's why Zyla is contorted over the bar of her stroller, moaning. She is trying to show me her boots. Red cowboy boots. To go with her yellow sundress.

"Great boots!" I exclaim, which the child takes as her cue to charge up and out of her stroller like a horse from a starting gate. Another thing I'd forgotten about 2-year-olds was how far and fast they travel. She is halfway down the block by the time Minna mobilizes to chase her and carry her back.

"Give her to me," I say. "You shouldn't be carrying her with that arm."

Minna hands Zyla over. "Should we get the sheets?" she asks.

We weren't planning to get sheets. We were planning to see paintings by Vermeer at the Met. But Minna called to say Zyla's big bed was being delivered, and she didn't have sheets. If she had sheets, then Zyla could sleep in it tonight, so did I mind getting sheets? Of course I did, but of course I didn't.

And so we proceed to Laura Ashley, Minna apologizing for the inconvenience, and me remembering how sweet it feels to walk down the street carrying a child who still hasn't lost her smell of angel dust.

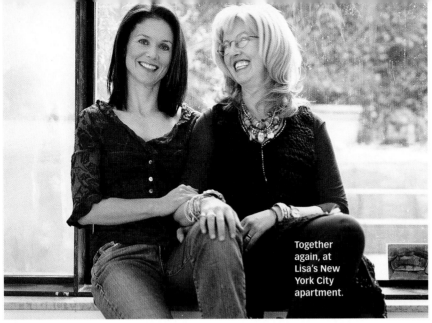
Together again, at Lisa's New York City apartment.

Maybe this is why nature makes you forget so emphatically what it feels like to have little kids—because if you remembered, it would break your heart.

"Are you okay?" Minna asks.

"Yeah, sure, I'm fine."

"Then why are you limping?"

"I'm not limping."

"Yes, you are. What's wrong?"

"Nothing. It's just that when I sit at my desk and write for long periods of time, then my hip hurts, that's all."

"Let me hold her," Minna says, reaching for Zyla.

wondering which sheets were right, and what if they weren't, and when would I find time to return them? Minna zeroes in on smoky rose with no hesitation, with the pizzazz to know that if the color is wrong, she'll simply throw something on the bed to make it right. Just as she is paying, her cell phone rings. "Shit!" she exclaims upon answering, which I don't think she should do in front of her kid.

"The delivery guys were supposed to come at 3, but they're on their way now. This screws everything up. The babysitter can't come till 3."

day has become far more urgent: making sure her daughter doesn't die in my care.

We have stairs, and another thing I'd forgotten was 2-year-olds and stairs. Zyla promptly reminds me by leaping down them as if into her mother's arms. How she survives, or doesn't at least split her head open, is a minor miracle, as well as a poignant reminder that I must not stray from her side. I follow her like a presidential bodyguard as she jumps on my bed, cartwheels across the kitchen, even climbs a few rungs of bookshelf. I chase her in circles around the coffee table until I realize I am limping from the pain in my hip.

Thankfully, I have a brainstorm: *Sesame Street.* I gave most of our tapes away years ago (when the boys became terrified someone might think they were babies) but saved one for occasions like this. I dig it out. I put it on. The logo of Children's Television Workshop appears on the screen, along with those three trademark swooshing sounds I used to know so well. Sounds I heard so many times a day for so many years and then, poof, not at all.

I watch Zyla watching Elmo, rubbing my hip. She is thrilled, Elmo is as cheerful as ever, but I start to feel very sad. Sad that

After our nights out together, I would invariably go home to read, and she would invariably go downtown to stage a drug intervention.

"But you have your wrist!"

"But you have your hip!"

Zyla resolves the matter by leaping into her mother's arms.

"Fun, isn't it, getting older?" I ask.

"Oh, yeah, it's great. I love it."

"The other day when I was at the doctor and I mentioned how whenever I get up fast the room spins, he smiled and said, 'Get used to it; that's how it goes now—and don't think it plateaus.'"

"'And don't think it plateaus?'"

"Yeah."

"He said that?"

"Yeah."

"You *paid* him to say that?"

Inside Laura Ashley, I marvel at how quickly Minna chooses her sheets. Faced with the same 40 or so color options, I would have wasted a pitiful amount of time

"Why do you need a babysitter?"

"To get Z out of the way. There isn't room in our apartment for movers and her." As if to illustrate the point, Zyla twirls from lampshades all the way to bedspreads.

"Can I help?" I ask.

"I feel so bad...."

"Don't feel bad. Just tell me what I can do." I happen to be having an easy week: My boys are visiting my parents in Toronto.

"Well, maybe if you take her to your place, then I can deal with the movers and come pick her up when they're done."

I TAKE ZYLA TO MY PLACE, BUT I lied—I mind. Even though I was nervous about spending time with Minna, I still wanted to spend it. I wanted to try to figure out what remained between us. But now that will have to wait. The goal of the

even though it took Minna and me 13 months to get together, we're still not even together. Sad that here I am with her daughter, whom I don't even know, just as she doesn't know my kids. Sad that the days of having babies are over now, like the days I used to hang out with Minna, and that a mere two hours of caring for a toddler is apparently all it takes to cripple me. Sad that time *does* in fact fly as fast as my grandmother always said it did, but who was paying any attention? That just when you're beginning to understand who you really are, what's worth your energy, and what can't possibly be worth your already too-limited time, you pick your kid up and your wrist snaps, you sit for too long and your hip hurts, and don't think it plateaus....

The doorbell rings. It's Minna. "Hey," she says. "I'm so sorry for dumping her."

"Don't be sorry. We had a good time."

Minna steps in and looks around, falling oddly silent. I imagine she's feeling the decorating equivalent of what I felt looking at her face in the sun: I can't believe how much has changed! When you see your friends regularly over the years, the evolution of their living space, like the evolution of their skin, occurs so gradually that you might not notice. But Minna has not been in any home of mine since the studio apartment whose kitchenette could have fit in the bathtub. I've acquired an obscene amount of stuff since getting married and having kids.

"Hey, Z," Minna calls to her daughter, who doesn't look up from Elmo.

"She seems happy," I say. "Why don't you have some tea?"

I lead Minna to the kitchen, where she heads straight to a pile of kids' art on the counter. She studies them as though they were the Vermeers, oohing, aahing, pointing out details in the work I never noticed myself. And I realize that even though the skin around her eyes has changed, the shine in them when she gets excited is still the same.

"Mamamamama!" Zyla calls. "Hungwy!"

"I should get home to feed her," Minna says. "Why don't you come, too?"

SHE WANTS TO SHOW YOU HER room."

"What?"

"She wants to show you her room."

So that's why Zyla is flipping over her high chair. She wants to show me her room. It's a pretty room, with burgundy walls, wooden floors, and dozens of dolls I'm advised to call babies. As Zyla arranges the babies on the smoky rose sheets, Minna and I sit on the floor and open some wine.

"It must really hurt," Minna says.

"What?"

"Your hip."

"No, it doesn't."

"Then why are you rubbing it?"

I didn't realize I was rubbing it. How embarrassing. Annoying. Even loathsome. "I hate it," I say. "Don't you hate it?"

"Hate what?"

"Getting older. How badly the body wants to decay. I mean, you can stave it off to a degree, if you have the time and the patience and the discipline as though you went to West Point. But I've become really conscious of it lately, the direction my body's being pulled in, and it's not exactly uphill."

"Me, too."

"You know, sometimes I look at my kids, running, getting faster, getting stronger, and I feel this burn of jealousy. Really, like a burn."

"I do know."

"I shouldn't feel jealous."

"Why not?"

"I don't know. They're my kids. I should feel happy for them."

"You do. But you also feel sad for you."

"I shouldn't feel this sad."

"Why not?"

"I'm a feminist! My body shouldn't matter so much. It's just the vessel. The more important stuff lies within...."

"But you enjoyed the vessel."

"Yeah."

"A lot."

We laugh. Only she knows how much. I wouldn't have trusted anyone else with some of those morning-after stories.

"Maybe this is so hard *because* you're a feminist. Because you were free to enjoy your body—and you did—it's harder to feel it change."

A good point. A really good point. So good my eyes fill with tears.

"Oh, *Lees,*" Minna says, moving closer and rubbing my back.

"I'm sorry," I say. "This is dumb."

"It's not dumb. It's honest. One of the things I've always loved about you is how honest you are with your feelings."

ONE OF THE THINGS I'VE ALWAYS loved about her is how positively she manages to spin every whiney/stupid/neurotic thing I say.

Zyla shrieks. A baby has gotten stuck between the big bed and the wall. I jump up to the rescue, but apparently too fast, because after all the sitting and chasing and carrying, my hip seizes and I lurch forward, planting my face into the smoky rose sheets.

Zyla laughs. And Minna. Then finally, but deeply, me. This aging thing turns out to be worse than I thought, but this friendship thing turns out to be even better. ●

THE TALKING CURE Feel better after a nice long chat with a friend? Everyone does. Here's why.

If you ever feel guilty (or unproductive or juvenile or gossipy) about your daily rap 'n' yap session with the girls, consider it cold cream for your well-being. Such talks are essential to emotional growth and mental health, according to Jean Baker Miller, MD, who cowrote the book on gal bonding, *The Healing Connection*, in 1997. Based on more than a decade of research and many decades of clinical practice, Miller concludes that not having at least one close woman friend can contribute to psychological dysfunction. "Eating and sleeping disorders, anxiety, certainly depression—all that can result from chronic disconnection," she says.

You can also add unhealthy aging to that list. One of the findings from the Nurses' Health Study—an ongoing investigation of more than 100,000 nurses since 1976—revealed that among the oldest women, those who didn't have at least one confidante showed the same decline in physical functioning and vitality as heavy smokers and the most severely overweight. Conversely, the more friends a woman had, the better shape she was in, "although the research suggests it's the quality of the relationship that counts," says lead researcher Yvonne L. Michael. She explains that close friendships "provide a buffer for stressful living that is likely to play out through your immune and endocrine systems, allowing you to age healthier." In Michael's opinion, having strong connections is just as important for health as exercise. But yes, you still have to hit the gym (and you were hoping you could replace your workout with a group hug).

—Chee Gates

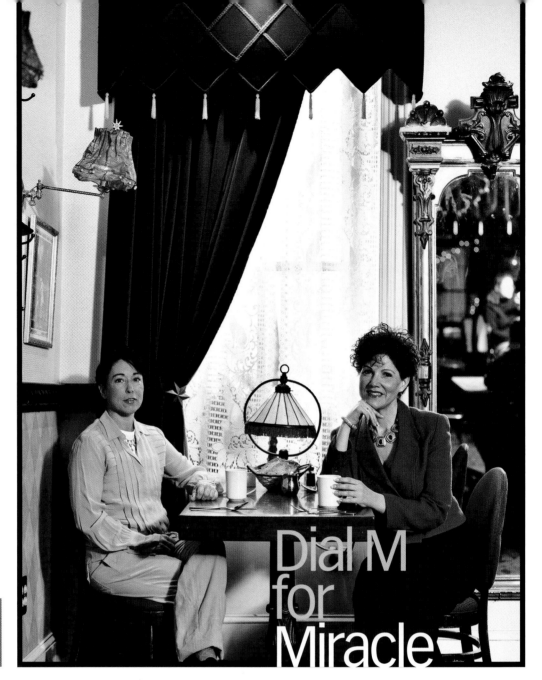

Tahoma (*left*) and Deborah at the White Dog Cafe in Philadelphia, December 2003.

Dial M for Miracle

She'd only read the stranger's name in a book; she couldn't have known the woman would save her life — could she? **LISE FUNDERBURG** reports.

OUT OF THE BLUE ONE DAY IN JULY 2002, Philadelphia psychotherapist Deborah Anna Luepnitz, PhD, received a phone message from a stranger. Tahoma Ironfeather was calling from a small island off the coast of Charleston, South Carolina, and said she needed to speak to Deborah after reading a book called *The Last American Man.*

Deborah was convinced Tahoma had made a mistake in contacting her but decided to return the call. Her efforts to clear up the confusion only made matters murkier. Was Tahoma calling in reference to Deborah's own just-published book, *Schopenhauer's Porcupines,* a study of intimacy and its dilemmas? Nope, Tahoma answered. Well then, perhaps Tahoma was trying to reach Deborah's friend and *Last American Man* author, Liz Gilbert? No. Gilbert's charismatic, nature-loving, self-involved subject, Eustace Conway, Tahoma explained, was a perfect double for Ronnie, a man who was breaking her heart. Oh, Deborah said, perhaps Tahoma wished to speak with Eustace? "Hell, no," Tahoma said. "I just spent three years with somebody like that—I don't want Eustace; I want some understanding."

Tahoma, a nurse practitioner and certified boat captain, had heard a radio interview with Gilbert, rushed out to buy the book, and devoured every page. The similarities between Eustace and Ronnie took Tahoma's breath away, and the thoughtful passages analyzing Eustace's psyche shed much-needed light on her feelings for Ronnie. Tahoma felt a second presence in those passages and, after sleuthing through the dedication and acknowledgments (both of which mentioned Deborah), decided she knew who it was. Tahoma, whose Chickasaw ancestors had great respect for the powers of the unseen, felt a ping each time she read Deborah's name. Call it a vibe, call it a voice, call it a moment of telepathic transcendence—Tahoma had learned to pay attention whenever it came along.

BEFORE THE INTERNET, TRACKing down Deborah would have been a challenge, since Tahoma lives on rustic Edisto Island, where many residents willingly forgo cable TV, dry cleaners, Starbucks, and a sewer system. But Tahoma had a modem, and Deborah—an author of three books, eloquent speaker, and member of the clinical faculty of the department of psychiatry at the University of Pennsylvania School of Medicine—was easily Googled.

Tahoma asked Deborah for help in understanding her own situation; they agreed to a onetime telephone consultation so that Tahoma could close her own book, the one with Ronnie as its main character. On the appointed day, they spoke frankly but also laughed at the funny bits that inevitably hover on the edge of heartbreak, and at the end of their hour Tahoma felt the clarity and closure she'd sought.

In September 2002, two months later, Tahoma felt woozy. Maybe it was the flu, she thought, or maybe this dull-mindedness was what it was like to get old—she was 48. Then she started having fleeting blackouts. She tried to count the episodes but kept losing track. One morning she woke up on the floor beside her bed

with extreme head pain. By the time the ambulance came, she was losing her vision.

Tahoma had suffered a grand mal seizure, and she spent the next two weeks in and out of hospitals in Charleston. Biopsy results indicated a rare, malignant brain tumor that had progressed to stage 3

Tahoma's prognosis was, simply put, scary: She'd likely die in two months.

(out of 4). Tahoma's prognosis was, simply put, crappy: The tumor was inoperable—too embedded in the brain tissue that controls speech, sight, hearing—and she would most likely die in as little as two months.

Two weeks after the biopsy, Tahoma sent Deborah an e-mail titled "Tahoma Update." She told Deborah of the tumor and the prognosis. Deborah wrote back asking if there was something she could do.

Tahoma recognized Deborah as both a talented counselor and an abundantly gracious person. Tahoma figured most people would have met that initial voice message with more of a "Screw you—get out of here!" than a return call. "Look," Tahoma responded, "I'm really sick. It seems like I'm going to die, and I want your support."

Deborah knew saying yes would eventually lead to great sadness and pain, but she also felt honored to share in such a momentous part of another person's life. She took a deep breath and said she'd be there for Tahoma. Deborah's commitment stemmed from a mix of generosity and curiosity: She was struck that Tahoma seemed to have no bitterness about her plight. "I would have been very mad at God," Deborah says, "but Tahoma never veered from her position that the illness was a gift. I just fell for her. I melted, and I felt I was to learn something, too, about the hard edges of my psyche."

For the next few months, Deborah sent an e-mail or a card or left a phone message every day. Tahoma couldn't always respond. Six weeks of radiation had knocked her on her butt, and she grew weaker and more nauseated with each treatment. She

stopped working and lay on her couch contemplating life and death.

As a spiritual companion, Deborah proved to be an excellent choice. She offered insight, compassion, and humor, and most important, she did not avoid talking about Tahoma's impending death.

"What's it like to have so little time?" Deborah asked at one point.

"Actually," Tahoma answered, "all I have now is time." Tahoma's life before the tumor was nonstop and jam-packed, like a Chinese acrobat spinning countless plates in the air. Now she relished the chasms of time and space each day brought. Tahoma's perspective reminded Deborah of a Roman philosopher. "Seneca said there are two choices in life," Deborah explains. "You can be led by fate, or you can be dragged by it. Tahoma ain't being dragged anywhere."

ON THE FOURTH MONDAY in December, Tahoma was at the tail end of radiation treatments. Up in Philadelphia, Deborah hiked over to her gym, settled into the recumbent bicycle, and read the local paper, as usual, browsing until she reached this headline, buried in the health and science section of *The Philadelphia Inquirer:* treatment shows promise in two forms of brain cancer.

Here was an experimental protocol, the only one of its kind in the world, at Drexel University's College of Medicine, a facility 20 minutes away from where she was pedaling. At Drexel radioactive iodine was attached to antibody extracts produced in mice and injected into patients. The antibodies had a particular affinity for tumor cells and so acted as an escort service, keeping the highly charged radiation from traveling to healthy cells in the body and brain. Fewer than 11,000 people are diagnosed with these types of cancer, but those who had undergone the MAb425 treatment were showing impressive results.

For an instant, Deborah felt hope. But then reason won out. "I thought, *Oh, surely Tahoma knows about this,*" Deborah remembers. "*She has been visiting brain tumor sites on the Internet, she has a great group of doctors—it would be impossible that she doesn't know.*" Also, what were the chances Tahoma had the "right" cancer?

Deborah finished biking, threw the paper in the trash, and headed for the showers. On her way out of the locker room, she reconsidered. She fished the paper from the trash, and when she got home, she checked an old e-mail to see what cancer Tahoma had. *Ping.* It was astrocytoma with anaplastic foci, one of the two in the study.

That night Deborah sent her daily e-mail to Tahoma, mentioning the article almost in passing. "I'm sure you know about this MAb drug," Deborah wrote.

"No," Tahoma answered.

The next day, Christmas Eve, Tahoma called Drexel. The clinic had shut down for the holidays, but a kind receptionist encouraged her to call back after the New Year.

Tahoma waited two weeks — *tick, tick, tick* — and called. Jackie Emrich, PhD, the lead author of the study's report, picked up the phone. She and Tahoma had a long talk, which led to good and bad news. Yes, Tahoma could be treated with MAb425, but each dose took an hour and a half of lab time to make, and the lab was getting calls from desperate people all over the world. Tahoma would be number 64 on the waiting list — not a reassuring position when your life expectancy is about the same number of days. On the other hand, Tahoma was thrilled that there was a list to be on. She also realized she needed time to recuperate from her weeks of radiation before trying something else.

You can tell a lot about Tahoma by her mottoes: "Try to understand" and "Keep moving." She doesn't own a lot of stuff, she doesn't earn a lot of money — she finds richness in canoeing and fishing and providing healthcare to people who need it even if they can't pay for it. Good for the spirit; not so good for the bank balance. And as anyone who's been around cancer knows, this disease is not a cheap date.

What Tahoma does have a wealth of, however, is some seriously good luck. "I could fall in shit and find a diamond," she would tell Deborah. Tahoma intended to hit the top of Drexel's waiting list, and she called Deborah to ask if she could stay with her in Philadelphia during the two-week treatment. *Hmm,* Deborah thought. She couldn't be happier about the prospect of

the trip, but her one-bedroom apartment doubled as her office, and Tahoma couldn't exactly settle into the futon couch that served as the patients' chair. Deborah offered to underwrite a hotel stay as a sort of guest room away from home.

Tahoma arrived on March 24, 2003, the night before her first MAb425 treatment. Deborah's nerves were on edge, thrill and

> "Seneca said you can be led by fate or dragged by it," says Deborah. "Tahoma ain't being dragged anywhere."

anxiety overlapping, and she arrived at Tahoma's hotel room armed with a toothbrush, pj's, a bag of fresh fruit, and no idea what to say. The door opened, they whooped each other's names, and the five-foot-tall Tahoma leaped at the statuesque Deborah, arms open for a hug. This powerhouse of a woman Deborah had been speaking to all these months was tiny. "You're just a little fidget!" Deborah said.

The women fell into slumber party mode instantly. They shared a slice of double-fudge cake from room service and watched TV, taking turns analyzing David Letterman's psyche. They talked about exercise and men and politics. The hotel arrangement turned out to be prudent after treatments made Tahoma dangerously radioactive; when lab workers ran a Geiger counter over her head and bladder, it sounded a furious *bang bang bang.* Nonetheless, throughout Tahoma's stay, whenever Deborah didn't have appointments, the women were inseparable. Tahoma's problems had brought them together, but Deborah found herself confiding things she'd never told another soul.

One more thing cemented their bond: The treatment worked. By April 2004, when this article went to press, Tahoma had lived 17 months beyond her diagnosis. She showed no signs of tumor in follow-up scans and was back to riding horses, working on a friend's farm, and filling in for other nurse practitioners. No one uses the

word *cure* with this kind of cancer, but as Tahoma says, "I've exceeded my expiration date."

The treatment came with its share of drawbacks. Tahoma sustained some neurocognitive damage. "When I get tired, I may start stuttering," she says, "and sometimes I can't do math. I'm not the most ego-driven person, but there are certain things, like my ability to remember things, that were a big loss for me. But really, death versus having a few neurological deficits — I'll take the deficits."

And she needs speech therapy. The trouble is, her insurance has run out. And the South Carolina Vocational Rehabilitation Department won't waste resources on someone with a diagnosis of "terminal." She's looking for an alternative she can pay for herself.

ANOTHER TWIST IS THAT Tahoma spent all that time preparing for death — and didn't die. She was jolted, as many people with terrible diseases are, into a greater appreciation for all the world has to offer. "That brightness of going 'Wow, I almost died' is starting to fade," Tahoma says. "The intellectual part of me understands that's appropriate, but the emotional part doesn't want to lose it."

Both she and Deborah see the story of their friendship as one of blessings and miracles and magic. Deborah also sees it as a testimonial to the power of the written word...and something more. "What can we call the thing that makes a person return a call to an eccentric stranger?" she asks. "Is it risk taking? Is it something spiritual — that sympathy outside us that bends the path toward we know not what? It is both of those, but the third thing is a faith in the goodness of other women. *Sisterhood* is a watchword of feminism, of course, and I learned it first in a Catholic girls' school in Cleveland, where the world was run by powerful women who — untrue to stereotype — were loving and reliable and fun. They taught us, against the grain, to form strong bonds with one another. I've loved a number of men in my life, but the thing that makes me feel safe is my trusty gaggle of girlfriends."

Ping. ●

Lisa and Brenda at Bergdorf's

Noon, a small café, every other month. Same players, same luscious dessert. Sound like a promising recipe for a lifelong friendship? According to **LISA KOGAN**, it is.

BRENDA ABRAMS HAD AN orange shag carpet and a thing for Elton John. My room was hot pink and my heart belonged to Cat Stevens. We both believed in Herbal Essence, Frye boots, and boys named Brad. We got our periods, our ears pierced, and our learner's permits—in exactly that order. All we knew of drugs was what we'd read in *Go Ask Alice*. All we knew of sex was what we saw in *The Way We Were*. We gorged on Twinkies and Fritos and red pop, never dreaming that cellulite could someday come between us and our Calvins. We were good girls. We were best friends.

Thirty years have come and gone. She's Brenda Josephs now, living with her husband, three kids, and nanny in a big suburban house outside Manhattan. I'm still me, living alone in a small prewar co-op inside Manhattan. She's on the board of trustees at her children's school, practicing law in her spare time. I'm on the computer writing this article, and my spare time is spent wondering how people find spare time. Most days I don't want her life. Most days she doesn't want mine—but we each have the occasional pang. We are still best friends.

There's an unspoken understanding that in case of an emergency we will always come early and stay late for each other, but our days of sharing a locker and nights of marathon phone sessions are behind us. We're down to meeting for lunch—it is an act of faith in faithless times.

On the first Monday of every other month, we take our latest assortment of absurdities, insights, outrages, and ironies to the little café on the fifth floor of Bergdorf Goodman and meet for the same meal we've been having forever. Brenda orders her standard, tuna salad on pumpernickel. She's a straightforward, no-nonsense eater. Her mother's desperate attempt to instill culinary diversity is still referred to as "the turkey tetrazzini incident of '74." I go with my usual open-faced-sandwich combo—three little toast discs topped with lobster in lemon mayonnaise, shrimp in brandy-chive dressing, and gravlax with dill. Though Brenda insists

I've got a Lipton monkey on my back, I always order iced tea. Though I insist she's got a death wish, she always opts for New York City tap water. Between bites we catch up on Jan, Sue, Gina, Jacqui, and Alison—friends now scattered across the Midwest. Sometimes we find ourselves aching for a past we couldn't wait to finish. Sometimes we study the very chic shoppers for signs of facelift. Sometimes we study each other. Brenda wears a simple black twinset and a silver chain around her neck. I wear burgundy lipstick and my heart on my sleeve. "I want a baby," I tell my friend, who has heard it all before.

"I know you do—I'm saving Lily's crib for when you have one," my friend answers in a voice that never fails to soothe.

"Can I have one of yours?" I ask.

"No."

"Then can I have your pickle?"

"No problem."

When the waitress offers us dessert, we simultaneously answer, "Just the check, please," then quickly reverse our decision and request one raspberry crème brûlée with two spoons. I crack through the burnt-sugar lid to the satiny custard below and complain that Brenda's half has all the berries. She wonders whether it's possible to actually feel one's arteries clogging, but I assure her that the egg yolks cancel out the heavy cream. "You'll see," I promise, "it'll be the raspberries that do us in."

The two women at the next table begin arguing over whose turn it is to pick up the check. They're 80 years old if they're a day. "Oh, for God's sake, Rosalie, I'm not calling you next time I'm in the city," says one as she grabs for the bill. "Joanne, your money's no good here," says the other as she snatches it right back.

And in a flash we taste our future memories. ●

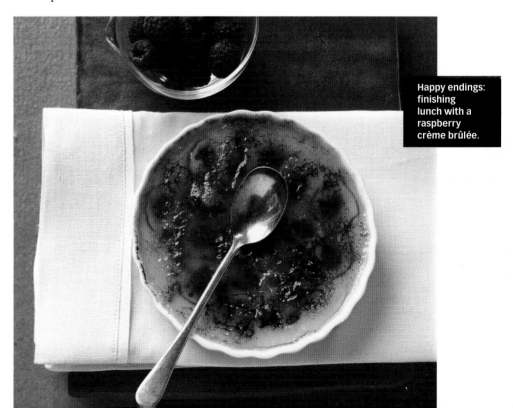

Happy endings: finishing lunch with a raspberry crème brûlée.

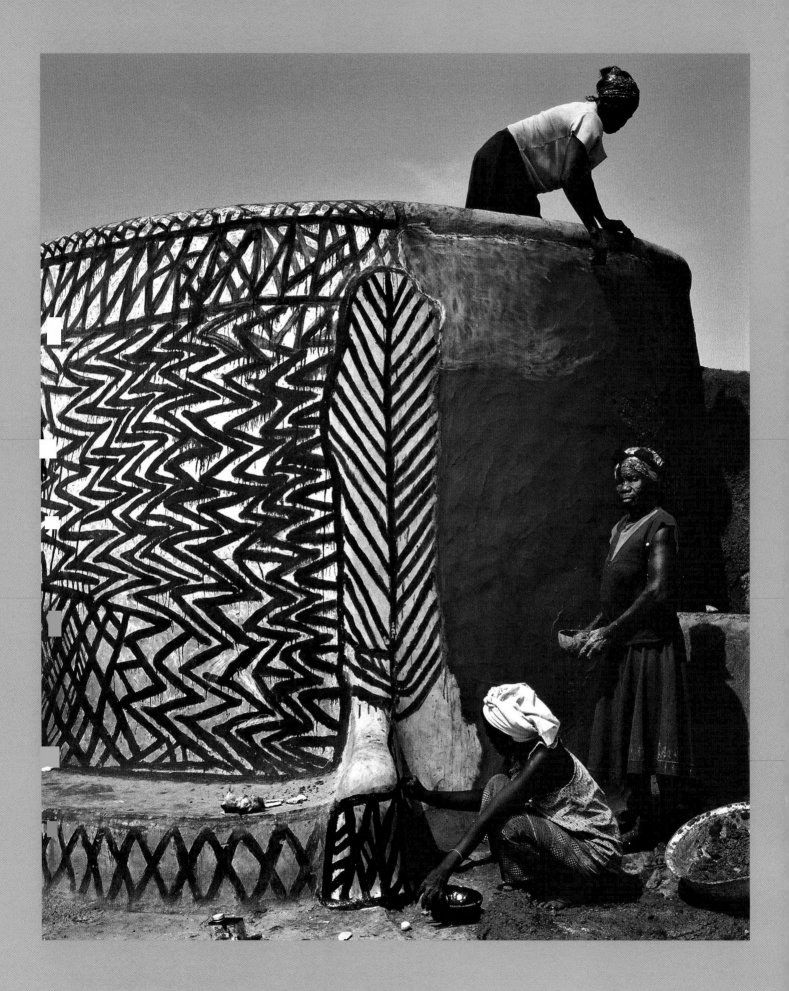

O

Living in the World

The final piece of a well-lived life is the difference
you make in the world. There's no shortage of
ways to give back—or stories to inspire you.

Everyday Heroes 252

———

Giving Back 279

———

Make a Connection 309

O

Everyday Heroes

Five years ago, Saranne Rothberg was diagnosed with cancer. Her rebel response was to reach for a Bill Cosby video and start a charity that brings laughter to, and from, those who need it the most. PATRICIA VOLK reports.

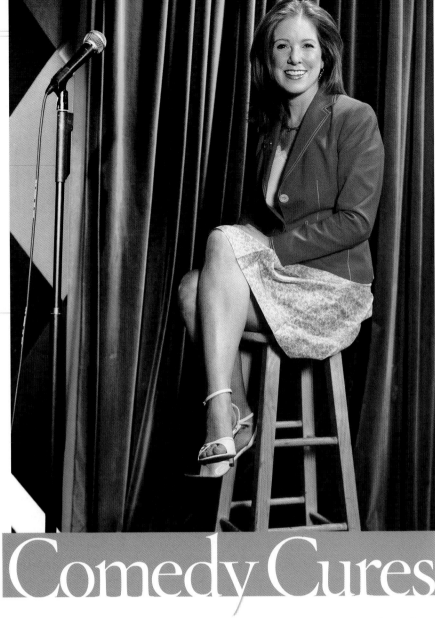

Comedy Cures

SARANNE ROTHBERG IS 41. SHE LOOKS 17. The woman is actually dewy. "Chemo exfoliates," she explains. "It's the chemo facial."

We crack up. After 11 misdiagnoses, three surgeries, four chemotherapy protocols, and 44 radiation treatments, the founder of Comedy Cures (a nonprofit that brings humor to people who really need it) laughs plenty. To her, it's therapy.

In 1993 Saranne gave birth to Lauriel. "I was breastfeeding," she says. "One duct wasn't draining." Over a period of 18 months, Saranne's internist, general surgeon, and endocrinologist all kept reassuring her that what she had was merely an infection. Four and a half years later, a lump poked up that was visible through her shirt. "I went to a new doctor and said, 'Say it isn't so.'"

It was so. Saranne had an aggressive, stage 2 carcinoma.

"All I could think was, I gotta get to Blockbuster and get every comedy tape they have," she says. "I've got to laugh. If it worked for Norman Cousins, I might as well start right now."

In 1964 Cousins, then editor of the *Saturday Review,* was diagnosed with ankylosing spondylitis, a painful, crippling disease. His doctor gave him a one in 500 chance of full recovery. Cousins checked out of the hospital and into a hotel. He watched *Candid Camera,* laughed himself silly, saw his symptoms slowly disappear. He

Saranne Rothberg aims for 100 laughs per person.

lived another 26 years. (Studies by Lee Berk, associate director of the Center for Neuroimmunology at Loma Linda University, support laughter's benefits, though no one claims it's a panacea.)

Saranne's goal that first night was to get Lauriel to bed as early as possible so she could absorb what happened. "After a while, I put an Eddie Murphy tape in. Laughing, I couldn't think about crying," she says. "My body couldn't constrict. I got hooked on the experiment. Bill Cosby? The episode where his wife sends him down to make breakfast and the daughter wants chocolate cake? Cosby says, 'Well, chocolate cake has eggs and milk. It has flour. That's breakfast!' Now I was really laughing." When Lauriel, who was 5, woke up, Saranne told her, "We're having chocolate doughnuts for breakfast. You'll be my humor buddy.

We'll make a list of fun things that make us laugh and do two of them every day."

Six weeks after her diagnosis, smack in the middle of a vitriolic divorce, Saranne had her first surgery. A week later, she needed a second operation. When her doctors found even more malignant cells, she told her medical team, "That's it. No more surgery. Deal me the strongest chemo you've got."

Adriamycin, a.k.a. the red devil, was prescribed. Saranne felt the instant the drug hit her brain: "At that moment my entire life made sense," she says. "As a kid, I'd raised money for muscular dystrophy. I studied broadcast journalism in college. I'd scouted and booked comics for prime-time TV. I'd been a news anchor and reporter, so I knew how to interview and write a press release. If you look at a life, every single thing seems scattered ➤

What's so Funny?!

COMEDY IS RARE AND essential and highly subjective. All we know with any degree of certainty is that the Three Stooges were never funny and never will be, the Marx Brothers were always funny and always will be. Dennis Miller and Eddie Murphy used to be funny, but not anymore. *The Simpsons* is incapable of being anything less than consistently hilarious, and Jerry Seinfeld makes American Express commercials worth sitting through. Here, in no particular order, are a few other thoughts:

1. **Richard Pryor is God.**
2. It is astonishing that evil genius Ricky Gervais and the team responsible for *The Office* are able to get through each scene with a straight face. Is this brilliant, lacerating look at working life better than *The Larry Sanders Show*? Better than *Mary Tyler Moore*? It's a close call, but the answer is yes. (Available on DVD.)

3. *The Daily Show with Jon Stewart* makes bad news good. Correspondent Stephen Colbert might be the funniest man on late night.

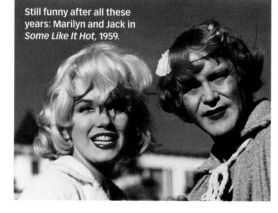

Still funny after all these years: Marilyn and Jack in *Some Like It Hot,* 1959.

4. If you missed *Never Scared,* Chris Rock's HBO special, it's out on video.
5. Riotous, ironic, melancholy, magical, Steve Martin's book *Pure Drivel* is the perfect blend of silly and smart.
6. If you read nothing else, read everything ever written by David Sedaris.
7. **Mike Nichols and Elaine May are God.**
8. We'll give you a subject: Mike Meyers—now talk amongst yourselves.
9. Christopher Guest (*This Is Spinal Tap, Waiting for Guffman, Best in Show, A Mighty Wind*) is a scream in front of and behind the camera.

10. Sure, playing chess with death is amusing, but forget Ingmar Bergman— Andrew Bergman writes and directs extraordinarily delightful films (*Blazing Saddles, The Freshman, Honeymoon in Vegas, Soapdish*).
11. **Albert Brooks is God.**
12. And speaking of Brooks—Mel Brooks and Carl Reiner's *2000 Year Old Man* is available on DVD.
13. *20th Century Masters— The Millennium Collection: The Best of Bill Cosby* really is Cosby at his best.

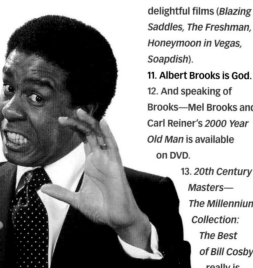

A Pryor engagement: Richard rules! 1977.

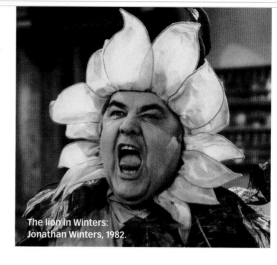

The lion in Winters: Jonathan Winters, 1982.

14. Spike Lee's hilarious concert film, *The Original Kings of Comedy* (particularly Steve Harvey's work), is a pleasure.
15. Stand-ups worth sitting for: Wanda Sykes, Mark Maron, Jim Gaffigan, Paula Poundstone, Mitch Hedberg, Bill Maher, Colin Quinn, Rich Hall, Steven Wright, Gilbert Gottfried, Denis Leary.
16. **George Carlin is God.**
17. *Dr. Katz, Professional Therapist* is one of the funniest cartoons ever made, and it's available on VHS.
18. Comedy Central's *Primetime Glick* series proved that nobody is faster on his feet than Martin Short.
19. If you don't know Eddie Izzard, get thee to a video store and treat yourself to *Dress to Kill.*
20. **Jonathan Winters is God.**
21. The first three seasons of the subversive wonder *Family Guy,* in which a toddler quests for world domination, are available on DVD, and sales of this loopy cartoon have been so successful that Fox is bringing it back as a series.

22. Scratch the mainstream surface of *Everybody Loves Raymond* and you'll find an edgy little sitcom with the show's unsung hero, Peter Boyle, wreaking comic havoc without ever leaving his La-Z-Boy.

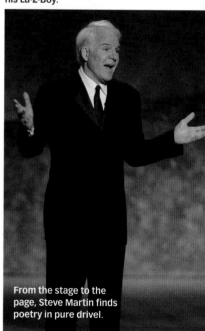

From the stage to the page, Steve Martin finds poetry in pure drivel.

23. *Some Like It Hot* is still crazy funny after all these years.
24. *Annie Hall* remains a funny valentine to love, life, and Manhattan.
25. Three words: *Club Comic View.* Black Entertainment Television's nightly stand-up will send you to bed smiling.

—*Lisa Kogan*

like stars until you have the map that shows you the constellations. It was my destiny," she says, "to redefine what it means to be a patient."

The day of her very first chemo treatment, Saranne sat with her head in a trash can. "I was throwing up, but I'd taken a notepad and I was writing, writing, writing. The whole charity came full-fledged—we'd have live shows for people who are dealing with illness and loss, a toll-free joke-of-the-day number: 1-888-HA-HA-HA-HA. I even had the name, Comedy Cures. I knew there was a place for humor in tragedy. I'm not promising laughter is going to cure you, although I'm sure it helped me. Even if you're not actually physically better, joy and laughter make you feel better," Saranne says. "Life is hard, and society is hard, and if you don't consciously prepare yourself each day to practice wonder and joy, you get really good at practicing stress and pain and anger and anxiety and fear. You know," she adds, "kids laugh 300 to 400 times a day. But grown-ups? Only about 15."

"What happens?" I ask.

"Taxes!" She laughs. "Wrinkles!"

Nine in the morning after her first red devil day, Saranne was on the phone. "I have a vision for a charity," she told a local attorney. He was a stranger, but she needed a lawyer and they had a mutual friend. She described the Laugh-A-Thons she wanted to produce—interactive performances that would include comic acts, joke telling, and education about humor's value. "We're going to transform the sound and look of a hospital," she told the lawyer. "Every patient will have the opportunity to laugh."

"You got it," he said.

An accountant volunteered to help Saranne get Comedy Cures nonprofit status. Somebody donated an office. Atlantic Telecom overnighted free phones. Comedy Cures was ready to roll.

"Don't you think you should wait till your treatment's over?" friends cautioned.

"I told them, 'If you stop me from doing this work, the cancer's winning,'" Saranne says. "Even when I was exhausted, I'd spend ten minutes a day pushing the dream forward."

Every time Saranne got infused, she threw a party from her chemotherapy chair. "I said, 'If I have to do this, I'm going to enjoy it. Chemo is going to bring me life, not kill me.' So I got friends and family together. We had party favors, little sandwiches, ice pops, and we sat and watched tapes and laughed."

While still on chemotherapy, Saranne staged the first Laugh-A-Thon at Lauriel's school. It was a test run. Three hundred kids and their parents showed up for a program that included a Laughter Symphony, with Saranne assigning different kinds of laughs to different sections, like an orchestra. She demonstrated her full body giggle, which starts at the toes. During the open mike session, a little boy with cerebral palsy rolled to the microphone. He had difficulty forming words. The audience waited. Saranne didn't know what to expect. "What did Tarzan say when he slammed into the tree?" the boy finally managed. "Who greased the v-i-i-i-i-i-i-i-ine?"

The feeling in the air was electric. Parents came up afterward and said they'd never seen their children so rapt.

Saranne knew she was onto something big. She began staging interactive Laugh-A-Thons for patients throughout the Northeast. But three months after she finished radiation, the cancer was growing with a vengeance and she was diagnosed with early stage 4 metastatic disease. Saranne needed yet another surgery and more chemo.

As soon as she was on her feet, Saranne took her programs on the road again. The goal of every show is 100 laughs. (The Comedy Cures brochure urges you to consult your doctor first if you have a hernia.) "If 200 people are in the audience, that's 20,000 laughs," Saranne says. Last year she performed at 54 live events for 34,000 people. She visits Gilda's Clubs (social clubs for anyone dealing with cancer, named after the late comedian Gilda Radner) and has brought Comedy Cures to Paul Newman's Hole in the Woods Ranch, the Girl Scouts, and United Way. Jackie Mason volunteered for a fund-raiser. After 9/11, the head of the Red Cross mental health division called and said, "Can you get here right away?" The next day, she was at Ground Zero,

armed with small, handmade Wellness Joke Books for the relief workers and their families. The books are created by volunteers, including terminally ill patients, who donate jokes and cartoons. "You can go to someone who has a prognosis of a week or a month and say, 'Would you like to do community service?' People always say yes. They give back before they check out."

Saranne keeps moving, keeps laughing. She's planning to host a day of laughter for up to 3,100 children who lost a parent or caregiver on 9/11. But she recognizes only too well that reconciling yourself to loss is a process. "First you have to mourn what happened. Then you can give pain the freedom to leave. It's hard to find your laughter until you've found your pain."

In 2001 two suspicious nodes appeared in Saranne's neck. Western medicine, she decided, was not the only option. "In my system," she says, "chemo is Kool-Aid."

Everywhere she went, Saranne stood up and asked, "Can anyone get me an appointment with the Dalai Lama's doctor?"

One morning the phone rang. It was a woman who'd heard about Saranne from their mutual hairdresser. "You have an appointment at 1 P.M. on Monday with the Dalai Lama's doctor," she said.

"A modest little man in a saffron robe examined me," Saranne says. "He took my pulse. He gave me herbs for tea. 'You are very well,' he said. 'In three months, your scans will show shrinkage.'"

Today Saranne has no visible sign of disease. "I think the whole universe is conspiring to give me an incredible journey," she says. "Comedy Cures can't expand fast enough to meet the need. Time is the greatest gift—to have enough time to serve as many people as I'm supposed to serve. I'm a poster child for spunk."

For spunk. And for invention, moxie, and resilience.

A Comedy Cures ballpoint has a rainbow fright wig and feet. It stands up so you can't lose it in the sheets when you're splayed in a hospital bed. "If we're going to give them a pen, we might as well give them a pen that makes them laugh," Saranne says.

Saranne Rothberg hands me a pen. I laugh. ●

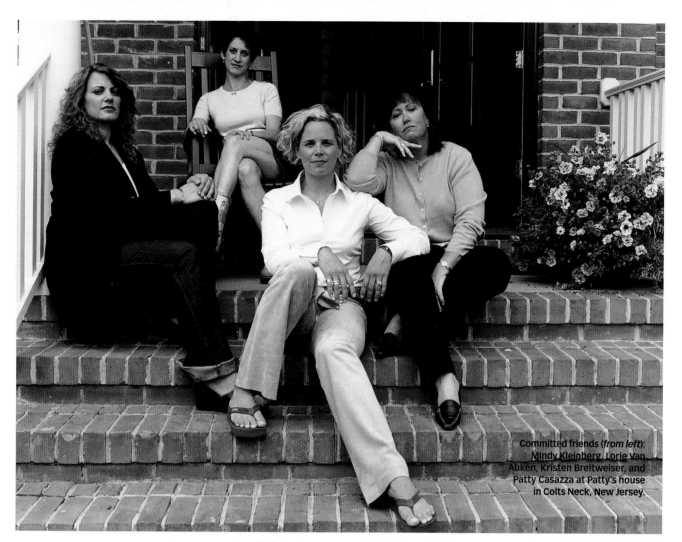

Committed friends (*from left*): Mindy Kleinberg, Lorie Van Auken, Kristen Breitweiser, and Patty Casazza at Patty's house in Colts Neck, New Jersey.

Hell's Angels

THE FOUR WOMEN SITTING AT MY table—passing cartons of Chinese takeout, cracking jokes, interrupting and finishing one another's sentences—could be any group of lively, attractive friends, come into the city from the suburbs to catch a Wednesday matinee. But in fact they've traveled from New Jersey into Manhattan to meet with a former director of the FBI.

These are the women who have come to be known, on Capitol Hill and in the media, as the Jersey Girls, the four September 11 widows whose energy, resourcefulness, and commitment have moved mountains—or in any case the Washington bureaucracy. They've held rallies, made phone calls, lobbied congressmen, appeared on radio and TV. And it's largely thanks to them that, despite the government's efforts to restrict the official inquiry to a series of perfunctory hearings, an independent commission investigated

Without their guts, persistence, pain, rage, and, above all, love, there would be no 9/11 commission, no Megan's Law, no Amber Alert, no Mothers Against Drunk Driving.

FRANCINE PROSE on "ordinary" women who became extraordinary when they turned helplessness into heroism.

the failures of September 11 and made crucial recommendations concerning our nation's security.

Lorie Van Auken rolls her eyes when I ask what new information they learned from their meeting this morning with the FBI chief. "You cannot believe...Nobody was talking to anybody...."

Unbelievable is a word that recurs in the women's conversation, and one that describes so much of what has happened since that September morning when Lorie Van Auken, Kristen Breitweiser, Mindy Kleinberg, and Patty Casazza saw their husbands off to work. All four men were executives who worked in the World Trade Center, three at Cantor Fitzgerald, one at Fiduciary Trust. None of them came home.

The women share so many private jokes and so much personal history, they know each other so well and so clearly enjoy one another's company that it's hard to believe they weren't always close friends. There are surface differences, of course: An age range of 16 years divides the youngest, Kristen Breitweiser—whose blonde good looks and unruffled eloquence have frequently cast her as the group's spokesperson—and the appealingly direct, wry Lorie Van Auken. Mindy Kleinberg has an earthiness reminiscent of Kirstie Alley, while Patty Casazza, the most reserved, has the ability to cut straight to the chase with quiet, on-target, funny observations. In the 2000 presidential election, two voted for Bush, two for Gore. But what they share is far more striking than their dissimilarities. All four are open, warm, down-to-earth, gifted with quick, saving senses of humor. And all of them are passionate about the mission that brought them together—and lifted them out of the numbing isolation that followed in the wake of September 11.

After the deaths of their husbands, the women sank into separate wells of grief, unsure about how they would live, how they would raise their children alone. "For the first month, I didn't leave the house," says Breitweiser.

"I was scared to death," Van Auken recalls. "I wasn't eating. I dropped 12 pounds pronto. I was barely breathing. You felt like you had a big hole right in your gut."

And they found it hard to communicate with people who hadn't lost family members on September 11. "We were in comas," Kleinberg says. "Everybody was an earthling, and now we were from Pluto. You needed to go to a support group and call someone so you could talk Plutonian."

It was through these support groups and their local churches that the women first met and discovered they all had questions that weren't being answered. "If our husbands and loved ones had been killed in a car accident," says Van Auken, "we would know everything. We would have a whole report on that accident. Right away. But with 9/11, we weren't being told anything." And as they slowly emerged from their "comas," they began to realize that if they wanted answers, they would have to find them on their own.

"Nobody was clarifying," says Casazza. "Nobody stood up and said, 'This is what happened.' So you're left to your own

devices. We used the Internet, contacted people we'd met, people who reached out to us."

Gradually, the women came to understand that what was needed was an independent investigation into the lapses in our security system that allowed September 11 to happen. And the turning point—the moment that galvanized them into action—occurred during a meeting of Van Auken and Kleinberg's support group, when one of the other members, Bob Monetti, whose son had been killed in the 1988 bombing of Pan Am Flight 103 over Lockerbie, Scotland, convinced them that they themselves had to take action.

> "I'm like a 14-year-old," says Mindy Kleinberg. "You say no to me, and I have to do it."

"We'd heard there was legislation on the floor to create an independent commission," says Kleinberg. "We assumed it would get passed. But Bob said, 'If you want something to happen, you have to have a rally, you have to lobby.' We walked out of that group, we called Kristen and Patty, we said, 'You know what? We have to have a rally.'"

They went to Home Depot, bought wood for posters, and made their own signs (3,000 deaths—3,000,000 questions!), which they carried, along with a huge banner, on the train to Washington, D.C. The first rally took place on a hot day, June 11, 2002—and their careers as activists had begun. Aided by the staff of New Jersey lawmakers Robert Torricelli and Chris Smith, they began to "stalk the halls and knock on doors" of other senators and congressmen, seeking support for the formation of an independent commission.

"We wouldn't go away," says Casazza. "We'd say, 'Nice talking to you. You're on our list of supporters.'" And despite fierce opposition from the White House, despite

the senators and congressmen who told the widows that governmental affairs were none of their business, they succeeded in their mission. "I'm like a 14-year-old," says Kleinberg. "You say no to me, and I have to do it."

FORMED AT THE END OF 2002, the bipartisan National Commission on Terrorist Attacks upon the United States held its first public hearing in late March 2003. And the Jersey Girls were present at every session, walking out in silent protest when it initially seemed as if Condoleezza Rice would refuse to testify. It's easy to see why, as the hearings progressed, the women became such a magnet for media attention. They are so engaging, and their passion for their cause is so fierce and infectious that after spending just a few hours in their company, I not only want to be their friend but I want to join them, to pitch in, to help in any way I can. It's all I can do not to offer to write all their petitions and press releases.

"All tragedies breed advocacy," says Kleinberg. "Look at all those people who have gotten through times of loss by doing something. That's how come we have Megan's Law, that's how come we have the Amber Alert. Those parents lost a child, and they realized that unsafe laws were putting children at risk. What really got to me was knowing that those Pan Am 103 people fought for years and years to get locked cockpit doors, and nobody fought along with them, including myself. And that made me feel terrible, because if I'd paid attention and helped them, maybe none of this would have happened."

ALL FOUR WOMEN TALK ABOUT the way that loss can serve as a wake-up call. "You're like Eve biting the apple," says Van Auken. "You're totally blind before, you have no idea that this even exists. You bite the apple, and this whole other thing opens up before you."

In the days that follow my meeting with them, I talk to other men and women who have suffered cruel, often violent catastrophes—and alchemized the intensity of their personal grief into public activism. In the agonizing process of repairing their own lives, they have found ways to save other lives, to remedy the failures that brought about the death of a family member. Everywhere on the Internet, in the halls of Congress, and in new bills passed by state and federal lawmakers is evidence of the efforts—and successes—of these "ordinary" heroes who have lost, or nearly lost, someone in a tragedy that should never have occurred. They've struggled against prejudice, negligence, faulty legislation. They've collected information, helped find cures, formed organizations dedicated to research, human rights, and grass roots politics.

One of the oldest and most visible of these organizations is Mothers Against Drunk Driving (MADD), which was started by Candace Lightner, a California mother whose 13-year-old daughter was killed, and Cindi Lamb, a Maryland mom whose infant daughter was paralyzed—both by drunk drivers. Wendy Hamilton, the current president of MADD, remembers how she began her career with the organization, as a volunteer.

"My sister and her baby were killed on September 19, 1984. After the funeral, I stayed around to help my brother-in-law and their surviving child. I was going through Becky's dresser drawer and found a bumper sticker for Mothers Against Drunk Driving. By then we'd found out that the driver who killed my sister had had a high level of blood alcohol. And around that same time, I read a magazine article about MADD that listed their phone number.

"Those two events were like lightning bolts. I felt that Becky was telling me to call. I felt that it was her way of saying to me, 'Get off your butt and do something.' She was a nurse, she'd had such a drive and passion to be involved in people's lives. I remember her talking about the drunk-driving victims she saw in her work, and how angry it made her. And then I called a minister friend, who said, 'You have two choices. You can choose to be bitter, or you can choose to be better.' It was a turning point in my life. I myself was the mother of three children, and I didn't ever want to get the kind of phone call my mother had gotten. I felt I had to do something to alert

people to why this violent, preventable crime was occurring."

Now, more than two decades after its founding, MADD is an international program with more than 600 chapters. It has worked to pass thousands of anti–drunk-driving and underage drinking statutes, as well as federal laws requiring states to raise their drinking age to 21 and to lower the threshold of impaired driving to a blood alcohol content of .08 percent or lose highway funding.

Other activists have carried on and widened the fight against drunk driving.

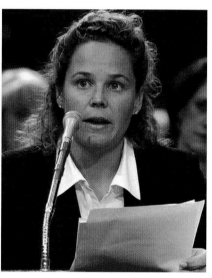

Kristen Breitweiser testifying on Capitol Hill.

After recent Naval Academy graduate John Elliott was killed and his girlfriend, Kristen Hohenwarter, seriously injured in July 2000 by a drunk driver who had been picked up by police and released into the custody of a friend just hours earlier, John's parents, Bill and Muriel Elliott, founded the Hero Campaign for Designated Drivers. Because of their efforts, the state of New Jersey has passed John's Law, which mandates that when police arrest a driver for DWI, the car must be impounded for 12 hours. Now when New Jersey police release DWI offenders into the custody of a relative or a friend, that person is notified that he or she may be held legally responsible if the drunk driver gets back behind the wheel.

Another critical piece of legislation that came out of victim advocacy is New Jersey's Megan's Law, which mandates that

communities be notified when a convicted sex offender moves into the neighborhood. In 1994, 7-year-old Megan Kanka was murdered by a neighbor, a sex criminal. Her parents, Maureen and Richard Kanka, began circulating a petition for the passage of such a law. Two years later, a similar proposal became federal law. "If we'd known that a twice-convicted pedophile was living in our neighborhood," says Maureen Kanka, "Megan would be here right now."

Much of the inspiration for the Kankas' work, says Maureen, came from their community. "We were so grief-stricken. But the outpouring of love and support was phenomenal. One Sunday a thousand people came through our house to pay their respects. They brought us food, they gave money. After a while, we had $30,000 sitting around the house. Someone said, 'You'd better put it in the bank.' And that was the start of the foundation. My husband kept saying, 'This could be really big.' But never in my wildest dreams did I think it would go as far as to change the law." The Kankas still remain actively involved in child-safety issues and awareness programs; their latest project involves giving nonprofit sports teams grants to do background checks on coaches and managers.

Subsequent crimes involving children have led to the founding of other child-safety foundations; working together, a number of those groups helped design the national Amber Alert program, named after yet another child victim, 9-year-old Amber Hagerman. Now whenever a child is kidnapped, the media is immediately notified, bulletins are broadcast, and many highways have photos of the child and signs instructing motorists on how to recognize the kidnapper's vehicle.

AFTER 21-YEAR-OLD MATTHEW Shepard was murdered in Laramie, Wyoming, in a much-publicized antigay hate crime, his parents, Dennis and Judy Shepard, started a foundation in their son's name to advocate acceptance and help end bias.

"While Matt was in the hospital and soon after he passed away," Judy Shepard remembers, "we received hundreds of thousands of e-mails and letters saying, 'Please use this opportunity to make a difference, use your voice,' which is now a national voice. It wouldn't have been fair to Matt not to do something to help his community."

Some survivors turned activists have not only forgiven the perpetrators of crimes against their loved ones but have dedicated themselves to bettering the conditions that, they feel, were partly responsible for their deaths. Linda and Peter Biehl's daughter, Amy, was murdered in 1993 by an angry political mob in South Africa, where she had gone to work as a socially committed Fulbright scholar.

"Within hours after what happened to Amy," says Linda Biehl, "we began receiving faxes and phone calls from people who lived in her township, people she worked with, white people as well as black, thousands of people. And what everyone said was: 'Please. Come see. Come help.' Amy had always shared with us her dreams and goals. There was no hesitance on our part. This was a part of what we felt we had to do. Two months after her death, we came to South Africa as guests of the township. We were brought into the environment where she was killed, shown the issues of the day. As time went on, people gave money and we set up a foundation."

The Biehls began to spend more and more time in the township where Amy had died, trying to understand the roots of the hatred that had killed their daughter, and in 1998, when two of her killers received amnesty and were released from prison, they came to work with the Biehls. Their foundation is aiding schools, funding music and arts programs, working to prevent violence, and helping to establish businesses in South Africa's poorest townships.

"It's a 24/7 responsibility to raise the money and sustain it—a huge commitment," Linda Biehl acknowledges.

All the survivors turned activists I spoke with emphasized the level of commitment and engagement that what they're doing requires, and the sense of mission that inspired them to get involved. For Lois Gibbs, the first president of the Love Canal Homeowners' Association, the wake-up call came in June 1978, as she sat in her son's hospital room. Her son Michael, who had been healthy when the family moved to the Love Canal area of New York State (where Gibbs's husband worked for Goodyear Chemical), was suffering from asthma, epilepsy, liver problems, a urinary disorder, and a depressed immune system. Her daughter, Melissa, born in the area, had a serious blood disease.

"My kids were sick," says Gibbs. "And we'd read in the paper that our neighborhood had a dangerous toxic-waste problem. So I put one and one together. But I was waiting for someone to do something, waiting for someone to come along and hand me a petition to sign.

"Our neighborhood had a dangerous toxic-waste problem, and my kids were sick," says Lois Gibbs. "But I was waiting for someone to come along and hand me a petition to sign."

"So there I was in Michael's hospital room, and I've always thought of myself as a responsible mother, as the best mom I could be. But if I didn't do anything, I realized, no one would. So how could I keep telling myself that I was a responsible mother?

"I don't know what I was so scared of. The unknown, I guess. I was afraid someone would slam the door in my face. But I got the petition together and knocked on the first door I came to, and they opened the door and said, 'We've been waiting for you!' After that I kept knocking on doors. I could no longer blame anyone else for not doing anything. I realized: I have a responsibility here."

One reason the homeowners' association was so successful, Gibbs says, was that it functioned as a true democracy. "That's because I was such a scaredy-cat," she says. "I was a high school graduate with a C average. I didn't feel I could make life-and-death decisions for other people. So anytime a decision had to be made, we turned it back over to the group. We had real respect for one another, and we had the group's support for every action we took."

Eventually, Gibbs left upstate New York for Washington, D.C., where her children's health improved, and where, in 1981, she founded the Center for Health, Environment, and Justice (CHEJ). The center's achievements have been extraordinary. Gibbs is often referred to as the mother of Superfund—the federal government program to clean up waste sites. CHEJ has initiated programs to help communities evaluate cleanup options. They have sponsored right-to-know legislation guaranteeing the free dissemination of information about environmental pollutants, lobbied against the establishment of new toxic dumps and for the regulation of how incinerator ash, solid wastes, and other pollutants are disposed of.

"If people want to win out over an environmental health risk, they need to organize and create political pressure," says Gibbs. "It's that fight that will change the outcome. You can save the world."

WHAT ALL THESE ADVOCATES AGREE on is that if you want to make a difference, you have to be willing to do it yourself. That was the life-changing advice that the Jersey Girls got from Bob Monetti, whose 20-year-old son, Richard, a Syracuse University junior, was returning from a semester in London on Pan Am 103. "My wife kicked me so hard for that [advice]," he says. "She knew what they were getting into. But it was frustrating to listen to them. They were saying the country doesn't give a damn, [and] the government doesn't want to know the truth." The women had no idea what to do. "I told them, 'If you don't do something, nobody's going to do it.'"

Like the Jersey Girls, says Monetti, his activism—and the formation of the Victims of Pan Am Flight 103—began with anger and frustration. "We wanted information about the crash, about the warnings that had come before it. And it was as if the State Department was hiding—they just weren't coming out and helping. We didn't make a conscious decision to do something political. We just kept hitting roadblocks, and we realized we had to get publicity and take political action."

In the process, Monetti's life changed completely. He phased out of his career as an engineer, and for 13 years he worked as a consultant on airline security for the FAA, along the way becoming a member of its Aviation Security Advisory Committee. Though he's less than optimistic about the current state of airline security, he still believes in the value of knowledge and information. "[Our] biggest recommendation was that the intelligence people should tell the airlines what the most likely problems are. You can't protect against something if you don't know what it is you're protecting against." He believes in matching bags with passengers and moving checkpoints closer to the gates.

Monetti cautions against the idea that advocacy is a substitute for mourning and grief. "It's a good thing to do in conjunction with all the other things you have to do to get through a disaster. But you have to deal with your own loss. Otherwise, three, four years down the road it comes back to bite you in the butt."

The Jersey Girls know this, too. None of them is pretending that activism is a way to "get over" their loss. Partway through our lunch, Kristen Breitweiser asks if we can take a cigarette break. "I started smoking after 9/11," she confides to me in the kitchen. "Maybe I thought my smoking would make my husband so mad, he'd come back and get me to quit. But so far it hasn't worked."

Still, their activism has given them a sense of purpose and sent them in a direction that was far from obvious in the dark weeks and months that followed the tragedy. They talk about the larger sense of responsibility they feel that extends far beyond their own families, their own losses, and that embraces the other families who lost the people they loved on 9/11—and all of us. Knowledge has brought not only empowerment but obligation. The fact that they have had such astonishing success means they can no longer sit

If you'd like to donate time or money to one of the organizations mentioned here, see below:

Amy Biehl Foundation
P.O. Box 2926
Newport Beach, CA 92659
949-650-5356
amybiehl.org

Center for Health, Environment and Justice (CHEJ)
P.O. Box 6806
Falls Church, VA 22040
703-237-2249, ext. 25
chej.org

HERO Campaign for Designated Drivers
The John R. Elliott Foundation

P.O. Box 700
Somers Point, NJ 08244
866-700-4376
www.herocampaign.org

Matthew Shepard Foundation
301 Thelma Dr., #512
Casper, WY 82609
307-237-6167
matthewshepard.org

Megan Nicole Kanka Foundation, Inc.
P.O. Box 9956
Trenton, NJ 08650
609-890-2201

megannicolekanka foundation.org

Mothers Against Drunk Driving (MADD)
511 E. John Carpenter Frwy., Suite 700
Irving, TX 75062
800-438-6233
madd.org

Victims of Pan Am Flight 103, Inc.
P.O. Box 903
Cherry Hill, NJ 08003
609-405-6169
web.syr.edu/~vpaf103

back and rely on anyone—their congressmen, their government, the intelligence network—to keep the nation safe. "It would be like knowing there was a fire in the room," says Patty Casazza, "and not telling anybody."

What motivates them, they keep saying, is the feeling that if another terrorist attack occurs on our soil, they would feel personally responsible for not having done even more.

"During all this," says Kleinberg, "we were still raising grieving, horribly sad, mind-bogglingly destroyed children. There were points along the way that we didn't want to do it anymore. But we couldn't quit. How could I go to sleep, how could I not go to Washington and ask them to fix things—knowing all the things I know?"

For all their impatience with the government's reluctance to uncover the truth, their experience has strengthened their conviction about the importance of being engaged, active citizens of a democracy. "Being an American gives us the right to ask questions and to have this commission," says Breitweiser. "Suffering the loss we've suffered has given us the passion to see this through."

"You don't need to get your wake-up call in the form of a body part," says Kleinberg. "You need to care about what's happening now. You go down there and find out what's

being voted on by our elected officials, things that affect all of our lives—and no one knows about them! The only way anything gets done is when the public cares, when constituents pick up the phone, call their elected officials, and say, 'I want you to vote this way!'"

MODEST, UNASSUMING GLORIOUSLY commonsensical, the women tend to see themselves as hard workers rather than as heroes. But the truth is that they are heroic, as are the other men and women who have used, and continue to use, their grief as a source of energy and drive as they work for a larger cause. They are models and inspirations, not least for their own families. Again and again, the Jersey Girls mention how much what they're doing has meant to their own children. "They looked at us, and they were scared," Breitweiser says about the kids in the immediate aftermath of 9/11. "They were looking at their mothers, who were flattened, totally smeared into the earth. I wanted to be able to say to them: You don't have to be victims—you could be survivors.

"It's been important for them to see us take charge of the situation. For the kids to see how much we've accomplished has taught them that even though you have the wind knocked out of you, you can still carry on. You can throw your shoulders back, take a deep breath, and carry on." ●

THE FIRST ANNUAL
Chutzpah Awards

These women have pushed, pulled, prodded, and persevered through thick and thin, poverty and wealth, hope and hopelessness, past naysayers and yes-men. Meet ten women whose chutzpah—audacity, nerve, boldness, conviction—has taken them to the most amazing places. Fasten your seat belts and prepare for uplift.

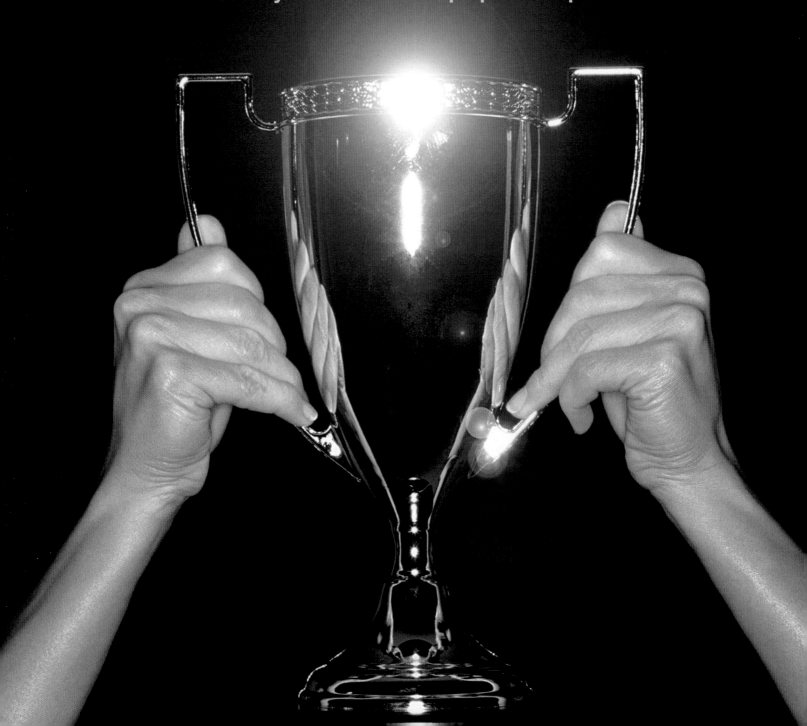

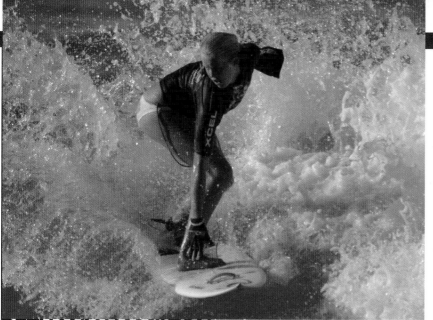

LATEEFAH SIMON
THE YOUNGEST FEMALE "GENIUS" AWARD WINNER.

In 2003, Lateefah Simon, 27, executive director of the Center for Young Women's Development in San Francisco, had $4,000 in the bank and a $15,000 payroll to make the following week. "It's going to be okay," she told her staff. "We cannot fail." Then Simon phoned every foundation she could think of until one finally sent her a check.

The center was founded in 1993 by Rachel Pfeffer and a collection of social service providers working to help young women living in poverty. It pays a living wage (plus medical and childcare benefits) while the girls learn job skills and trains them to become youth advocates in their communities. Simon began doing street outreach for the center when she was 17. In 1997, when Pfeffer and some of the service providers moved on, Simon's passion and leadership qualities were recognized and she became executive director.

A 19-year-old single mother, Simon didn't have so much as a handbook to help her. "Everybody *knew* we were going to go down," she recalls. "There's no way that the ghetto girls were going to make it." But she taught herself everything from bookkeeping to grant writing; in the process, she revamped an organization run solely by young women of color, most of whom had been homeless or incarcerated. Today the center has doubled its budget (to around $600,000 annually) and the number of girls it serves—nearly 2,000. It has employed more than 180 young women to run its programs, 98 percent of whom go on to college or employment. "We even have one Centerite at Harvard," Simon says. In 2003, she received a $500,000 MacArthur "genius" award, the youngest woman so honored. Simon plans to go to college and then continue her life's work: "To change the way the world sees poor young women."

BETHANY HAMILTON
A TEENAGE WAVE RIDER RETURNS TO THE WATER AFTER A SHARK ATTACK.

Halloween 2003: Thirteen-year-old Bethany Hamilton was riding the waves on Kauai's North Shore, as she did most mornings. An amateur surfing champion ranked among the top five in the world, Hamilton was paddling with her best friend and her friend's dad when a 15-foot tiger shark suddenly loomed in the water. Before she knew what was happening, the creature had bitten off most of her left arm just below the shoulder, shaking her as she clung to the surfboard with her other arm, before it swam off. Hamilton, who relies on a strong Christian faith, stayed calm as her friend's father tied a tourniquet around her arm and brought her back to shore,

and she didn't cry during the attack.

Although many people wouldn't go ankle deep in the ocean again—or in a mud puddle, for that matter—Hamilton was back on her surfboard one month later, and insisted that she receive no special treatment from surfing officials when she entered competitions. "I just wanted to be normal," she says. "It was definitely hard, and it felt weird, but I was glad to be back out there." To keep up her courage while she's in the ocean now, Hamilton prays, or calls to her friends nearby, or sings. "I don't know why singing works," she says. "Maybe it takes your mind off things." When it comes to fear, Hamilton says, "Just get over it."

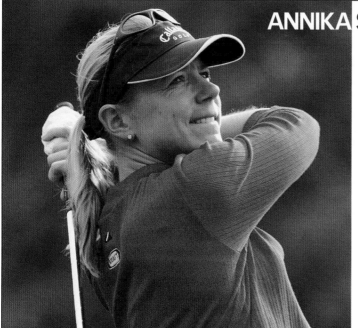

ANNIKA SÖRENSTAM
A FEMALE COMPETES ON THE PGA FOR THE FIRST TIME IN 58 YEARS.

After winning 53 tournaments worldwide, Annika Sörenstam looked around for a challenge. She found it in the 2003 Bank of America Colonial, a tournament on the men's tour. She wasn't attempting to break gender boundaries (Babe Didrikson Zaharias played a PGA event in 1945). She wasn't aiming for headlines (though she got loads of them). She accepted the sponsors' invitation to play on the PGA tour, she told CNN, "because I like to test myself.... I'm looking for ways to take my game to a different level."

Then every sportswriter, sportscaster, and armchair duffer weighed in. A number of men on the PGA tour, including the number two golfer, Vijay Singh, said that she didn't belong there. Sörenstam withstood the hoopla with grace and a shy smile that won people over—if not perfect putting. She missed the cut by four strokes (placing ahead of 11 men). She told the crowds, "I'm living my dream, and that's what it's all about." But it ended up being about more than that: When 14-year-old Michelle Wie entered the PGA Sony Open seven months later, *The New York Times* put the story not on the front page but on the bottom left of its sports section. Thanks to Annika, competing with the men is suddenly no big thing.

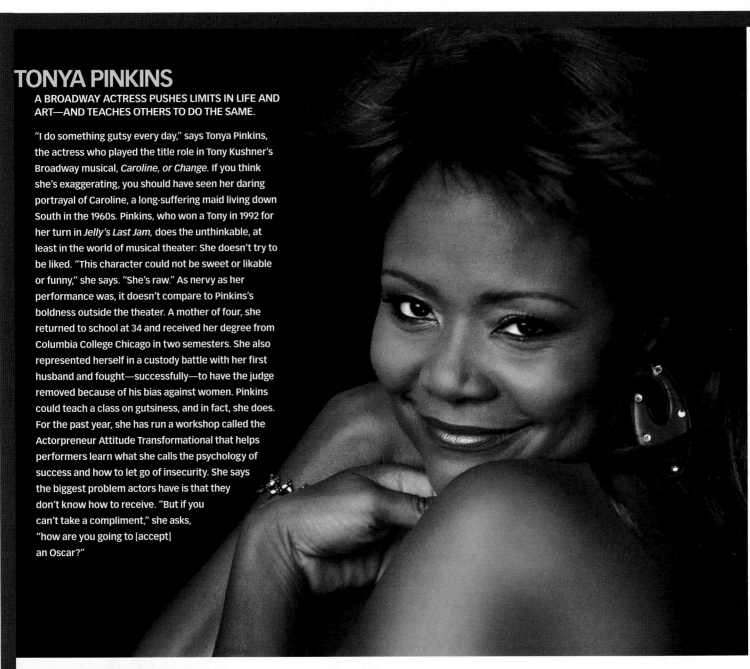

TONYA PINKINS

A BROADWAY ACTRESS PUSHES LIMITS IN LIFE AND ART—AND TEACHES OTHERS TO DO THE SAME.

"I do something gutsy every day," says Tonya Pinkins, the actress who played the title role in Tony Kushner's Broadway musical, *Caroline, or Change*. If you think she's exaggerating, you should have seen her daring portrayal of Caroline, a long-suffering maid living down South in the 1960s. Pinkins, who won a Tony in 1992 for her turn in *Jelly's Last Jam,* does the unthinkable, at least in the world of musical theater: She doesn't try to be liked. "This character could not be sweet or likable or funny," she says. "She's raw." As nervy as her performance was, it doesn't compare to Pinkins's boldness outside the theater. A mother of four, she returned to school at 34 and received her degree from Columbia College Chicago in two semesters. She also represented herself in a custody battle with her first husband and fought—successfully—to have the judge removed because of his bias against women. Pinkins could teach a class on gutsiness, and in fact, she does. For the past year, she has run a workshop called the Actorpreneur Attitude Transformational that helps performers learn what she calls the psychology of success and how to let go of insecurity. She says the biggest problem actors have is that they don't know how to receive. "But if you can't take a compliment," she asks, "how are you going to [accept] an Oscar?"

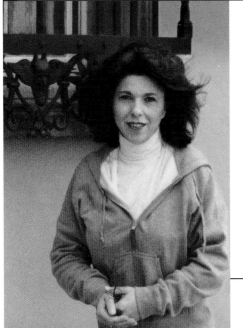

RESHO O'NEILL

BRIDGING THE GAP: A TRANSLATOR LEAPS FROM OHIO TO THE WAR IN IRAQ.

When the United States went to war with Iraq in March 2003, Fadya Resho O'Neill was minding her own business: the General's Chop House, a steak and seafood restaurant in Waterville, Ohio, that she co-owns with her husband, Dave. Born in Syria, O'Neill, 50, emigrated to the United States at 21. Not long after the war started, a cousin mentioned that the State Department had approached him to become an Arabic-English translator for the military.

"Why don't you go?" O'Neill asked him.

"Why don't *you* go?" he responded.

This, it turned out, was a life changer of a question. Before O'Neill could say, "*Limaza la?*" ("Why not?"), she was in a war zone, bouncing around in the open back of a Humvee as a civilian contractor. Since arriving in Iraq in September 2003, O'Neill has interpreted everything from interrogations of Iraqis accused of crimes to discussions between Americans and Iraqis seeking supplies, aid, or information.

Like anyone who lives and works side by side with the military, she has come under hostile fire. Sometimes it's of a verbal nature, and she fires right back in Arabic or English. One day, for instance, she was obliged to interview a 15-year-old boy who had been

DONNA DEES-THOMASES

THE MOM BEHIND ONE OF THE BIGGEST PROTEST MARCHES IN U.S. HISTORY.

Five years ago, Donna Dees-Thomases, a publicist for *The Late Show with David Letterman* and a mother of two, saw a report on a deadly shooting at a California nursery school. She felt outrage, then a kind of helplessness, and anger again. This particular shooting hit home: It had taken place at a Jewish community center similar to the one her children attended near her home in New Jersey. "That shook me deeply," she says, "I decided to put my publicity skills to use. I thought I could publicize the gun violence epidemic and find ways to empower other moms to get involved."

Her next act was deceptively simple—she contacted five friends. But those calls would lead to the 2000 Million Mom March, one of the biggest protest marches in U.S. history. "We have single people and dads in our organization, too," she says, "but the glue that held it together was really the moms."

After the 1999 announcement of the march, Dees-Thomases summoned courage she didn't know she had: Angry gun owners flooded the organization's Web site with threatening e-mails and powerful National Rifle Association lobbyists started a smear campaign, branding her "a loony leftist." Three months later, Dees-Thomases's husband asked for a divorce. "When that happened, I thought about quitting," she says, "but the march became such a life force that I couldn't."

On Mother's Day in 2000, more than 750,000 people marched on the National Mall in Washington, D.C., and for the movement's fourth anniversary, moms from all over the country mobilized again. "The NRA's goal is to intimidate. And sometimes they do, but the stakes are too high to back down. Failure," Dees-Thomases says, "is not an option."

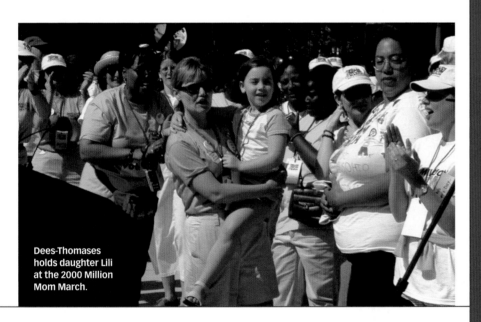

Dees-Thomases holds daughter Lili at the 2000 Million Mom March.

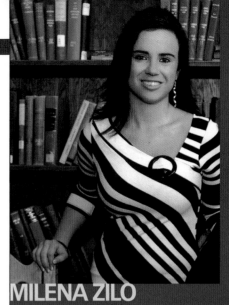

MILENA ZILO

SHE DIDN'T TAKE NO FOR AN ANSWER.

Growing up in Albania, Milena Zilo had mapped out her career. "I wanted to be a finance major," she says. "I just had a passion about it." When she and her family moved to Denver, Zilo fixated on the University of Denver's highly regarded finance program. Three years later, at 18, Zilo felt pretty confident she'd be accepted, with her 3.5 average, two internships, and enrollment in "every single club." But a rejection letter arrived, and a devastated Zilo hid it from her parents. "My big dream was shot," she says. "I worked so hard in high school, and I felt like such a failure."

Then she took action. She skipped school one day and drove to the office of the university's then vice chancellor of enrollment, John Dolan, vowing that she wouldn't leave until he admitted her to the school. Dolan's secretary stonewalled Zilo. Undeterred, she grabbed a brochure with his photo and tracked down Dolan on campus as he hurried into a meeting. "I told him I only needed five minutes," she says. "I said they had made a terrible mistake." Dolan brought her back to his office. He listened and flipped through the notebook of recommendations and achievements she had brought. Then he stepped out for a few minutes. When Dolan returned, he said she was right. They'd made a mistake. He was so impressed with her drive that he even offered her a scholarship. (Other students will benefit from her persistence, too: The school's application process has been altered to include a personal interview.) Now in her junior year, Zilo says. "If there's one thing I've learned, it's don't stop at the first letter of rejection; if it's something you believe in, you have to go for it."

arrested in the Sadr City (formerly Saddam City) quarter of Baghdad for harboring quite a cache of illegal weapons. O'Neill asked the boy to write his name, and he scoffed, saying he couldn't, because under Saddam there was no reason to become literate. "What do you mean? Saddam came to your house and told your parents not to send you to school?" she retorted. "You can blame a lot of stuff on Saddam, but there's no reason not to learn the basics." Another day a man told her that if a certain Iranian ayatollah directed him to kill himself, he would, because he wanted to get to heaven. "If someone told me to kill myself, I'd say, 'You go first,' " she told him. "How do you know what heaven is like? Has somebody come back down from there and told you?"

One Iraqi asked her, "Tell me honestly, which side are you on?" She said she was on the American side, but that the Americans were on the side of the Iraqi people. He said the Americans were coming to take Iraqi land and buildings. "Are you crazy?" she said. "These people have their own buildings. Do you think anyone who had a chance to live in the United States would come live here?"

It's not just O'Neill's talk that is tough. She's working to renew her contract. "I want to stay at least a year," she says. "I really want to see what happens."

IRSHAD MANJI

A WRITER WHOSE BOOK LED TO DEATH THREATS STILL SPEAKS HER MIND.

When 35-year-old Irshad Manji sat down to create the engaging and lively *The Trouble with Islam,* she knew that her book would be bigger, much bigger, than girl meets God. As Manji writes, Islam is the only major religion where extremists hold such complete sway over the mainstream. Given that modern interpretations of the faith still call for women to be stoned for adultery, and being homosexual is just cause for murder (Manji is a lesbian), she was aware that she would come to the attention of Islamic bullies and terrorists.

Her book is an open letter to Muslims and non-Muslims alike, a letter that begins, "I have to be honest with you. Islam is on very thin ice with me...." She confronts her fellow Muslims on their blatant anti-Semitism, for the misleading clarion call against American imperialism, for silence in the face of terrorism, for the abuse of Muslim women in conservative Islamic communities. She challenges the

literalism with which even intellectual Western Muslims interpret the Koran—a literalism that leaves the floodgates open for terrorists to "hijack" the faith she holds so dear.

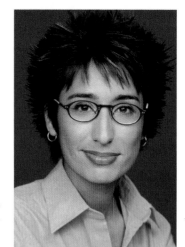

Manji has become the target of death threats and must travel with what she calls "appropriate security." She has to check her e-mail daily and forward threats to the police; she cannot carry a cell phone when traveling because GPS systems could make her an easy target to track. She has been called "the nonfiction Salman Rushdie." Shortly before her book came out, Manji met with Rushdie and asked him why she should publish a book that would invite the kind of havoc into her life that has been wreaked on his. Manji says he told her, "Once you put out a thought, it

cannot be unthought. A book is more important than a life."

Muslim women and men the world over have responded by sending Manji letters and e-mails of praise, thanking her for her appeal to liberalism in Islam. Her own mother, a devout Muslim woman who lives in western Canada, heard discreet whispers of praise for her daughter's bravery in the community mosque. During Manji's last visit to her childhood home, her mother tucked a card into her suitcase. The author discovered it when she returned to eastern Canada, where she lives. Her mother wrote to thank her for speaking up, for not abandoning her faith but challenging it. The letter concluded, "Bravo. You go, girl."

KATHRIN JANSEN, PhD, AND LAURA KOUTSKY, PhD

THUS IT IS PROVED: DESPITE MASSIVE SKEPTICISM, SCIENTISTS CREATE A VACCINE FOR CERVICAL CANCER.

Kathrin Jansen, PhD, is used to skepticism. When she began research in 1993 to create a vaccine to prevent cervical cancer, she wasn't surprised that some of her colleagues raised their eyebrows. But when an applicant for a position on her research team told her flat out that her idea wouldn't fly, she realized how few people believed in her work.

Still, Jansen, executive director

for microbial vaccine research at Merck Research Laboratories in West Point, Pennsylvania, felt she was onto something. A fellow researcher put her in touch with Laura Koutsky, PhD, an epidemiologist at the University of Washington, and the two started working together. They knew that nearly all cervical cancers are caused by the human papillomavirus (HPV). Jansen made a vaccine by introducing a

viral gene into yeast, which produces a protein that stimulates the immune system to fight the virus. Then came the tough part— years of research despite limited resources and doubt from within the organization about Jansen and her colleagues' proposed methods of testing. "The naysayers put up barriers, or tried to direct the team in what ultimately would have been the wrong direction," recalls Jansen. The detractors

were silenced when the proof-of-concept clinical study was published in the *New England Journal of Medicine* in late 2002. There are still questions to be answered about the vaccine (how long it's effective, for instance), but it's clear that it will affect women's health around the globe. "This outcome was the absolute high of my scientific career," says Jansen, who estimates the vaccine could be available within five years.

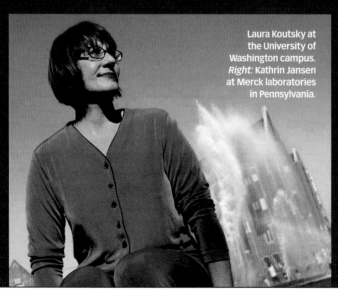

Laura Koutsky at the University of Washington campus. *Right:* Kathrin Jansen at Merck laboratories in Pennsylvania.

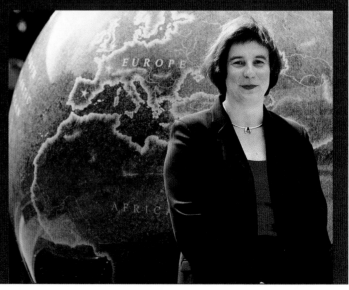

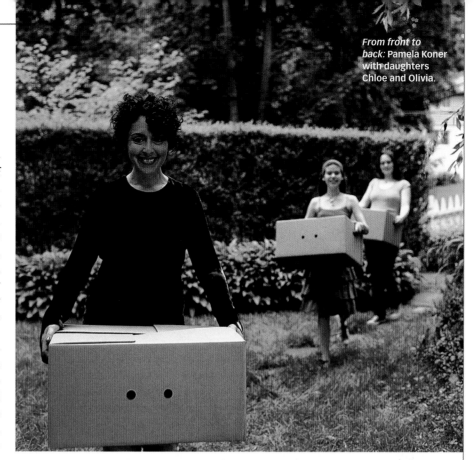

From front to back: Pamela Koner with daughters Chloe and Olivia.

THE TOWN OF HASTINGS-ON-Hudson, New York, 18 miles north of Manhattan, is as picturesque as its name. Men and women with good jobs as television reporters, documentary filmmakers, and jazz musicians (the nonstarving kind) patronize the Tower Ridge Yacht Club, Galápagos Books, and the Village Balloon & Flower Shoppe. Children spend birthday money at the Toy Cottage and put new shoes from the Hastings Bootery in the closets of pristine homes.

Pembroke, Illinois, is one of the poorest places in the country, and its homes barely qualify as houses: Plastic and plywood cover the windows of dirt-floored shacks topped with tires to keep the roofs from blowing away. There is no bookstore, no drugstore, no bank in this township 70 miles south of Chicago. The unemployment rate is more than three times that of the state, and the mostly unskilled residents have a tough time trying to reach any available jobs in dilapidated cars on gravel roads. Children sleep on bare mattresses and eat meager meals of neck bones and spaghetti cooked on propane-fueled stoves.

There would seem to be no connection between such disparate communities. But in the fall of 2002, Pamela Koner sat on the deck of her pretty house in Hastings, reading an article in *The New York Times* about children going hungry in Pembroke, and she couldn't bear it. "People were living in third-world conditions right outside Chicago," she says, "and I thought, *I have to do something.*"

What she did was create Family-to-Family. With the determination of a bloodhound, she tracked down allies: Lisa and Jon Dyson, pastors at Pembroke's Church of the Cross, which sponsors a food pantry, and Rodney Alford, MD, who runs a clinic in the town. Next Koner sent letters to parents of children in the Homework Club, an after-school program she operates. With gratifying speed, more than 60 Hastings families made a commitment to send monthly cartons of food to families in Pembroke. Soliciting some corporate help, Koner got a local manufacturer to donate

"I Have to Do Something"

Hastings-on-Hudson was blessed. Pembroke, Illinois, wasn't. So a group of concerned citizens cooked up an extraordinary movement that feeds whole families as well as the soul of a community. AIMEE LEE BALL reports.

packaging supplies, and Food Emporium kicked in $1,200 worth of coupons. With suggestions from an outreach worker in Pembroke, Koner creates a grocery list for a week's worth of menus and dispatches it to her Hastings team, who each shop individually at a cost of roughly $25. "People enjoy putting food in the cartons and

knowing that the next hand to touch that food will be 'their' family," she says.

Through letters and photos exchanged between Hastings and Pembroke, it's easy to see the impact of F2F, as Koner calls it. The recipients are overwhelmingly relieved that their kids don't go to bed hungry. And they're given a chance to broaden their palate. Christine Woods says her four grandchildren stuck up their noses at beans for dinner, but when she added canned tomatoes and garlic from the monthly package, the aroma was enticing. "They had two bowls each," she says. Jean Harrison is trying to connect the unexpected bounty with a lesson for her eight children and 26 grandchildren. "I don't want them grabbing," she says. "You ain't gonna have luck if you're a hog."

Even as the effort broadens—there are now monthly drives for coats, blankets, over-the-counter medicines, and children's books—Koner believes that F2F could be easily replicated in other communities. "I don't expect mountains to be moved," she says. "But maybe if you've got enough food for three weeks out of every month and you get that carton for the last week, you can think about something else. All of us should get to realize the possibilities of our lives." ●

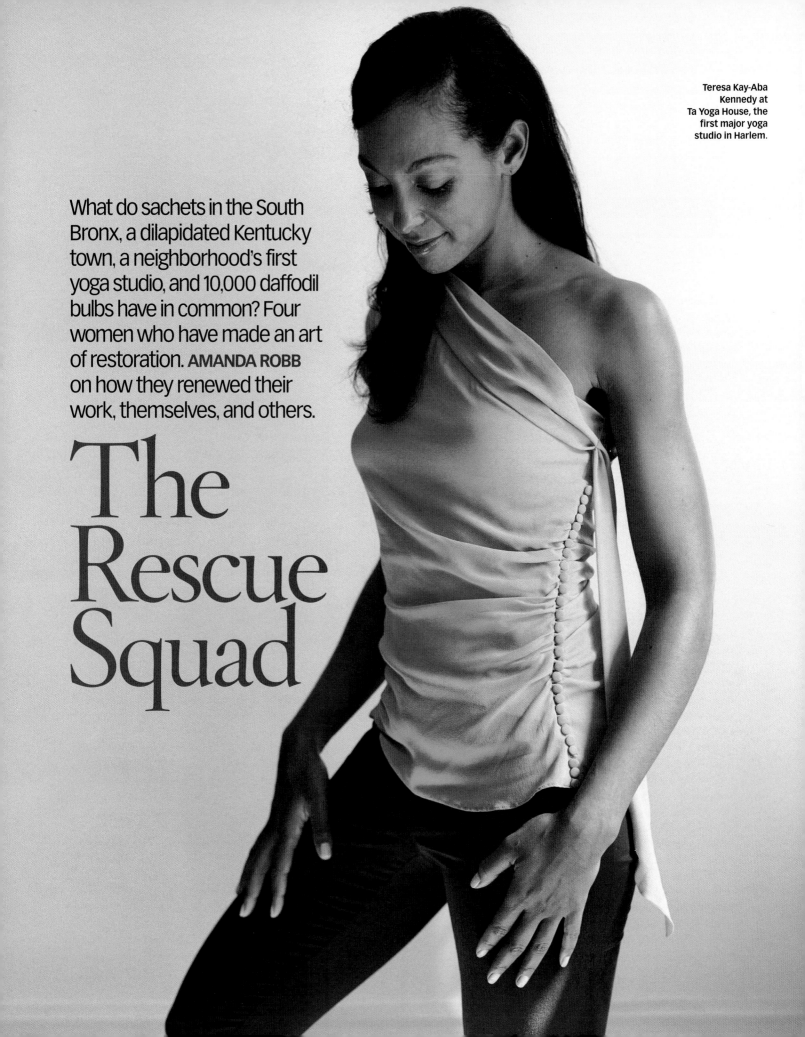

What do sachets in the South Bronx, a dilapidated Kentucky town, a neighborhood's first yoga studio, and 10,000 daffodil bulbs have in common? Four women who have made an art of restoration. **AMANDA ROBB** on how they renewed their work, themselves, and others.

The Rescue Squad

Teresa Kay-Aba Kennedy at Ta Yoga House, the first major yoga studio in Harlem.

Teresa Kay-Aba Kennedy

After graduating from Wellesley College with a double major in sociology and studio art, Teresa Kay-Aba Kennedy earned an MBA from Harvard Business School. At 24 she went to work for MTV—often working until 1:30 in the morning—and quickly became a vice president. Everyone was impressed, except Kennedy's parents.

"My mom kept saying, 'Honey, ease up.' My then boyfriend said, 'You need balance.' But I thought that was an evil word." Then Kennedy's body gave out. First she lost 20 pounds because of Crohn's disease (an inflammatory bowel disorder). Once she recovered from that, she visited Brazil, where she took an aerobics/martial arts class and injured a disk in her back. After conventional medical treatments put Kennedy back on her feet, she tried a gentler approach to maintaining her health: practicing yoga and eating natural foods, both of which her mother had done since the 1970s. She challenged herself with her father's three-question mantra: "Who am I? Where am I? And what must I do to be me?"

Soon Kennedy began feeling well instead of just successful. She abandoned corporate life to pursue a new career. She discovered that New York City had more than 100 yoga centers but not a single major studio in Harlem. Kennedy approached empowerment zone leaders to secure a debt commitment for her idea—a yoga and wellness center. It was a tough sell, she says: "I had to convince them that black people do yoga." She told community leaders that many African-Americans took classes elsewhere in Manhattan and that the few yoga classes then offered in Harlem—at a church and at a hospital—were well attended.

Kennedy opened the Ta Yoga House in 2002 (*ta* means "earth" in Egyptian). "At first I taught all the classes," she says, "but I realized I was becoming a type A yogi, so I hired a staff." The center serves about 500 people, many for free. To make money, Kennedy teaches wellness techniques to corporate executives at company retreats. "My dad now suffers from Alzheimer's disease, but he still challenges me with his three questions," Kennedy says. "Finally, I'm in balance enough to answer."

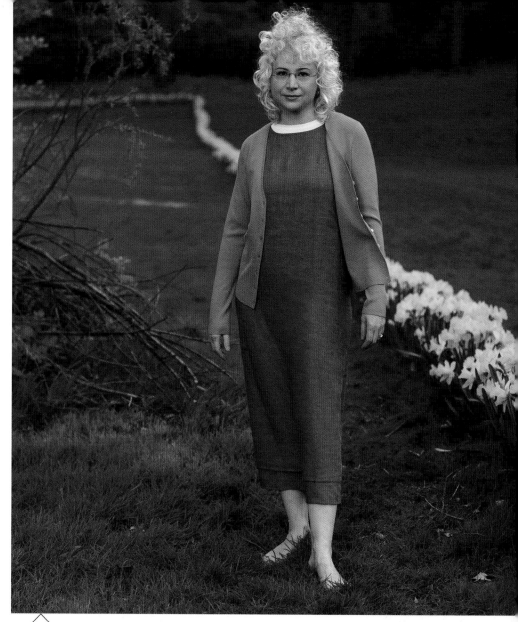

Susan Skarsgard

In the fall of 2003 Susan Skarsgard was worried about the state of the world. The 49-year-old General Motors designer and graduate student felt a sense of unease every time she heard about the war in Iraq, the larger Mideast situation, terrorism. She thought, *What could I do about any of it?*

As Skarsgard began preparing a thesis project for her MFA at the University of Michigan, she read about the security wall Israel is building in and around the West Bank. She had an idea to replicate that line for her project—in flowers at the University of Michigan's Nichols Arboretum.

"It's not about Israel specifically," she says, "but about how we as human beings impose a line on a natural place. How the place becomes different from what it was. And how the line can go away just as the Berlin Wall did."

Skarsgard's art has included print-making, calligraphy, and expressive lettering. She's never had to rely on anyone else to make her projects happen, but for *Imagine/Align*, she needed thousands of flowers, dozens of volunteers, and permission to dig a half-mile-long ditch in the arboretum.

The arboretum director eventually agreed to the project. A flower wholesaler offered 10,000 daffodil bulbs for $3,430. And in October 2003, more than 150 people showed up for eight days of planting. Daffodils are perennials; they bloom every spring, though they're affected by the elements and the care they receive—which means the line will change over time.

Skarsgard is still concerned about the state of the world, but now she has hope that people—friends, strangers, even enemies—will come together and create peaceful solutions. "I never thought I could make this happen," she said in April 2004. "But now the flowers are starting to bloom."

The GM designer and her half-mile line of daffodils in Ann Arbor, Michigan.

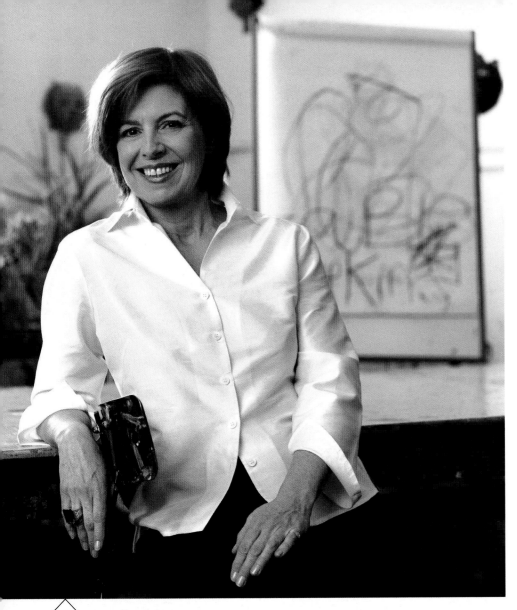

Gail Nathan

When artist Gail Nathan was a girl in the Bronx, the borough was full of tree-lined streets, small shops, and charming parks—one with the Bronx River curving through it. By the time Nathan was an adult, President Carter spoke of the devastation of the South Bronx. Like others, Nathan fled. She eventually settled in Virginia.

"As idyllic as my life in the South was," she says, "I knew I wouldn't stay forever." In 1998 Nathan fell in love with a Bronx-based artist and moved back to New York City. Their only problem was that she needed a job. The week Nathan unpacked, the Bronx River Art Center, which offers art and environmental programs to borough residents, advertised for an executive director. Even though she had no corporate financial experience, Nathan applied. "All I could tell the interview committee was that I'd never been in debt or bounced a check," she says.

She got the job and discovered the center's budget would challenge her penny-pinching abilities. To cheer herself up, Nathan went to a fancy boutique. In the linens department, she had a eureka moment: "Sachets!"

Nathan asked her staff and art students to photograph the Bronx River, which is a lot cleaner than many people imagine. They transferred the images onto fabric and filled the sachets with herbs from a Cape Cod distributor. (Volunteers now plant lavender, chamomile, and spearmint in the community garden on the banks of the river each spring; they use the harvest in the sachets.)

The center's product line—which has already expanded to include eye pillows—is available through its Web site (bronxriverart.org), and Nathan plans to expand to spas, salons, and specialty shops. She'll use the profits to employ residents; offer more classes in printmaking, ceramics, and environmental studies; and, as she says, "change the mind-set of anyone who still thinks the Bronx is a wasteland."

The Bronx River Art Center's executive director with a drawing by one of its teachers.

Linda Bruckheimer

Linda Bruckheimer moved from Kentucky to California when she was 15 years old. She adapted quickly: She became an art dealer and later married a big-shot movie and television producer. But she went back home at least once a year to visit her grandmother.

During one of those trips in 1993, she became enchanted by an antebellum house and its tiny, partially shuttered town, Bloomfield. Back in California, she had nightmarish flashes of super-stores and subdivisions gobbling up Bloomfield. Bruckheimer decided to buy the house—and eventually nine other nearby buildings (in various states of disrepair). She splits her time between Los Angeles and Bloomfield, and has restored a building that is now the Olde Bloomfield Meeting Hall and opened an antiques shop. Today several residents work in the new businesses operating in the renovated buildings.

Bruckheimer can't really explain why she has put so much time, effort, and money into bringing Bloomfield back to life, except that "fixing up" was a major pastime of her childhood. "At my grandmother's house on Honeysuckle Way, we were always planting flowers or vegetables and painting fences," she says. "We never even left the furniture in one place for long." (Her second novel, *The Southern Belles of Honeysuckle Way,* is dedicated to her grandmother, who died in 2002 at age 103.)

"My grandmother, like many women, had an innate need to take care of things," Bruckheimer says. "A lot of major historic sites—Mt. Vernon and the Alamo, for example—have been threatened by the bulldozer. It was always a woman or a group of women who saved them. I guess I'm just trying to do my share."

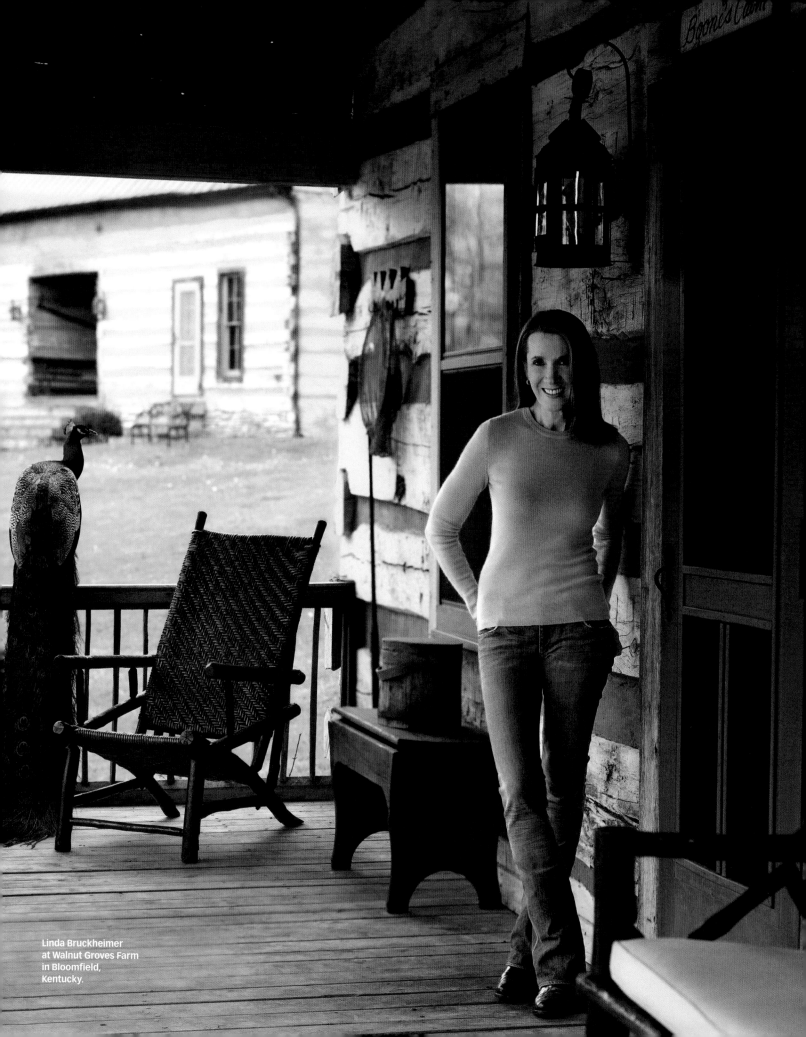

Linda Bruckheimer at Walnut Groves Farm in Bloomfield, Kentucky.

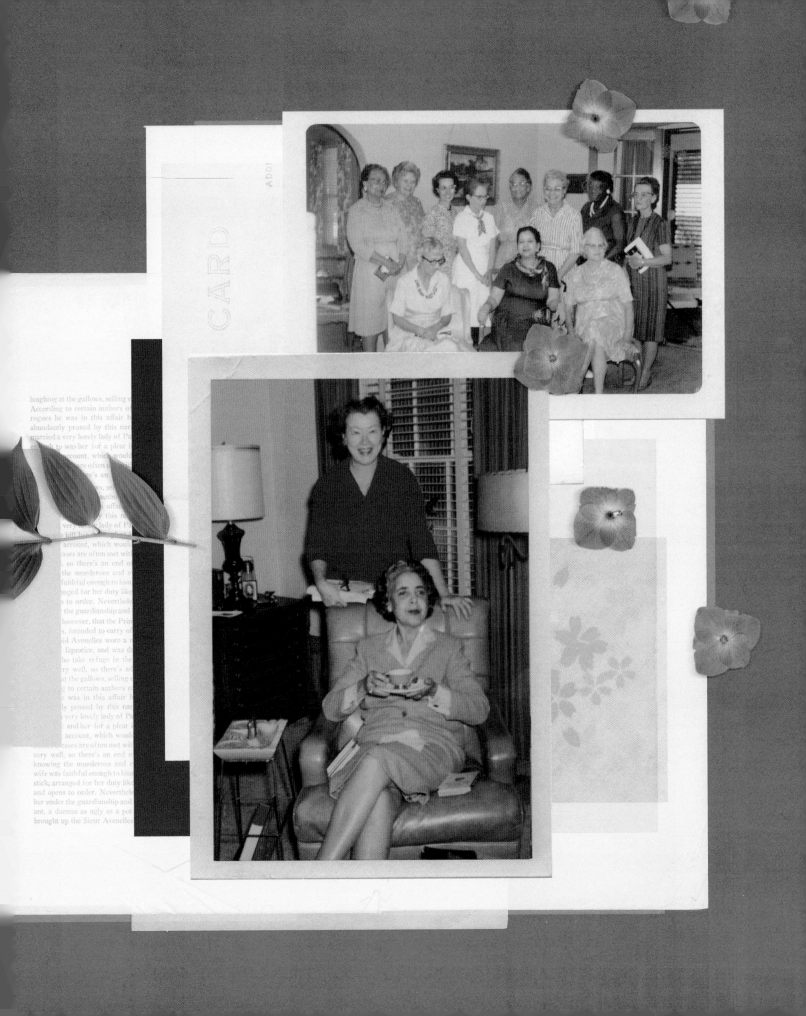

In a segregated city traumatized by a brutal, race-based riot, a group of women, black and white, got together for strong tea, lace cookies, and great books. Thirty-nine years later, their remarkable conversation is still going on. CLAUDIA KOLKER listens in.

The First Wednesday Reading Club

ONE-HUNDRED-YEAR-OLD JEANNE GOODWIN isn't answering my question. ● We're sitting in her airy Tulsa parlor, dotted with fresh flowers and stacks of books. A giant hydrangea fills the patio outside. I've come to ask Goodwin, who is black, about the interracial book club she helped found in 1964. For its time, First Wednesday Reading Club was revolutionary. Maybe equally remarkable, the group still meets faithfully today. ● "We historians tend to concentrate on big signpost events," Scott Ellsworth, a Tulsa-born race-relations scholar, has told me. "We study the Freedom Rides, the March on Washington. But the truth is that these women, talking books over cookies and tea, are just as much a part of that story." ● Goodwin, the club's sole surviving founding member, presides over her friends and family like a head of state.

Opposite page, top: An early gathering of First Wednesday Reading Club. *Back row, far right:* Norma Burkitt, one of the founders. *Bottom:* Members Jewel Markham (*standing*) and Jeanne Goodwin in the early sixties.

When she wants a fact, she dials a friend from memory on the phone poised on her lap. A former schoolteacher, she still polices her kin's grammar and reads insatiably. That big hydrangea? She grew it from a cutting when she was 96. Naturally I have questions for this vigorous woman. I am 39 years old, used to reading groups with all the social risk of a Cobb salad at the club. I'm fascinated by the brio it took to start an interracial reading group at a time when blacks and whites couldn't even eat together in a Tulsa restaurant.

"So what did First Wednesday Club teach you?" I ask Goodwin, leaning close.

She stares quizzically at me for half a second.

"It didn't teach me anything," she says.

I stare back. It will take another week, till the first Wednesday of the month, before I understand.

ON THE MORNING OF THE BOOK club, I take a taxi to the house of Hortense Johnson, a retired librarian. The middle-aged white driver asks what brings me to town.

"A book club?" he says doubtfully. "Because, you know—we're in a largely black part of town." There's no malice in his voice, just encrusted ignorance: residue of a lifetime in the confines of one race. In Tulsa, though, the words have special resonance. For 60 years here, polite segregation hid one of the worst incidents of racial violence in U.S. history.

In the 1900s Tulsa was a haven for blacks fleeing the South, according to local historian Eddie Faye Gates. So many blacks had found success here by 1921 that Tulsa's black neighborhood, Greenwood, was dubbed Black Wall Street. Underneath, though, postwar-America's demons were seething. In 1921 a black teenager was accused of trying to molest a white teenage girl (she later refused to press charges). White rioters attacked Greenwood, reducing Black Wall Street to rubble. Historians say between 100 and 300 people, mostly blacks, were killed. Eventually black Tulsans would rebuild their homes. But in white Tulsa the riot was barely spoken of again. Only in the 1990s did the tragedy and the question of reparations become a

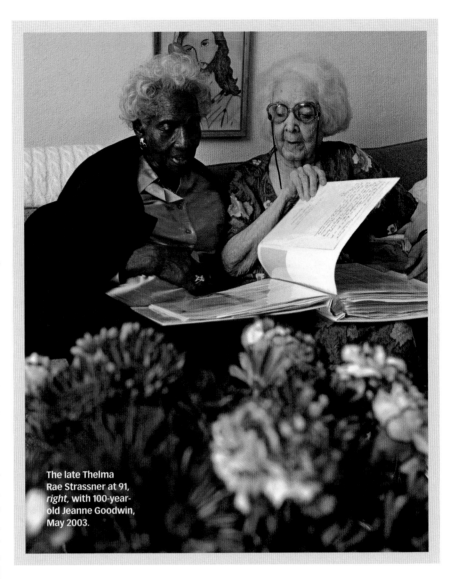

The late Thelma Rae Strassner at 91, *right*, with 100-year-old Jeanne Goodwin, May 2003.

public issue, one that is being intensively examined today. In 2003, a team of civil rights lawyers, including Johnnie Cochran, filed a class action lawsuit against Tulsa and the state of Oklahoma.

In 1964, in the depths of Tulsa's silence about Greenwood, a white YWCA president named Norma Burkitt envisioned the First Wednesday Reading Club. The public library had compiled a list of books on "human relations"—anthropology, sociology, psychology. Why not gather black and white women, Burkitt wondered, to discuss the texts.

"Social interaction between blacks and whites was zippo," Scott Ellsworth says. But this university town had a healthy population of women activists intent on living

differently. It was from this pool that Burkitt invited her first guests.

"I believe they wore hats," Burkitt's son, 78-year-old William Burkitt, recalls. "Meetings were always in somebody's house—one of their goals was seeing how each other lived. But from the very beginning it was a tea party. It was social."

They were educators, social workers, and librarians. And to a woman, they were booklovers—like white-haired Hortense Johnson, now opening her door for me.

INSIDE, THREE DOZEN WOMEN, mostly middle-aged or older, are finding seats. A white woman in an embroidered Guatemalan dress is wedged beside a black woman in a kente cloth jacket on a rose-colored couch; another black woman in a suit chats with a pale woman in a tailored blouse. On one side of the room, a table holds casseroles, green beans, lacy cookies, and domed biscuits.

Thirty-nine years after its founding, First Wednesday Reading Club has scarcely changed. With a membership of some 30 women, it is still about half black, half white. There are no bylaws, no required reading, no dues. Sometimes a club member reviews a book. Just as likely the group invites a guest speaker, like Clifton Taulbert, author of a series of books on pre-integration Mississippi, or the late great cook and caterer Cleora Butler, who finished writing her cookbook, *Cleora's Kitchens,* at the age of 84.

"I always said that after Cleora came, the reading club became the eating club," Jeanne Goodwin tells me dryly.

"Sit here!" my hostess, who is 93, whispers forcefully. She hauls a heavy chair my way.

Facing us are club member Florence Reed, a black woman with cropped hair, and her guest, Maribeth Spanier, who is white. Reed, it turns out, is a librarian beset by Crohn's disease and clinical anxiety. Spanier is the therapist who helps her navigate. Together they describe the process to the rapt audience.

"It's amazing how your mind can just go bonkers," Reed says. "Before my illness, if I faced a problem where race or ethnicity was an issue, I'd deal with it. Then suddenly you hear yourself saying, 'I'm supposed to take yoga, but black people don't take yoga!' Every morning when you look in the mirror, you see a roadblock. You try to see if it's a reality or a [mis]perception."

Spanier nods with empathy. A woman in a flowing muumuu lifts a hand. "I don't know you," she tells Spanier cordially, "but I would like to."

Anecdotes and questions drift through the rosy room. The mood is candid, casual yet decorous. When Hortense Johnson announces that it's time to eat, I grab my chance. I want to ask each woman the question Jeanne Goodwin eluded. I corner 79-year-old Erika Hill, a pink-cheeked Latvian-American in a girlish frock. When she first moved here in 1948, she tells me, her black housekeeper tried to come in through the back door. "'Don't do that!' I tell her," Hill says. "And my in-laws tell me not to say this." When I ask Hill what First Wednesday has meant to her, she just

They were educators, social workers, and librarians. And to a woman, they were booklovers.

waves. "Oh Lordy," she replies. "We are very human and we love each other."

Retired white social worker Talva Lacey nibbles a green bean. "It's just very loose. We enjoy each other," she suggests.

Catherine Nielsen, in the tailored blouse, finally offers me a clue. "There's a huge difference between the way we are now and the early days, when there was a much more intentional blending," she says. "In 1964 Tulsa was a very segregated city. But a small cadre of people moved toward integration."

First Wednesday members all belonged to that vanguard. Jeanne Goodwin was married to the publisher of Tulsa's black newspaper; her social circle included George Washington Carver and Martin Luther King Jr. Hortense Johnson mentored generations of black students. Jewel Hines, now 84, was a social worker who spent ten years in Liberia.

The women of the Tulsa reading club, I realize, already were pathbreakers. First Wednesday wasn't an experiment. It was a statement: a manifesting of the kind of world they chose to live in. "Maybe it's because we came out of a Tulsa that had a race riot," says Nielsen. "Those scars were there. The club was a very soft, gentle healing."

Modern Tulsa, while still cautious about race relations, is a far more open place. Its citizens discuss the Greenwood riot bluntly and don't need clubs to associate with whomever they want. Why then, I ask Nielsen, years after more structured clubs have faded, does First Wednesday live on?

Like the others, Nielsen fumbles for words. "There's just deep affection."

She sounds to me like club member Jeanne Goodwin declaring crisply that First Wednesday had not taught her a thing. Then I have a revelation.

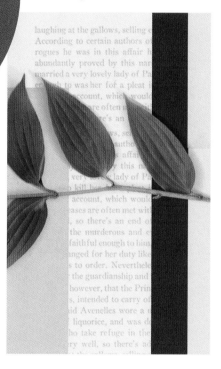

People flail for words, I think, when they're trying to express something profound. Try to summarize a sibling, or explain a marriage decades old. What is there to say? Even the most ritualized relationships, after a lifetime, become organic. Inexplicable. Deeper than a definition. I think of the hydrangea in Goodwin's yard. She'd grown it from a cutting, with intention. But at some point, when the stem poked out a branch, when the roots spread deep into a map, Goodwin must have let that slip alone to grow itself. It no longer was a project to be studied. It was, like a long friendship, simply a living thing. ●

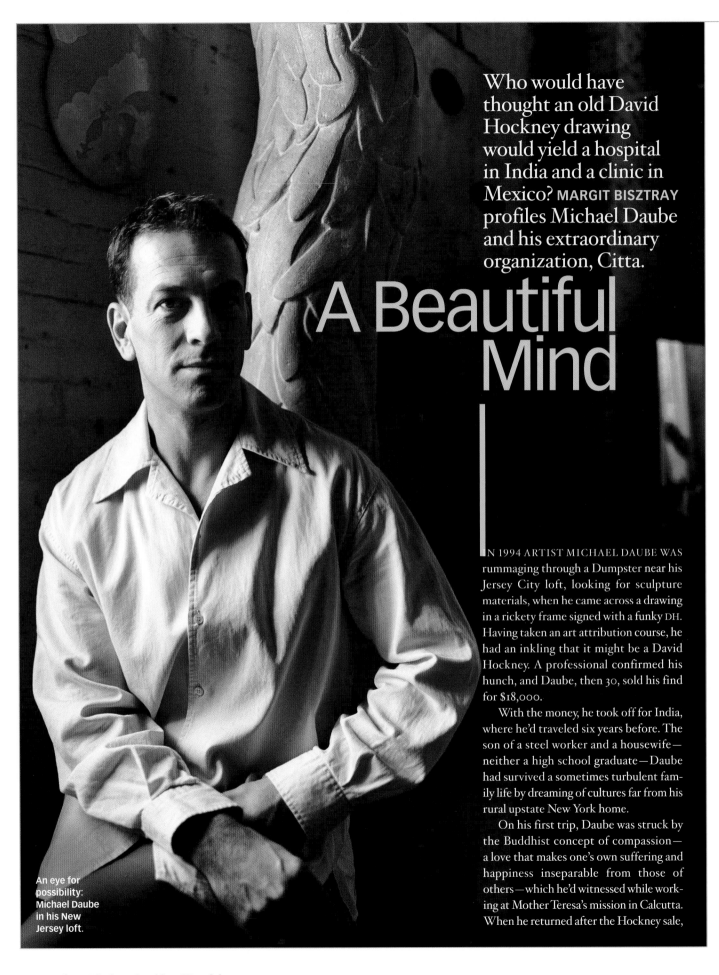

Who would have thought an old David Hockney drawing would yield a hospital in India and a clinic in Mexico? **MARGIT BISZTRAY** profiles Michael Daube and his extraordinary organization, Citta.

A Beautiful Mind

IN 1994 ARTIST MICHAEL DAUBE WAS rummaging through a Dumpster near his Jersey City loft, looking for sculpture materials, when he came across a drawing in a rickety frame signed with a funky DH. Having taken an art attribution course, he had an inkling that it might be a David Hockney. A professional confirmed his hunch, and Daube, then 30, sold his find for $18,000.

With the money, he took off for India, where he'd traveled six years before. The son of a steel worker and a housewife—neither a high school graduate—Daube had survived a sometimes turbulent family life by dreaming of cultures far from his rural upstate New York home.

On his first trip, Daube was struck by the Buddhist concept of compassion—a love that makes one's own suffering and happiness inseparable from those of others—which he'd witnessed while working at Mother Teresa's mission in Calcutta. When he returned after the Hockney sale,

An eye for possibility: Michael Daube in his New Jersey loft.

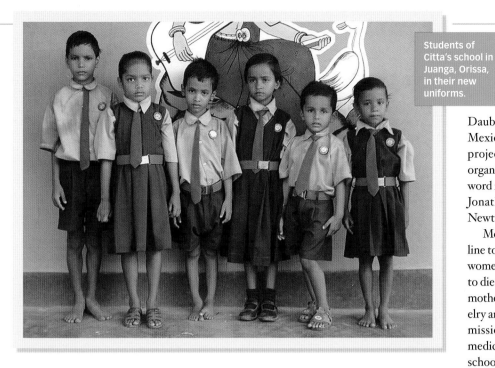

Students of Citta's school in Juanga, Orissa, in their new uniforms.

he went back to Mother Teresa and asked her how he might practice compassion $18,000 richer. She suggested opening a school in the country's poorest, most heavily tribal state, rural Orissa. Prone to floods and cyclones, it's an area about which even devoted aid workers ask, "Why would you go there?"

Daube soon found out what they were talking about. "In Orissa, people with extremely sick babies approached me begging for any kind of medicine, even aspirin," he says. "I saw a man in a basket hanging from bamboo poles held by two skinny men who intended to carry him

more than 18 miles through mud to the nearest hospital. Instead of building a school, I began to build a hospital."

It quickly became clear that Daube would need more money to complete the project, so he returned to New York in search of work. In a stroke of good fortune, a friend introduced him to musician David Byrne and artist Adelle Lutz, who ended up giving him odd jobs. ("They knew I could help with art projects as well as fix a fence," says Daube.) Over the next two years, he would work for Byrne and Lutz until he'd saved enough money, then travel back to Orissa to add a floor or roof to the hospi-

tal. In 1995 Byrne performed a concert to raise funds for a clinic he and his assistant convinced Daube to help them build, in Chiapas, Mexico, to serve the Mayans. With both projects to manage, Daube formed an organization he named Citta, the Sanskrit word meaning "mind-heart"; soon director Jonathan Demme and actress Thandie Newton lent their support.

Most recently, Citta has thrown a lifeline to the poorest regions of Nepal, where women used to leave newborns in the snow to die rather than watch them starve. Now mothers support their families making jewelry and doing bead- and needlework commissioned by New York designers. More medical centers, as well as orphanages and schools, may follow. "After we are involved in a region, it usually becomes apparent what else is needed," says Daube. "Our approach is holistic. There is never just one aspect that allows a community to emerge from poverty."

These days Daube is on the road most of the time, but he's become the unofficial big brother to Babu, an 8-year-old Orissa boy. Abandoned in a temple as a child, Babu now hangs out at the Citta hospital in Orissa, which serves 60,000 people, and he's learning to read at the newly completed school. From that original discovery of the Hockney, Daube has opened up an entire world of beauty and possibility. ●

The Show Goes On

"DID WE MISS THE TURN?"

It's easy to lose your bearings in this part of South Dakota. Road straight as a slide rule; flat, parched prairie; no scenery to hang the eye on. Only sky, and the occasional tourist sign. YOU ARE ALMOST EAR! reads one for the Corn Palace.

"Did we miss the turn?" Arlowene Sandau again asks her husband, Ed, an hour after leaving home in Sioux Falls. With their 19-year-old daughter, Briannan, they're driving west toward the Yankton Sioux reservation, ribbing each other over the prospect of getting lost. At the same time, Mitchell Newman and Carl

Erika Schneider— a winner of *O*'s Big-Dream contest— starts a theater on a troubled South Dakota Indian reservation that unites generations, changes lives, and brings down the house. LIZ BRODY reports.

Occhipinti, both from Chicago, are heading up to the reservation from Omaha in a rental car. All five, and several others, have responded to *O*'s call for connections that could help one of our Big-Dream contest winners, Erika Schneider, a six-foot-one, 32-year-old blonde who lives on the reservation with Sherwyn Zephier, the son of a chief. Schneider hopes to start a community theater—an ambitious project for an area where few people have seen a play, much less acted in one.

And things have been a little tense. Her first show, *Tunkasina, We Are All Related*, opens in a week, and she's short a few

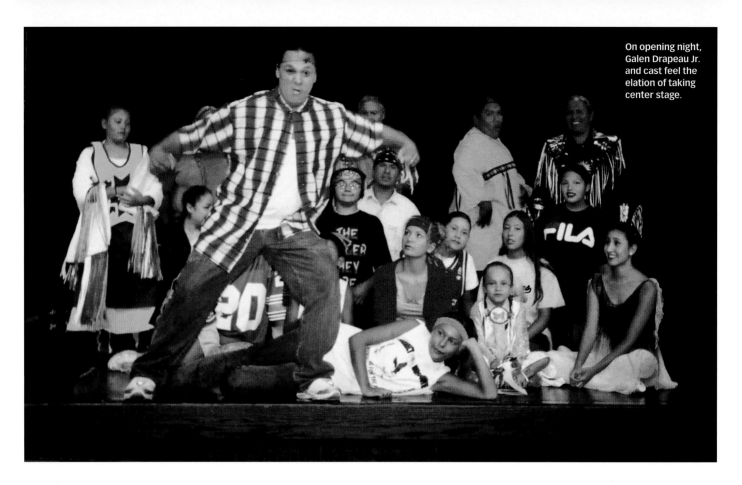

basics—like mikes and lights and actors who know their lines. Thankfully, Newman, the artistic director of Thirsty Theater, and Occhipinti, a veteran theater director, are here to help coach the cast. And the Sandaus, who own A&E Sound & Lighting, have dropped everything to lug in equipment and operate it for the week. No matter what, Schneider insists, the show will go on.

THE YANKTON SIOUX RESERVA-tion, about 40,000 acres of tribal lands, is a place where the buffalo roam, along with Crips, Bloods, drugs, and alcohol. The town of Marty, one of several on the res, is a despairing clump of government housing, broken down and boarded up—feeble protection against the 20-below winters. The Marty Indian School, however, has offered an unused detention hall as a theater. And days of clearing, cleaning, and painting have turned the room into a respectable stage, especially after donated curtains and scenery arrived from Scenic View, of Chicago, through a Big-Dream connection to the League of Chicago Theatres. "This is one of the first arts projects in our area that involves the white and Native Ameri-

can communities working together," says Schneider. "And that is a big step here." The tensions between the two groups along the reservation's borders have led to an uneasy segregation.

A FEW DAYS BEFORE OPENING night, two girls in the cast, from different gangs, are edging for a fight. "Didn't you read the script?" Schneider asks them. The play is about a Native American gang leader who discovers that the spiritual wisdom of his ancestors offers a more fulfilling path than the violent ways of his partying homies. The theme was welcomed by tribal elders, who have been grappling with how to shake the community out of its lethargy. Elder Henry Selwyn, a man of solemn words, whose 17 children include a gang leader ("He's sitting today someplace he should not be"), has witnessed the slow drip of apathy that has numbed the young to the vibrancy of their own culture. "The play's healing words are medicine to our ears," he says with some hope. "People are coming alive."

In fact, by opening night the two gang members are joking. The lights and sound are working on cue. As the audience files

in, backstage the cast forms a circle and the play's lead, Galen Drapeau Jr., a tribal spiritual leader, breaks into a piercing Dakota prayer song. The whole group joins in. The fierce pull of thousands of years of tradition yanks away any bothersome stomach butterflies. Charged and centered, the actors walk out to the stage, and Morning Star Community Theatre is born.

As the three-night run proceeds, more Big-Dream connections secure the theater's future. Steven and Cindy Noble, who own Flood Music in Sioux Falls, donate a soundboard; TMG, an electronics store, offers spotlights. And other futures take hold: Julia Marshall, 20, a cast member who'd dropped out of high school, decides to go back. Being in the play inspired her to "get involved again," she says. "I'd like to study drama at college."

Everyone is fired up. After the last show, Drapeau bounds over to Schneider. "I want to do it again," he shouts. "Here, at other Indian schools, anywhere!" Exhausted, Schneider and Zephier pick up costumes. "It started out as our dream," she says, beaming. "Now it's their dream." ●

O

Giving Back

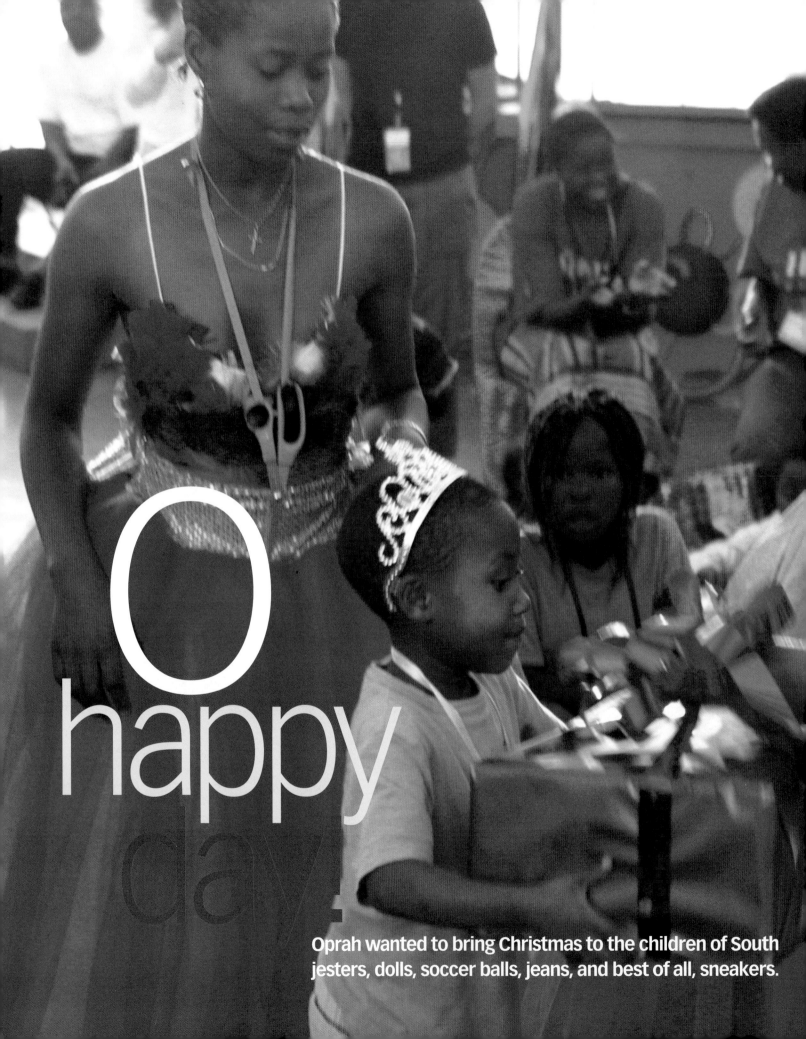

O
happy
day

Oprah wanted to bring Christmas to the children of South
jesters, dolls, soccer balls, jeans, and best of all, sneakers.

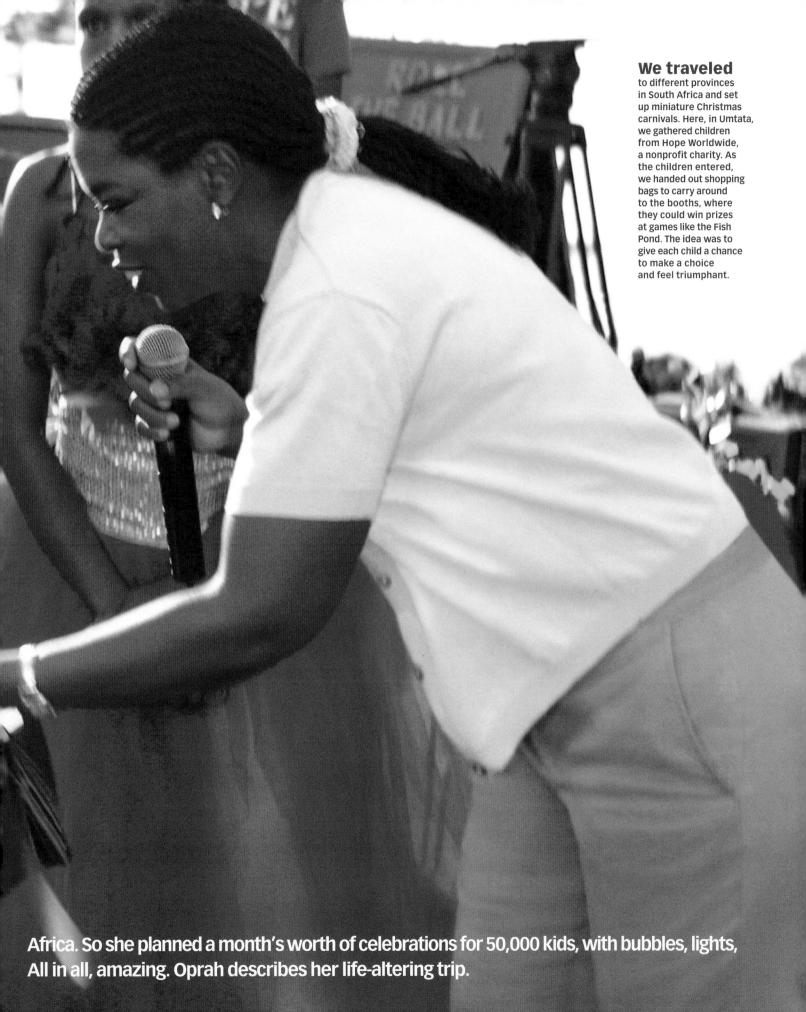

Africa. So she planned a month's worth of celebrations for 50,000 kids, with bubbles, lights,
All in all, amazing. Oprah describes her life-altering trip.

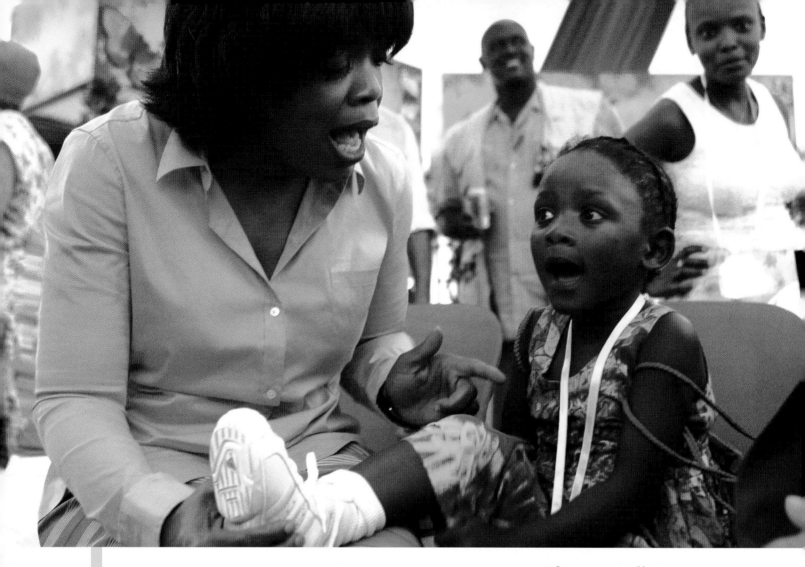

I'LL NEVER FORGET THE YEAR I was 12 and living with my mother in Milwaukee. We were on welfare, and a few days before December 25, she announced to me and my half-brother and half-sister that we wouldn't be receiving Christmas gifts. My sadness wasn't so much about not having toys as it was about facing my classmates. What would I say when the other kids asked what I'd gotten? That Christmas, three nuns showed up at our house with a doll, fruit, and games for us. I felt such a sense of relief that I'd been given something. That I wasn't forgotten. That somebody had thought enough of me to bring me a gift.

For Christmas 2002, as a gift to myself, I wanted to create that same feeling for someone else. My intention was to do for the South African children what those nuns had done for me. I wasn't trying to eradicate AIDS, end poverty, or stimulate economic development. I simply wanted to create one day that the kids could remember as happy.

All we ever hear about African children is how hungry they are, how poor they are, how sick they are. The worst thing about being poor, as I recall, is that it makes you feel abnormal. I've always encouraged giving. Using your life. Teaching what you learn. Extending yourself in the form of service. So I put the challenge to myself: Using the abundance I've been blessed with, what could I offer that would be meaningful to someone else? I wanted to reach a million children in South Africa; time allowed for only 50,000.

I put together a team made up of the Oprah Winfrey Foundation, staff members, and friends. I then partnered with the Nelson Mandela Foundation, and I talked with orphanage caretakers about gifts that would be culturally acceptable. I was told that none of these children had ever seen a black doll—most were dragging around blonde, naked Barbies. Wouldn't it be a wonder if each girl could see herself in the eyes of a doll that looked like her? It became my passion

There wasn't a kid there who didn't think she wore a shoe size smaller than she did. Most had never had their feet measured. They were so used to tight shoes that when you gave them a pair that fit, they'd think it was too big. After we measured one little girl for sneakers, she came up to me and said, "Ma'am, can I keep the shoes?"

and mission to give a black doll to every girl I met.

The most exciting part of planning the trip was choosing the dolls and all the other presents. At one point, I got a little thrill out of seeing 127 sample dolls filling my office! After I'd picked the one I would have wanted when I was a girl, I called up the manufacturer and asked that its barely brown dolls be double-dipped to darken them. We chose soccer balls for the boys, solar-powered radios for the teens, and jeans and T-shirts for everyone. And I wanted every child to receive a pair of sneakers. In South Africa, where many of the children walk around barefoot in the blistering sun, shoes are gold.

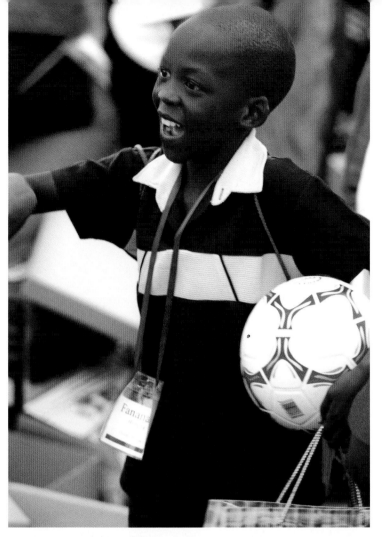

The joy
wasn't just
about toys. It was
the feeling: *Somebody
thought of me. I matter.
I wasn't forgotten.*

I loved choosing the presents for the children. I spoke with Nelson Mandela about gifts that would be culturally relevant, and I learned that soccer is one of South Africa's most popular sports—so I spent days searching for the perfect soccer ball.

At first the kids seemed to have no idea what the word *fun* means. I'd say, "I came from America to see you because I heard stories about how brave you are, and I wanted you to know that people in America love you. I wanted you to have one happy day that you could remember—so this is for you to have *fun!*" They'd just stare at me, even after I repeated the word in their language. But once the kids opened the presents, they definitely got it. I'd say, "Wasn't that fun?" and they'd say, "Yes!"

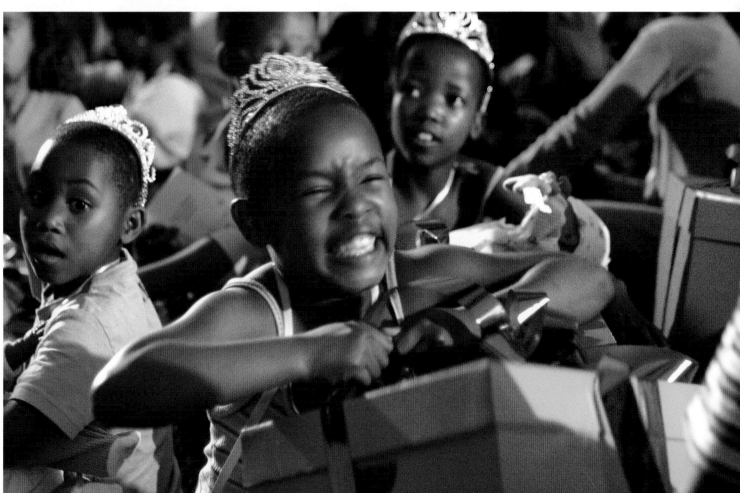

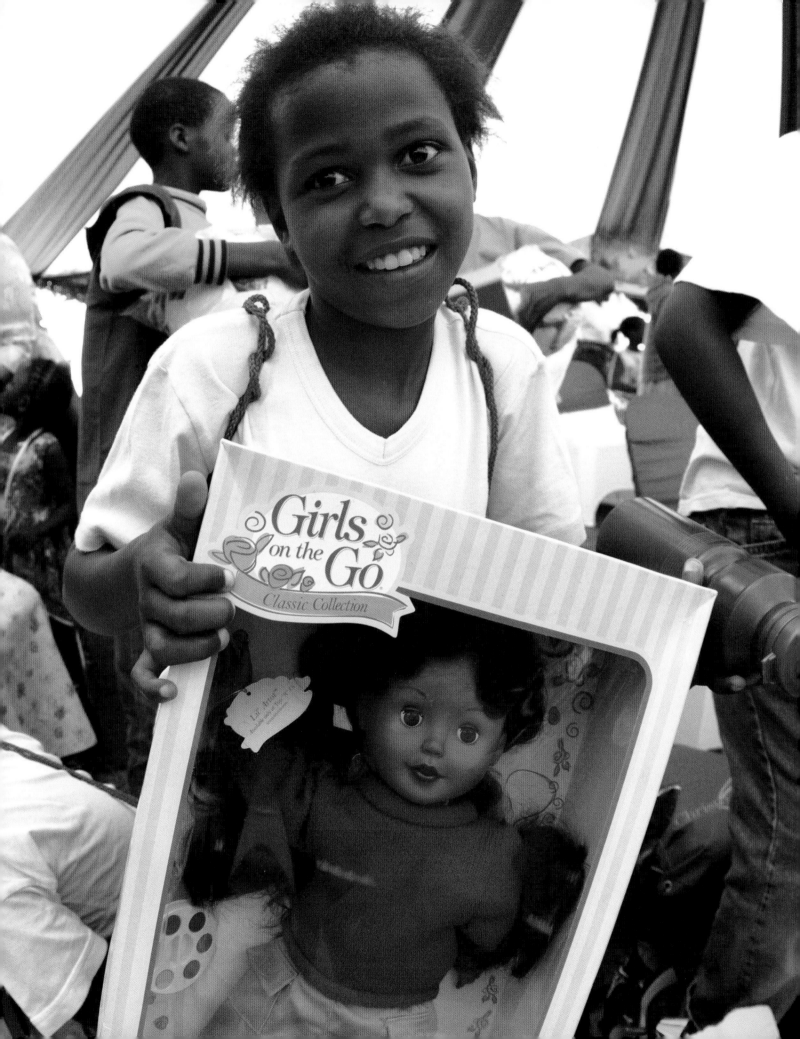

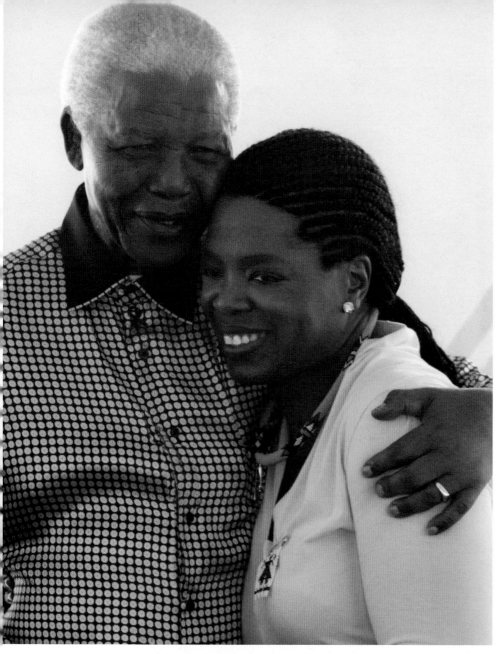

Nelson Mandela made me feel strengthened, deepened, broadened, and more loving and forgiving.

❮ **During my** time in South Africa, I shared 29 meals with my strongest living mentor—Nelson Mandela. With every story of courage he shared, I'd think, *How did this happen to me—how did I get the chance to sit and talk with Nelson Mandela? Absolutely unbelievable!*

∨ **My idea** is to bring hope to South Africa, because where there is no hope, there is no vision—and where there is no vision, the people perish. I believe that the only way to make a lasting change is through education, so that people can better themselves. In rural Umtata, thousands of school children lined up to receive gifts, just miles from where Mandela grew up. Two weeks earlier, Mandela and I broke ground on a school to open in January 2005 in Johannesburg—the Oprah Winfrey Leadership Academy for Girls South Africa. One teenage girl said at the groundbreaking, "Men have always ruled the world, but this is all over now because we girls are coming, and believe me, we are coming in a storm! Who knows, maybe one of us can find a cure for this disease that is killing us. To my sisters, I say, 'Let's please try for the best!'"

❮ **Most of** the girls had never seen dolls that look anything like them. You should have seen the expressions on their faces when they tore off the wrapping paper to find black dolls.

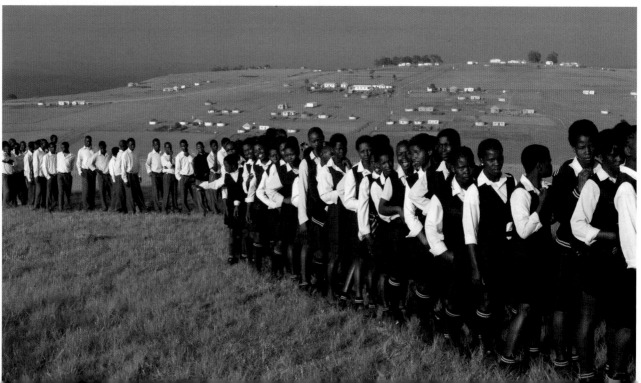

what one person–you–can do

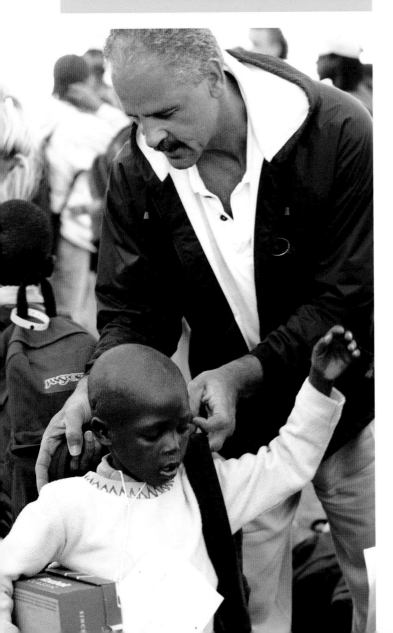

◁ In this shot, Stedman is helping a boy strap on his backpack full of gifts. As much as the children enjoyed receiving toys, many seemed more excited about the sneakers and the clothes. That's because clothing makes you feel like you belong to the rest of the world.

My first stop was in Johannesburg, where I met a group of orphans. There and in the villages I visited every day of the three weeks after that, the staff from my show created carnivals and parties for the children, who'd traveled from miles around. The kids were simply told that they were coming to a party, and many had borrowed shoes just to get there. One girl had lost her mother the day before and was coaxed to come only by the promise of riding in a car for the first time. As the kids entered, I could see their eyes light up and their sorrows and burdens fall away while they took in the wonder—jesters, fairies in lavender tulle, and silver bubbles floating everywhere. I have no words to describe the looks on their faces when I announced, "Everybody can open their presents at the count of three!" One girl who couldn't get the wrapper off her doll fast enough began kissing its face through the plastic! Yet the joy wasn't just about toys. It was the same feeling I'd had when the nuns came to my house so many years ago: *Somebody thought of me. I matter. I wasn't forgotten.* In that moment in Johannesburg, I thanked God that I was born to see this—to touch, hear, and feel that kind of happiness. In every village we visited, that joy just came from someplace above and below the ground and completely filled me. It was the single greatest experience of my lifetime.

Before my trip, I was shut down about the AIDS story in Africa. Like you, I'd heard the numbers—millions of children homeless, one in three people ravaged by the disease in some countries—but I was numb to what those figures represented. The statistics had just stopped registering for me—until I met a 14-year-old who'd lost her mother to AIDS and I followed her back to the shack where she and her 8-year-old sister are prey to a drunken uncle. Until I held up the head of a 10-year-old girl who'd been raped so many times while fetching water for her blind grandmother that when she finally arrived in the safety of an orphanage her only request of the caretaker was "Please, ma'am, don't make me fetch water." Until I measured the feet of a boy who insisted he wore shoes three sizes smaller than he did because he hadn't been fitted for a pair in years.

"Our society has failed," Heather Reynolds, a nurse who started an orphanage called God's Golden Acre outside Durban, told me. "We've landed a man on the moon, we've got every technology—yet children are starving around the world. What sort of society are we?" I walked away from my conversation with Heather feeling a profound sense of resolve to do even more—beginning with a pledge I've made to feed a village of South Africans for a year.

Toward the end of my trip, I received a gift from a 12-year-old that far surpasses any I gave. "Mother Oprah," her letter began, "thank you for making me feel normal—for giving me self-esteem and my humanity. I am convinced that God provides." It was as if she was saying what I'd felt that Christmas so many years ago: *Thank you for acknowledging that I exist. Thank you for not forgetting me.* I've always believed that when you give, you get a whole lot back—that life is sweeter when you share what you have. In South Africa that Christmas, my life was sweetened 50,000 times over. ●

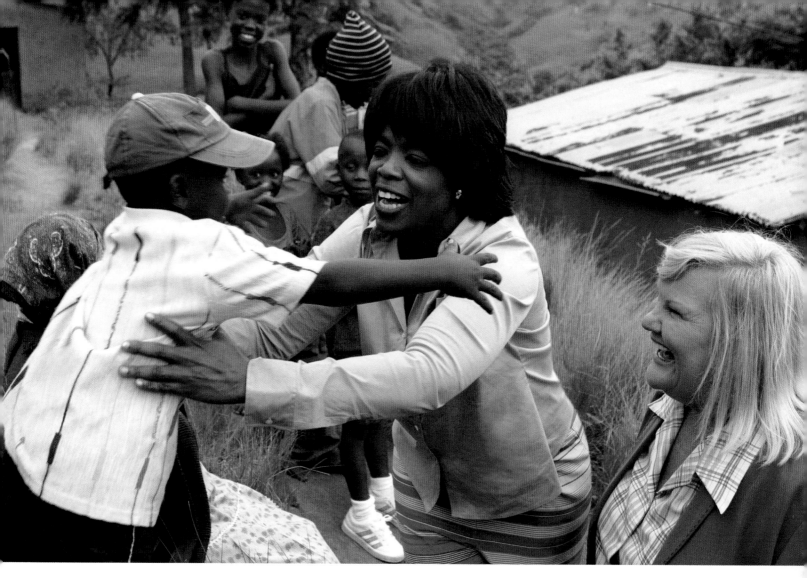

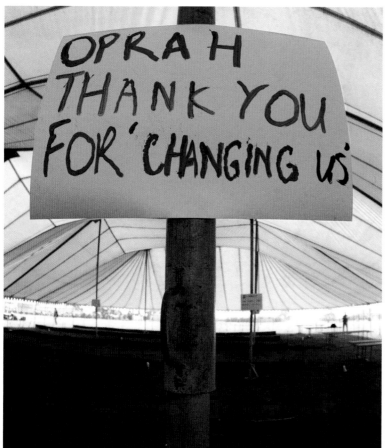

∧**There wasn't** a child I met whose life wasn't touched by the HIV/AIDS crisis—either through losing parents or being born with the virus. Because of a myth that has spread throughout the country that the cure for HIV/AIDS is to have intercourse with a virgin, hundreds of children have been sexually violated, even as babies. Here, Heather Reynolds, a nurse who began an orphanage called God's Golden Acre near Durban, introduces me to some of her beloved children.

<**Teachers and** children at a school near Durban gave me a warm send-off—a gift far greater than any I could have given myself. Before I visited the children of South Africa, I didn't even know the kind of joy I felt there even existed.

I thanked God that I was born to see this—to touch, hear, and feel that kind of happiness.

OPRAH TALKS TO BARACK OBAMA

The riveting young Illinois state senator who brought the house down at the 2004 Democratic National Convention (people are still talking about him) takes a rare break from his 16-hour workday to tell Oprah about his multicultural upbringing, his political plans and priorities (are we talking White House?), the saving grace of his wife and daughters—and what all Americans can do about today's "empathy deficit."

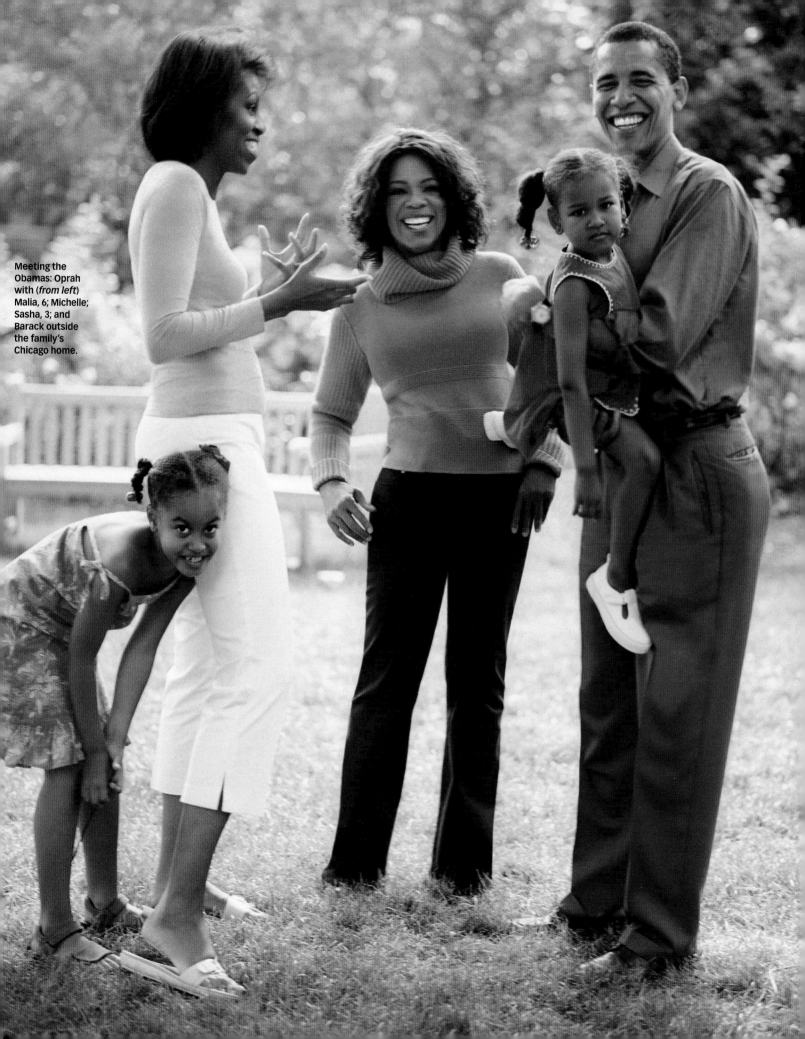

Meeting the Obamas: Oprah with (*from left*) Malia, 6; Michelle; Sasha, 3; and Barack outside the family's Chicago home.

IT'S A SPEECH I'LL NEVER FORGET: Barack Obama, the Illinois state senator from Chicago, addressing the nation at the 2004 Democratic National Convention. "I stand here knowing that my story is part of the larger American story, that I owe a debt to all of those who came before me, and that in no other country on earth is my story even possible," he said with a fervor that could be felt through the airwaves. "Tonight we gather to affirm the greatness of our nation, not because of the height of our skyscrapers or the power of our military or the size of our economy," he continued. "Our pride is based on a very simple premise, summed up in a declaration made over 200 years ago: 'We hold these truths to be self-evident, that all men are created equal.'"

The man whose name means "blessed" in Arabic is the son of a Kenyan father, Barack Obama Sr., and a white mother, Ann Dunham, from Kansas. The two met as college students in Hawaii in 1959 (Barack Sr. was the first African to enroll at the University of Hawaii), and two years later, when Ann was just 19, their child was born. At the time, miscegenation was still a crime in many states, and it was also unwelcome in Kenya. Under that pressure, Barack Sr. left the marriage when his son was just 2 years old and went to Harvard to pursue a PhD. Later, after he had returned to Kenya to work as an economist, Ann married an Indonesian man, and when Barack was 6, the family moved to a town outside Jakarta, where Maya, Barack's sister, was born. After four years, the family returned to Hawaii and Barack began corresponding with his father and trying to understand his African heritage. His father's death in a traffic accident in Nairobi in 1982 prompted Barack to travel to Kenya and meet the rest of his family for the first time.

Following his graduation from Columbia University, Barack attended Harvard Law School and became the first African-American president of its law review. In 1992 he married Michelle Robinson, also a Harvard-educated lawyer. The couple has two daughters: Malia, 6, and Sasha, 3.

Barack's autobiography, *Dreams from My Father: A Story of Race and Inheritance,* was

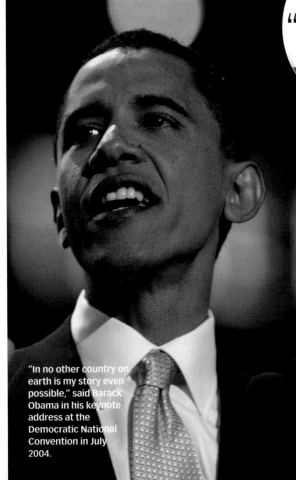

"In no other country on earth is my story even possible," said Barack Obama in his keynote address at the Democratic National Convention in July 2004.

published in 1995, when he was 33. The following year, he won a seat in the Illinois state senate, representing Chicago's poverty-stricken South Side. Still, Obama wasn't exactly a household name when he stepped into the race for the U.S. Senate last year. But then he won the primary with 53 percent of the vote and captured the attention of John Kerry, which landed him on the world stage for one of the most extraordinary speeches I've ever heard.

OPRAH: *There's a line in* The Autobiography of Miss Jane Pittman *[a 1974 TV movie based on Ernest J.*

Gaines's novel] when Jane is holding a baby and asking, "Will you be the One?" While you were speaking, I was alone in my sitting room cheering and saying, "I think this is the One."

BARACK: That's so nice. I think I'm one of the ones. I fight against the notion that blacks can have only one leader at a time. We're caught in that messiah mentality. As a consequence, a competition is set up. Who's the leader of the Korean-American community or the Irish-American community? The reason we don't know the answer is that they've got a collective leadership—people contributing in business, culture, politics. That's the model I want to encourage. I want to be part of many voices that help the entire country rise up.

OPRAH: *How do you define yourself as a leader?*

BARACK: Though I'm clearly a political leader now, I didn't start as one. I was skeptical of electoral politics. I thought it was corrupting, and that real change would happen in the grass roots. I came to Chicago [after college graduation] to work with churches organizing job-training programs. I thought the way to have an impact was through changing people's hearts and minds, not through some government

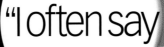

"I often say we've got a budget deficit that's

program. So I did that for three and a half years, went to law school to become a civil rights attorney, then wrote a book.

OPRAH: *You were so young when you wrote* Dreams from My Father. *Why did you decide to write a memoir at 33?*

BARACK: I had the opportunity. When I was elected president of the *Harvard Law Review,* people were willing to give me money to write. That's a huge luxury. I thought I had something interesting to say about how our cultures collide as the world shrinks. My family's story captures some of the tensions and evolution and cross-currents of race, both in this country and around the globe. One of the contributions I thought I could make was to show how I came to terms with these divergent cultures—and that would speak to how we all can live together, finding shared values and common stories. Writing the book was a great exercise for me because it solidified

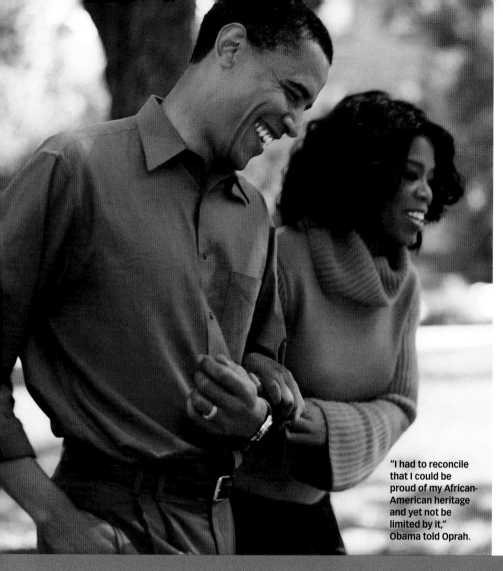

"I had to reconcile that I could be proud of my African-American heritage and yet not be limited by it," Obama told Oprah.

and yet not reject the love and values given to me by my mother and her parents. I had to reconcile that I could be proud of my African-American heritage and yet not be limited by it.

OPRAH: *That's now my favorite Barack Obama quote! There's another line you delivered in your speech at the convention that still resonates with me: "Children can't achieve unless we raise their expectations and turn off the television sets and eradicate the slander that says a black youth with a book is acting white." I stood up and cheered when you said that.*

BARACK: That's something I went through personally. Bill Cosby got into trouble when he said some of these things, and he has a right to say things in ways that I'm not going to because he's an older man. But I completely agree with his underlying premise: We have to change attitudes. There's a strain of anti-intellectualism running in our community that we have to eliminate. I'm young enough to understand where that opposition culture, that rebellion against achievement, comes from.

OPRAH: *Where does it comes from?*

BARACK: Fear—at least for me and a lot of young African-Americans. There's a sense in which we feel that the only way to assert

important, but what I worry about most is our empathy deficit."

where I'd been and set the stage for where I was going.

OPRAH: *When did you first realize that you were a little black kid? Was it the incident you wrote about, in the seventh grade, when someone called you "coon"?*

BARACK: Because I grew up in Hawaii and then lived in Indonesia for a while, I understood my affiliation to Africa and black people from an early age, but only in positive terms. I became aware of the cesspool of stereotypes when I was 8 or 9. I saw a story in *Life* magazine about people who were using skin bleach to make themselves white. I was really disturbed by that. Why would somebody want to do that? My mother had always complimented me: "You have such pretty brown skin."

OPRAH: *In the book, you eloquently describe what it's like to be out playing basketball and talking about "white folks," then coming home to the white folks you lived with—the people*

who loved and cared for you. That must have been confusing.

BARACK: It was. One of the things I fell prey to during my teen years was this need to separate myself from my parents and grandparents and take on this macho African-American image of a basketball player talking trash. The other day, somebody asked me, "Why do you think you ended up embracing all the stereotypes? You tried pot, coke." Back in the seventies, we had Shaft and Superfly or Flip Wilson and Geraldine. If you had to choose between those, it was pretty clear which direction you'd go. But you're right: As a teen, I had this divided identity—one inside the home, one for the outside world. It wasn't until I got to college that I started realizing that was fundamentally dishonest. I knew there had to be a different way for me to understand myself as a black man

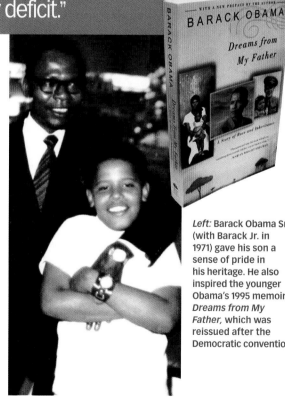

Left: Barack Obama Sr. (with Barack Jr. in 1971) gave his son a sense of pride in his heritage. He also inspired the younger Obama's 1995 memoir, *Dreams from My Father,* which was reissued after the Democratic convention.

strength is to push away from a society that says we're not as good. It's like: Instead of trying to compete, I'm going to have my own thing, and my own thing may be the streets or rap music.

OPRAH: *Do you think we've lost the belief that we can succeed? I was talking with Skip Gates [Henry Louis Gates, scholar of African-American history and culture], and he was saying how ironic it is that our parents believed that their little nappy-headed boys and girls could grow up and be somebody if they worked twice as hard.*

BARACK: We no longer operate that way, but we should be working twice as hard, because we still have challenges and barriers other communities don't have.

OPRAH: *Let's go to the night of the Democratic convention. How were you chosen to deliver the keynote speech?*

BARACK: We won our primary in a way that shocked people. In a seven-person field, we got 53 percent of the vote. People's assumption had been that if I won, I'd get 90 percent of the black vote, then maybe a little of the liberal white vote. We did win the black vote by 90 percent, but we also won the white vote—both on Chicago's South Side and up north. That created a sense of hopefulness among Democrats. I debunked this notion that whites won't vote for blacks. Or suburbanites won't vote for city people. Or downstate Illinois won't vote for upstate Illinois. That was the bedrock of my campaign: People may look different, talk different, and live in different places, but they've got some core values that they all care about and they all believe in. If you can speak to those values, people will respond—even if you have a funny name.

OPRAH: *When I was working at a news station in Baltimore, the manager wanted me to change my name to Suzie. He said, "Nobody will ever remember Oprah."*

BARACK: I was told, "People will remember your name and won't like it." You can have one African name, but not two. You can be Barack Smith or Joe Obama—but not Barack Obama.

OPRAH: *I loved reading where you said, "People don't know whether it's Osama or Yo' Mama."*

BARACK: Alabama, Bahama, or Barama.

OPRAH: *I think the name is working for you now.*

BARACK: Absolutely. Yours turned out okay for you, too. So anyway, John Kerry came to town for an event a few weeks after the primary. He and Teresa and I were all sitting at the same table, and I gave a speech before he did—and I can talk pretty good! [*He and Oprah laugh.*]

OPRAH: *When did you know that about yourself? I've known since I was 3, when I was speaking in church.*

BARACK: I didn't grow up in a setting where I had a lot of formal training, but I always knew I could express myself. I knew I could win some arguments. I knew I could get my grandparents and mom frustrated! Anyway, because of the five-minute speech I gave at the Kerry event, he thought it would be good for me to speak at the

> I want to make real the American ideal that every child in this country has a shot at life.

convention, but I didn't know in what capacity. About two weeks before the convention, I was asked to give the keynote address.

OPRAH: *I remember the first time I got called to do* The Tonight Show. *I was like, "My God—Johnny Carson!" We were jumping on the tables. The convention was your Johnny Carson moment. Did you dance a little hula?*

BARACK: I said, "This will be big."

OPRAH: *Did you start thinking about what you'd say?*

BARACK: The best move I made was to begin writing the speech that night. After I'd scribbled some notes, I wrote it in about three nights and sent it to the Kerry staff.

OPRAH: *It was really smart to write it when it was flowing and hot.*

BARACK: Exactly. By the time the speech had been edited for length, I was no longer particularly nervous. I was just making sure I didn't get up on the podium, open my mouth, and have nothing come out.

OPRAH: *Did you rehearse?*

BARACK: It turned out that there was a mock podium backstage where I could practice. I'd never used a teleprompter before.

OPRAH: *No? Get out!*

BARACK: I usually speak extemporaneously.

OPRAH: *Well, the speech was perfection.*

BARACK: I appreciate that.

OPRAH [to Barack's wife, Michelle]: *Were you nervous for him?*

MICHELLE: We're pretty low-key, but I was on the edge of my seat. He's a terrific speaker; he delivers in so many high-pressure moments. My question was: Will he really knock it out of the park? When he walked out onstage, all those OBAMA signs went up, and we just felt the energy of people being with us. That's when I was like, "Yes, he's going to do this."

OPRAH: *You could feel it. Barack, during the speech, there was a moment when you locked in and got your rhythm. I said, "He's gone!"*

BARACK: And it's in that moment that you know it's not just about you. It's about the audience and their energy and their story being told through you. The news coverage was very flattering. But the best sign came when we were walking down the street in Boston and the hotel doormen and the cops and the bus drivers were saying, "Good speech."

OPRAH: *That's when you know you hit the ball out of the park and it's still flying.*

BARACK: It's when you know you've gone beyond the political insiders.

MICHELLE: And that obligatory "You did a good job."

BARACK: When we came back, we went on a downstate RV tour—39 cities, five days.

MICHELLE: With the kids.

OPRAH: *Isn't politics fun?*

BARACK: Even in conservative Republican counties, 1,200 people would just show up at 9 on a Sunday morning.

OPRAH: *Did that response solidify your message?*

BARACK: It confirms the instincts that got me into politics. I believe the American people are decent people. They get confused sometimes because they get bad information or they're just busy and stressed and not paying attention. But when you sit down and talk with them, you're struck by how tolerant and loving they are.

OPRAH: *Most people honestly want to do as well as they can in their lives.*

BARACK: Exactly. They've got their struggles and heartaches, but they're basically good.

OPRAH: *What do you want to do with your politics?*

BARACK: Two things. I want to make real the American ideal that every child in this country has a shot at life. Right now that's not true in the aggregate. Of course, lightning can strike, and someone like you or me can do well. But so many kids have the odds stacked so high against them. The odds don't have to be that high. We can be sure that they start off with health insurance, that they have early childhood education, that they have a roof over their heads, and that they have good teachers. There are things we can afford to do that will make a difference. Part of my task is to persuade the majority in this country that those investments are worth it, and if we make better choices in our government, we can deliver on that promise.

For my second and companion goal, I'm well situated to help the country understand how we can both celebrate our diversity in all its complexity and still affirm our common bonds. That will be the biggest challenge, not just for this country but for the entire planet. How do we say we're different yet the same? Of course, there will be times when we'll argue about our differences, but we have to build a society on the belief that you are more like me than different from me. That you know your fears, your hopes, your love for your child are the same as what I feel. Maybe I can help with that because I've got so many different pieces in me.

OPRAH: *I think you're uniquely situated at this time. You know what? When I went to Africa with Christmas gifts, my prime goal was to show African children as happy and responsive and loving so that people could see, Oh, these children are just like my children. When people see children with distended bellies and flies on their eyes, they block it out and don't relate. When I got an e-mail from a white South African lady saying, "For the first time, I realize these children have birthdays," I thought, We won.*

BARACK: That's great. I often say we've got a budget deficit that's important, we've got a trade deficit that's critical, but what I worry about most is our empathy deficit. When I speak to students, I tell them that one of the most important things we can do is to look through somebody else's eyes.

People like bin Laden are missing that sense of empathy. That's why they can think of the people in the World Trade Center as abstractions. They can just crash a plane into them and not even consider, *How would I feel if my child were in there?*

OPRAH: *We Americans also suffer from an empathy deficit, because we often feel that the woman in Bosnia or Afghanistan who loses her child is somehow different from us.*

BARACK: They become abstractions.

OPRAH: *Would you define what you're doing as a new kind of politics? I don't consider myself political, and I seldom interview politicians. So when I decided to talk with you, people around me were like, "What's happened to you?" I said, "I think this is beyond and above politics." It feels like something new.*

> I want to be a part of many voices that help the entire country rise up.

BARACK: I hope it's new. Many of the moments that become "history" happen when politics expresses our deepest hopes. Both of us grew up in a time when there were so many reasons to be cynical: Watergate, Vietnam....

OPRAH: *And the politicians themselves. That's why you didn't want to be one.*

BARACK: When I speak, the first thing I confront is people's cynicism. I understand it. It seems like politics is a business and not a mission. Some of our leaders have been long on rhetoric, short on substance—power is always trumping principle. That's why we withdraw into our private worlds and lives, and we think politics can't address the things that are most important to us. But the civil rights movement was a political movement. The movement to give women the vote was political. We are all connected as one people, and our mutual obligations have to express themselves not only in our families, not only in our churches, not only in our synagogues and mosques, but in our government, too.

OPRAH: *How do you actually get people to be more empathetic?*

BARACK: Your story about South Africa was

terrific. Images, actions, and stories always speak the loudest. That's why I see my book as part of my politics. And I'll write more books. Policy has to be guided by facts, but to move people you have to tell stories.

OPRAH: *You think you'll have time to write more books?*

BARACK: I wrote the first one while I was getting married and running a voter registration project. I'll find time.

OPRAH: *There was a moment during the eighties, after I'd come to Chicago and my show had been national for a while, that I just felt like all the planets had lined up for me and it was my moment. Do you feel that for yourself?*

BARACK: There's been an interesting confluence of events over the last year that have Michelle and me looking at each other and talking.

MICHELLE: We're clear on the fact that we have to stay humble and prayerful. We have to dig down deep to our roots. When things come together, we know some of it is Barack, some of it is us—but a lot of it has nothing to do with either of us.

OPRAH: *When your opponents fall by the wayside based on scandal you didn't create...*

BARACK: It's an interesting moment. It makes me feel that much more determined and that much more responsible. It makes me think I've got to make sure that I don't...

MICHELLE: ...screw it up.

OPRAH: *When I had the same moment, I literally went to my knees. You're either humble or you're not. If you were a jerk before the fame, you just become a jerk with a bigger spotlight. Whoever you are really comes through.*

BARACK: This platform is an enormous privilege. And it's not for me. It's for the people I meet in these little towns who have lost their jobs, don't have healthcare, are trying to figure out how to pay for their child's college education, are struggling and occasionally slipping into bitterness. It's not easy solving these problems. There are big global issues—the shift in the economy, the decline in manufacturing, the threat of terrorism, and complicated healthcare concerns. There will be conflicts and difficulties, and I don't pretend that everybody is going to agree with me all the time.

MICHELLE: I would want Barack as my senator. I know this man. He is brilliant, he is decent, he is everything you'd want.

OPRAH: *How important a role does your family play?*

BARACK: They're everything.

OPRAH: *When I heard you deliver your primary speech, I actually believed you when you thanked your wife. You're right: She has held this family together.*

BARACK: I love this woman. We've had our rough patches....

MICHELLE: There were many....

BARACK: The best quote so far in the campaign was in *The New Yorker.* The interviewer sat down with Michelle and said, "This must really be tough." She said, "This is crazy. He's never home, the schedule's terrible, and I'm raising two kids and working." Then Michelle pauses and says, "That's why he's such a grateful man."

OPRAH: *That's great.*

BARACK: The hardest thing about the work I do is the strain it puts on Michelle, and not being around enough for the kids. Then there are the financial worries after you've come out of Harvard Law School....

MICHELLE: It's Harvard, Princeton, and Columbia combined.

BARACK: So there's a lot that my family has had to sacrifice.

OPRAH: *What's a day like for you? How often are you away from home?*

BARACK: I've had ten days off in the last three years, and that includes weekends. My workdays are often 16 hours.

MICHELLE: And more people are making requests for his time.

OPRAH: *How do you decide what to do?*

BARACK: That has gotten harder. If you don't show up, people feel hurt. You get this beautiful letter from a school in South Carolina, and the teacher writes, "These kids would be so inspired if you came."

OPRAH: *My letters start out with, "Dear Oprah, we know you love children...."*

BARACK: Right now I still have an excuse: I haven't been elected yet.* After the election, handling the requests will require discipline. That's how Michelle has been a rock for me. She supports me by being a corrective. My instinct is to do everything. I don't want to disappoint anyone. Michelle is a little more sensible.

OPRAH: *Somebody has to say "Enough!"*

MICHELLE: The first people we don't want to disappoint are our kids. Barack is a great father. Even when he's away, he calls every night. People will suck you dry, and they don't think about the fact that you have two kids. He has to go to the kids' ballet events and their parent-teacher conferences. And he enjoys that.

BARACK: One of the wrestling matches I'm always having with my staff is getting my kids' events onto the schedule. I have to make sure they understand that's a priority.

MICHELLE: Now, if people can't get Barack to speak, they're like, "Michelle can come. She seems nice and smart, too." But I can't be gone every night. And I can't do something every Saturday from now until election day—that's when we go to the park or on playdates. It's up to the staff to figure out which Saturday they want me to do something, because there will be just one. My desire is to make sure that my kids are sane, happy, and healthy—which they are.

OPRAH: *At this point in the campaign, are you excited?*

BARACK: I think we'll win as long as we stay focused and don't get complacent. We have to continue to work hard. But I want to do more than just win. I want to win in a way that sustains the hopefulness we've carried since the primary. Not engaging in negative attacks, not being dragged into the mud. Steady. That kind of politics is harder, not easier.

OPRAH: *When you had that guy [a tracker from Barack's opponent's campaign who was following Barack everywhere] in your face every day, how could you not punch him?*

BARACK: Michelle will tell you that I generally have an even temper.

MICHELLE: If I had been there, I would've punched him! [Michelle laughs.]

BARACK: Initially, I tried to talk with him. I said, "Listen, I don't mind you following me, but please be 15 feet away. I'm on the phone with my wife." He would plant himself in front of our office....

MICHELLE: ...and then chase you into the bathroom.

BARACK: Well, he wouldn't actually go into the bathroom. He'd stand outside and watch me come out.

OPRAH: *God don't like ugly.*

BARACK: Those slash-and-burn tactics have become the custom in Washington politics. But we will not play that game. People don't want to hear folks shouting at each other and trying to score political points. They want to solve problems. I'm determined to disagree with people without being disagreeable. That's part of the empathy. Empathy doesn't just extend to cute little kids. You have to have empathy when you're talking to some guy who doesn't like black people.

There's a level of viciousness in politics because power is at stake. Fortunately, most of my past mistakes are ones that people already know about. That's one of the nice things about writing a book.

OPRAH: *I'm surprised you were so candid about having used drugs.*

BARACK: I think the biggest mistake politicians make is being inauthentic. By writing about my mistakes, I was trying to show how I was vulnerable to the same pitfalls as American youth everywhere.

OPRAH: *Right. Is there anything about Washington that frightens you?*

BARACK: The things that concern me have to do with my family. I want to make sure we're spending enough time with one another and drawing a circle of common sense around what can be a very artificial environment. That's where I rely so much on Michelle.

OPRAH: *What do you know for sure?*

BARACK: I know that I love my family. I know that people are fundamentally good. I know that, in the words of Dr. King, "The arc of the moral universe is long but it bends toward justice." I know that there is great suffering and tragedy in the world, but ultimately, it's worth it to live.

OPRAH: *Do you think you'll be the first black president?*

BARACK: A bunch of people have started talking about that. Listen, if you're in politics, at a certain point you think about where to take your career. But at this stage, it's way too premature. Politics is a marathon. So many things can change. You can't plan 12 years ahead. But what I will say is this: We can win the race we're in now. I think I have the aptitude to be a terrific U.S. senator. And if, at the end of my first term, the people of Illinois say, "This guy's been serving us well," then I'll be in a strong position to have a lot of influence in this country for a long time to come—whether or not I'm president. ●

*Since this interview, Barack Obama was elected U. S. Senator from Illinois.

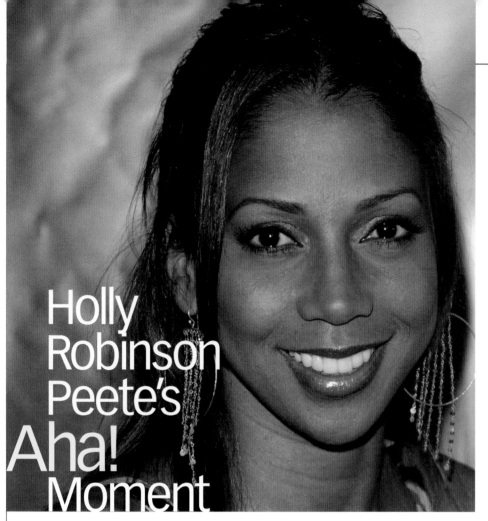

Holly Robinson Peete's Aha! Moment

The actress felt scared, helpless. Then a great athlete's courage filled her with passion and purpose.

THE YEAR WAS 1982, AND I WAS about to enter my first year of college, excited but scared about moving from Los Angeles to New York. My parents, divorced for many years, put aside their differences and escorted me to school. It made me so happy to see the pride in their eyes. "Okay," their expressions seemed to say, "maybe we sucked at marriage—but what a great daughter we raised!"

When we hugged goodbye and I watched them walk to the car, I noticed a strange hitch in my father's step. "Hey, Daddy, why are you walking like Fred Sanford?" I hollered, half-jokingly. "Oh, don't worry about me," he called back. "Just go to your classes or you'll be living in a junkyard, too."

My freshman year was typically fabulous and tumultuous. By Christmas I was homesick and couldn't wait to see my parents. But the moment my father answered the door, I knew something was wrong. The left side of his face was slack, his limbs trembled, and that slight limp had turned into a dragging leg.

Like a lot of women, I worshiped my father. When I was a little girl, he played Gordon on *Sesame Street*—what more could a 4-year-old want? I mean, I hung out with the Cookie Monster! Later he was a writer and producer on *The Cosby Show*. He had always been my rock and my protector. But I saw a first that day—fear in my strong father's eyes. He told me he had been diagnosed—at the young age of 46—with Parkinson's disease, which I'd never heard of. He described it to me as a "debilitating neurological disease for which there is no cure."

So I cried. And cried. And then I scoured six libraries to find out everything I could about Parkinson's. There wasn't much information, and the word *incurable* popped up constantly. Convinced there was nothing I

> The TV actress says she sees each day as a chance to "get off my butt and make a difference."

could do, I just pretended it would go away. For more than a decade I felt helpless as I watched my father become more debilitated, unable to perform simple tasks like buttoning his shirt or holding a fork. Sometimes his medication made him confused; sometimes he couldn't move or communicate. He wasn't yet 60 years old.

The year was 1996, and I watched on television as Muhammad Ali lit the Olympic flame in Atlanta, undaunted by his parkinsonian tremors. I called my father to see if he was watching. He was, and we talked about how proud and hopeful Ali made us feel. I knew then that my life would never be the same. How could I sit around feeling sorry for myself and my father when Ali's actions proclaimed, "I am not going to let Parkinson's disease steal my life"? He lit a fire under me that day. Along with my wonderful husband, Rodney Peete, a quarterback for the NFL's Carolina Panthers, I founded the HollyRod Foundation in 1997 to help people with Parkinson's. I wanted desperately to create a comfort zone for PD patients, their families, and caregivers, providing financial, physical, and emotional support. We recently started the HollyRod Compassionate Care Program at the University of Southern California's Keck School of Medicine in Los Angeles to assist people who have little or no health insurance and limited financial resources.

In 2002, Mr. Ali accepted our foundation's Matthew T. Robinson Award of Courage, named in honor of my father, who never lost his spirit or sense of humor through pain, the awful side effects of his medicine, and intrusive procedures. Dad even rallied enough to walk me down the aisle at my 1995 wedding to Rodney. Sadly, though, he wasn't well enough to attend the award ceremony, and two months later, in August 2002, he passed away. I miss him very much. Like Ali, he was a fierce fighter, and that memory empowers me to keep battling to help people become active in the fight against Parkinson's disease. I see each day as another opportunity to get off my butt and make a difference in someone's life. Hey—thanks, Champ. ●

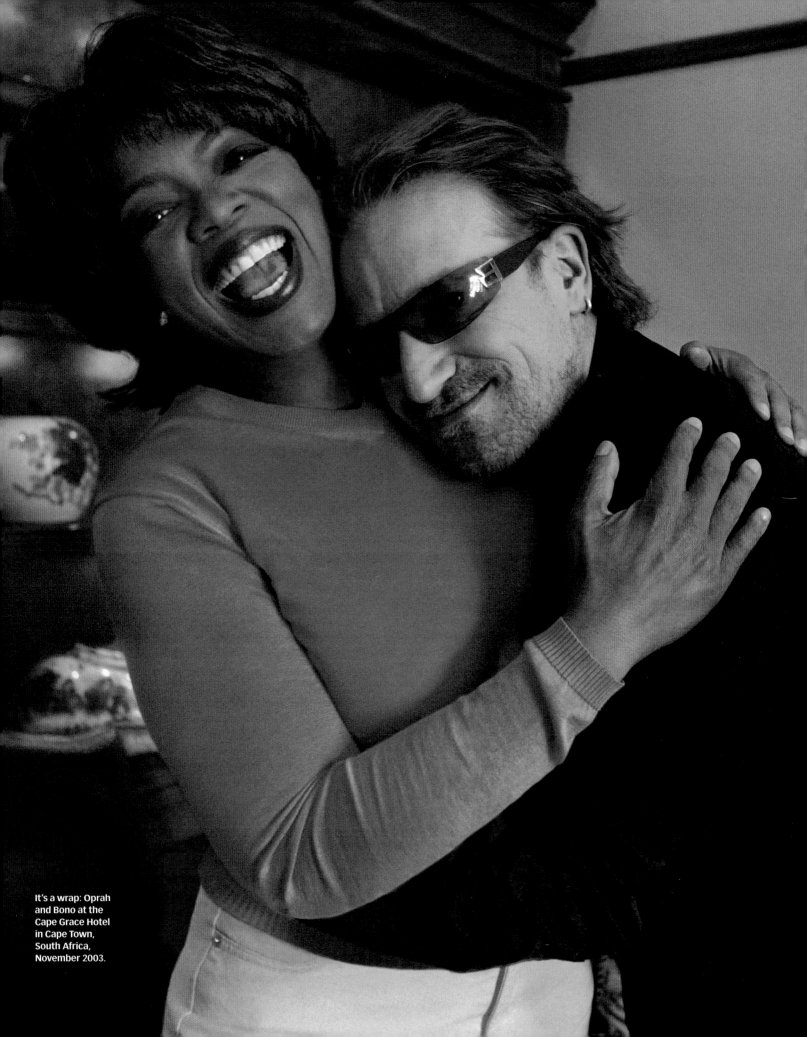

It's a wrap: Oprah and Bono at the Cape Grace Hotel in Cape Town, South Africa, November 2003.

OPRAH TALKS TO BONO

The superstar U2 front man talks about his excellent marriage, his Irish gloom, his commitment to Africa, how truth unlocks creativity, and his fear of being "interesting."

HE'S THE COOLER-THAN-COOL ROCKER, THE LEGENDARY FRONT man of U2, husband of 22 years, and father of four, who's singing his heart out to shine light on a crisis devastating a continent. By the time the sun sets this evening, AIDS will have claimed the lives of 6,500 more people in Africa. Before you finish this sentence, another mother, father, or child will succumb to the virus. We've all heard the numbers, shaken our heads at the horror, and moved on to whatever we had to do next. Bono, on the other hand, takes the AIDS epidemic personally.

"Our generation will be remembered for the Internet, for the war against terror, and for how we let an entire continent burst into flames while we stood around with watering cans—or not," he said when I sat down with him on my show. He compared the situation to watching Holocaust victims being put on trains while the rest of the world did nothing. Determined to take action, Bono launched a nonprofit organization, DATA (Debt, AIDS, Trade, Africa). One of DATA's goals is to reduce African debt, which would free up billions of dollars for healthcare and education. Who else could have used rock 'n' roll to get us to feel the impact of Third World economics?

I caught up with Bono again in Cape Town, South Africa, after he'd given a riveting performance in conjunction with World AIDS Day. Born Paul Hewson to a Protestant mother and a Catholic father in 1960 in Dublin, this man with a social conscience and a contagious fervor makes being a pop star a part-time job. When we talked in Chicago, he left me with his own blue wraparound sunglasses—such a hot gift. This time he left me with an even greater treasure—his wisdom. We talked about everything from songwriting to raising kids to working to save Africa. I have the ultimate admiration and respect for him.

OPRAH: *How does the music come to you? Quincy Jones once told me that he can sometimes see* melodies.

BONO: I've never seen the music. For me it's a puzzle. I hear strains of a melody, and only when I work it out to its end can I be at peace. Until then it's like a twitch.

OPRAH: *I got it.*

BONO: It just comes out. No choice. It's sort of embarrassing because it happens when you don't really want it to. You're writing a song on the back of an Air India sick bag, and you're not writing it because you need a hit—you're writing it because you need some sleep. You have to put it on paper so you can quiet the nagging.

OPRAH: *Can you set out to write a hit and then actually write one?*

BONO: Well, one of the things that hits have and that great music always has, you know—the music feels like it was already there.

OPRAH: *Like your song "Beautiful Day."*

BONO: I don't know if that's great. But when you stumble on certain melodies, you think, *That was already there.*

OPRAH: *It's like what Michelangelo said: The sculpture was already in the stone.*

BONO: And I don't think he was just being clever. The hit—what might be called eternal music, if you want to be high-minded—is a song that most people feel familiar with. And the most extreme end of that spectrum is music...

OPRAH: *...that resonates on a level that's indescribable.*

BONO: Right. Like "I've got sunshine on a cloudy day." Or my favorite song, "Amazing Grace." My second favorite song is "Help Me Make It Through the Night." What I like about pop music, and why I'm still attracted to it, is that in the end it becomes our folk music. In the seventies, when we were growing up and all the rock criticism was going on, disco was supposed to suck. But you listen to some of that music now—"I Will Survive"...

OPRAH: *And the Donna Summer stuff.*

BONO: Yes. It's like folk music now. That other stuff with the guitar solos? Who cares? The great music for so many

artists—the Beatles, the Rolling Stones—was always at the moment when they were closest to pop. It would be easy for U2 to go off and have a concept album, but I want us to stay in the pop fray.

OPRAH: *Do you have anxiety every time you release an album?*

BONO: Yes.

OPRAH: *You do?*

BONO: Of course. It's much easier to be successful than it is to be relevant. The tricks won't keep you relevant. Tricks might keep you popular for a while, but in all honesty, I don't know how U2 will stay relevant. I know we've got a future. I know we can fill stadiums. And yet with every record, I think, *Is this it? Are we still relevant?*

OPRAH: *Well, you haven't been invited to play a Bat Mitzvah yet.*

BONO: No. I just don't want to go through what I call the Interesting Music Phase. That really means "We just don't get it."

OPRAH: *So would you stop first?*

BONO: Yes. Our idea in the band is this: Two crap albums in a row and you're out. That gives us two to go. One crap album is fine, because you can pull back and try again. But after two, you're forever "interesting."

OPRAH: *I was watching you up onstage last night, and I said,* God, this just makes me want to go put on a pair of sunglasses and a leather jacket. *Is there anything better than*

"What I like about pop music, and why I'm

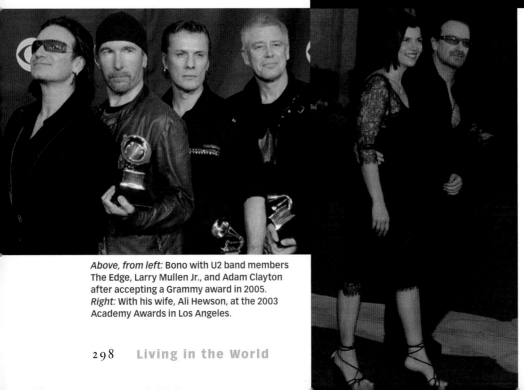

Above, from left: Bono with U2 band members The Edge, Larry Mullen Jr., and Adam Clayton after accepting a Grammy award in 2005.
Right: With his wife, Ali Hewson, at the 2003 Academy Awards in Los Angeles.

being on that stage in that moment and being you?

BONO: Wow—I don't remember feeling that good. You certainly have moments when the music dwarfs you, brings you to your knees, and you're only a tiny part of it. But most of the time, unfortunately, you're a very large part of it. And you're self-conscious, or something's irritating you, or you're underrehearsed. So, yes, there are moments like last night when we're standing out there singing a melody—"It's a long, long walk to freedom"—and the crowd starts singing with us, though they've never heard the song before. I had just watched this extraordinary man, Nelson Mandela, who taught us all a lesson, take that long walk to the podium. As everyone sang, I realized we were guests of the nation of South

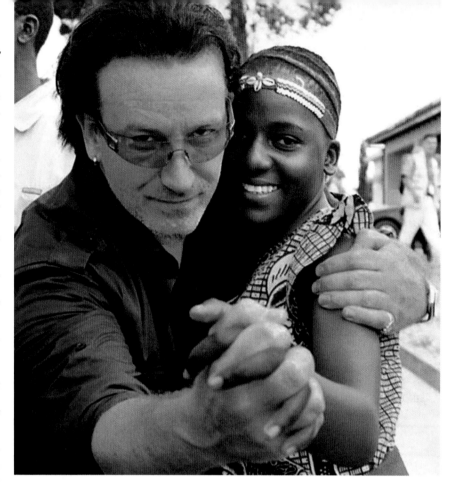

Dancing with an HIV-positive orphan in Kampala, Uganda, on a 2002 tour of Africa with then-U.S. treasury secretary Paul O'Neill to study poverty.

Africa. They were singing the hymn, he was smiling to the crowd—and we were in between.

OPRAH: *I felt that, too.*

BONO: It was even more poignant because it was a predominantly white audience singing to him. I'm standing there thinking, *This might be a big miracle we're witnessing.*

OPRAH: *The sea of white faces, singing that song to him.*

BONO: And there was no patronizing from either side.

OPRAH: *I agree. I was happy to be a witness to it.*

BONO: I was pretty knocked out. I wished my entire band were there. With the band, we would have pulled that house down, because there was a lot of energy in that crowd.

OPRAH: *So when do you really have a good time?*

BONO: When I'm playing with the band. As a soloist, I'm average at best. But with the band? There's nothing better, I promise you. I'm sorry, but I can say that. Two weekends ago, I was in New York with my wife, and we had a great time. My wife and I surfed our jet lag.

OPRAH: *What does that mean?*

BONO: When you have kids, you have to go to bed and get up at a certain time. But if

BONO: Oh, yeah. She's quite a character. And she has a very strong sense of herself. She's capable of extraordinary things. Right now she's working on a new way of doing business in apparel. It involves fair trade practices in which people in Third World countries get paid properly and get

couple of years. You may get the impression I'm always out there, but I'm usually home driving my kids to school. I like morning better than night.

OPRAH: *I thought all musicians kept those crazy "Quincy hours"—working late at night.*

BONO: I peak early in the morning. It's

still attracted to it, is that in the end it becomes OUR FOLK MUSIC."

you don't have the kids with you—which we didn't—you can go to bed when you're sleepy and stay up when you're not. That means you can stay out until 4 in the morning.

OPRAH: *I've got to learn how to surf my jet lag. How old are the kids now?*

BONO: The two girls are 14 and 12; the two boys are 4 and 2. They're great. I don't know why I have the life I have. I don't deserve it. I think the family is as strong as it is because of my wife, Ali. She is just really so cool.

OPRAH: *How long have you been married?*

BONO: Longer than I haven't been. We married when we were kids. We couldn't have known what we were getting involved in.

OPRAH: *And after all these years, you still think she's cool?*

health insurance—and you still make a fortune. It may be one of the biggest brands in the next years, so watch out. It's called Edun.

My wife is not ambitious in any way you may be familiar with. For her, ambition is a slow kind of burning. If each partner wants the other to realize his or her potential, the relationship will probably be okay. If one has to sacrifice for the other, which is so often the case, I don't think it's as good as two people trying to outdo each other [with support]. I think she has sacrificed more than I have, so I'm trying to balance that now.

OPRAH: *How often are you home?*

BONO: I'm home a lot. Because I live in Ireland, we can live under the celebrity radar. I might go missing for a whole year. As it happens, that might have been the last

downhill from there.

OPRAH: *Are you a full participant in parenting?*

BONO: Yes, except when I'm on tour. Even then I'm never away from Ali and the kids for more than three weeks.

OPRAH: *What have your children taught you about yourself?*

BONO: I have very little memory of my childhood, so as I raise my kids the memories come back in the most bizarre ways. Like you're singing your baby a song, and you don't know why you remember it, but somehow you do. You don't even know the tune, but you sing it anyway and think, *How am I singing this song?*

OPRAH: *There's a theory that whatever stage your children are at, it reminds you of that stage of your own childhood. Like if you have a 7-year-old and something traumatic happened* *to you when you were 7, that's when all your stuff comes up. Has that been true for you?*

BONO: I certainly thought my 20s were turbulent, but I didn't realize that the real turbulence comes later in life, when you get a chance—whether it's through your own children or others—to revisit what made you who you are.

OPRAH: *And brought on your rage.*

BONO: Yes. I wrote a piece called "Rage Is Not a Great Reason to Do Anything, but It'll Do." It's a story of me learning to write songs as a kid. I didn't go to music school, because I wasn't from that kind of family. And I remember the frustration of hearing a melody in my head but not being able to quite put it down. So you learn to rely on other people, the band, and you start thinking that's a weakness. But it's a strength to rely on others.

OPRAH: *You have a gift, though. Does it come from a place you can't really describe?*

BONO: Before I answer you, I want to say this: I think God gets annoyed with the gifted. We should know that our work is no more important than a plumber's or a carpenter's. And here's what I love about hip-hop artists: They set up the brand and start selling T-shirts. It's like, "Here's my chair. I built it. How many do you want?" Whereas with some other musicians, it's like, "I don't know anything about my record contract. I'm not involved in that stuff." That's such bullshit. That's one reason hip-hop is walking all over rock 'n' roll right now. In what I would call alternative music, there has been a bunch of lies—which meant that you couldn't own up to your ambition. You couldn't own up to the idea that art and commerce are certainly cousins, if not brothers. So where does all music come from—be it hip-hop or rock 'n' roll? I don't know. But I do know that all music is praise.

OPRAH: *I'll be quoting you on that.*

BONO: It's praise to the god of your making. Which, in the case of a rock star, might be oneself. Or a woman. Or an idea.

OPRAH: *I love that.*

BONO: When I was 10, I learned what unlocks creativity. We were studying William Butler Yeats, one of the great poets of the 20th century, and my teacher explained that there was a period when Yeats had writer's block. I put my hand up in class

and asked, "Why didn't he write about *that?*" It was like, "Oh, shut up." I've since learned that there's something to being truthful. The Scriptures say the truth will set you free. The truth is at the root of every piece of creativity. So if you're truthful about your situation, whatever it is as an artist—whether it's despair, whether it's hope, whether it's ambition—suddenly you're *there.*

OPRAH: *Isn't that what all real art is—truth?*

BONO: Yes. Truth is beauty. That can be a hard thing to say, because some things are not so attractive on the surface. But by owning up to them, we change them—just by speaking them. The first line on the page can be "I have nothing to offer. I'm empty today." That's why public confession—whether it's part of religious practice or on your show—is so important.

OPRAH: *Yes. Twenty years ago, people were living dysfunctional lives, but they thought they were the only ones living that way. I grew up thinking that people really did live like* Leave It to Beaver. *I thought,* Gee, if I had a mom who made me milk and cookies, my world would be okay.

BONO: In my music, I try to be as truthful as I can. I'm not sure I can be as honest in my life as I can be in my music, because with manners comes insincerity. Like "How are you?" "I'm very well." But I'm not. I have a massive hangover. Truth is sometimes difficult.

OPRAH: *What makes you happy?*

BONO: I'm not the happiest person, and I'm certainly not happy-clappy. There's a bit of "woe is me" that comes with melancholy, the Irish thing, and it's draining.

OPRAH: *Okay, so what gives you joy? Joy is a better word anyway.*

BONO: Joy is the hardest possible thing to contrive as an act. It's easy to describe anger, rage, happiness. But joy is difficult.

OPRAH: *Is joy elusive for you?*

BONO: I don't know. Our band has it when we're going off. There's a joy vibration there. It's not miserable-ism.

OPRAH: *Joy is a very high energy field.*

BONO: I'm grumpy. You seem to have a level of joy. Are there months when things aren't going right for you, when you're in a trough, or do you have just, like, one bad day a week?

OPRAH: *Not even a bad day a week.*

BONO: Really?

OPRAH: *Absolutely not.*

BONO: Well, I have a couple of bad days a week.

OPRAH: *So tell me this: Where do your commitment and passion come from? For as long as I can remember, you've been using your voice to make a difference in the world.*

BONO: Growing up in Ireland was part of it—the simple, practical life of Irish people. Wherever you go in Africa, you find an Irish priest or a young nun. They're everywhere! And then, of course, Bob Geldof [formerly of the Boomtown Rats] is my friend, and we did the whole Live Aid thing together. [Held simultaneously in the United States and the United Kingdom in 1985, Live Aid was the biggest benefit concert in history, raising millions of dollars for famine relief in Ethiopia.] Around that time, my wife and I lived in Ethiopia for a month, in a tent in a feeding station in the middle of nowhere. It was extraordinary. That royal Ethiopian thing is in these people; that Solomon and Queen of Sheba thing is all around. At my site, there was barbed wire, like a concentration camp—but the wire was meant to keep people out, not in. A man walked up to me, gave me a child, and said, "You take my son. He'll live if you take him." And I couldn't take the boy. But that really formed my commitment. I remember coming home on the plane saying, "We'll never forget this."

OPRAH: *And did you forget?*

BONO: I did. Yet somewhere inside me, I'll always remember it. Somewhere there was a prayer to say, and there will be a way to help. What I saw in Ethiopia wasn't just about people falling on hard times. It was a wider problem—political, not just social. So in this work, the circle is becoming a bit completed for me now. And my people have been supportive. The Irish can be annoying—and I'm one of them—but they really are good. Here in Africa, I'm the anomaly. It's an odd and freakish thing that I, an Irish guy, am sitting here and that you're even asking me questions. Yet the people we'd choose to describe the condition of the world are not often the people God would choose. The chosen may be punk rockers or hip-hop people. But nonetheless, the state of the world will be described. ●

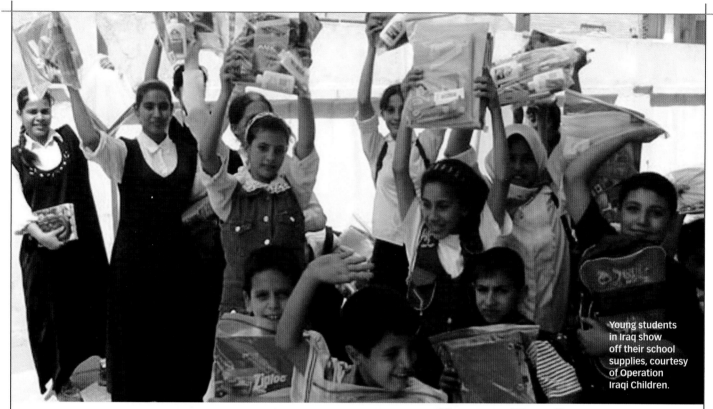

Young students in Iraq show off their school supplies, courtesy of Operation Iraqi Children.

How Do You Spell *Relief*?

Actor **GARY SINISE** tells how he and *Seabiscuit* author Laura Hillenbrand are racing to get school supplies into the hands of Iraqi children.

IN THE WINTER OF 2003, MY friend Laura Hillenbrand, author of the best-selling book *Seabiscuit,* got an e-mail from an American soldier in Iraq. He had just returned from visiting a rural school for girls where he and a translator had been reading Laura's book. Taught in a squalid, one-room building, with almost no learning tools and fewer books, the students were thrilled at the sight of the *Seabiscuit* paperback. An attached photo showed a soldier in full desert camouflage standing in a sea of smiling Iraqi girls, with one child clutching Laura's book as if it were a magical treasure. Looking at the picture, Laura cried. A few months earlier, while touring Iraq with the USO, I made a detour to visit an elementary school. American soldiers had transformed the place from a fetid shack to a clean, bright building, but children huddled four to a notebook, three to a pencil. Half a world apart, Laura and I made the same resolution: We had to get learning tools to these children.

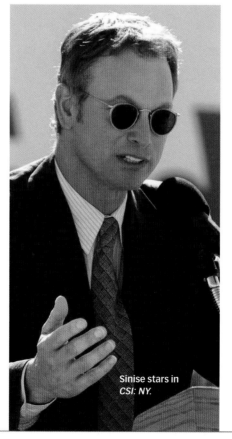

Sinise stars in *CSI: NY.*

When I returned to the States, we rolled up our sleeves and created Operation Iraqi Children (operationiraqichildren.org). In a few breathtaking and exhausting weeks, we had a Web site up and running from which donors could get instructions on what to buy for a school supply kit (colored pencils, scissors) and how to assemble it and send it to our Kansas City warehouse—where FedEx would deliver it gratis to an American base in Iraq. Soldiers would then distribute the kits to schools.

Operation Iraqi Children has supplied tens of thousands of kids with the tools of childhood. American soldiers laden with bulging Ziploc bags pull up to schools and are engulfed by gleeful children. Our goals are to bring the gift of learning to kids and to foster goodwill between the Iraqis and our troops. Is it working? At a recent distribution event, children sang and danced while their parents hugged the soldiers. As one Iraqi parent put it, "We shall never forget this day." ●

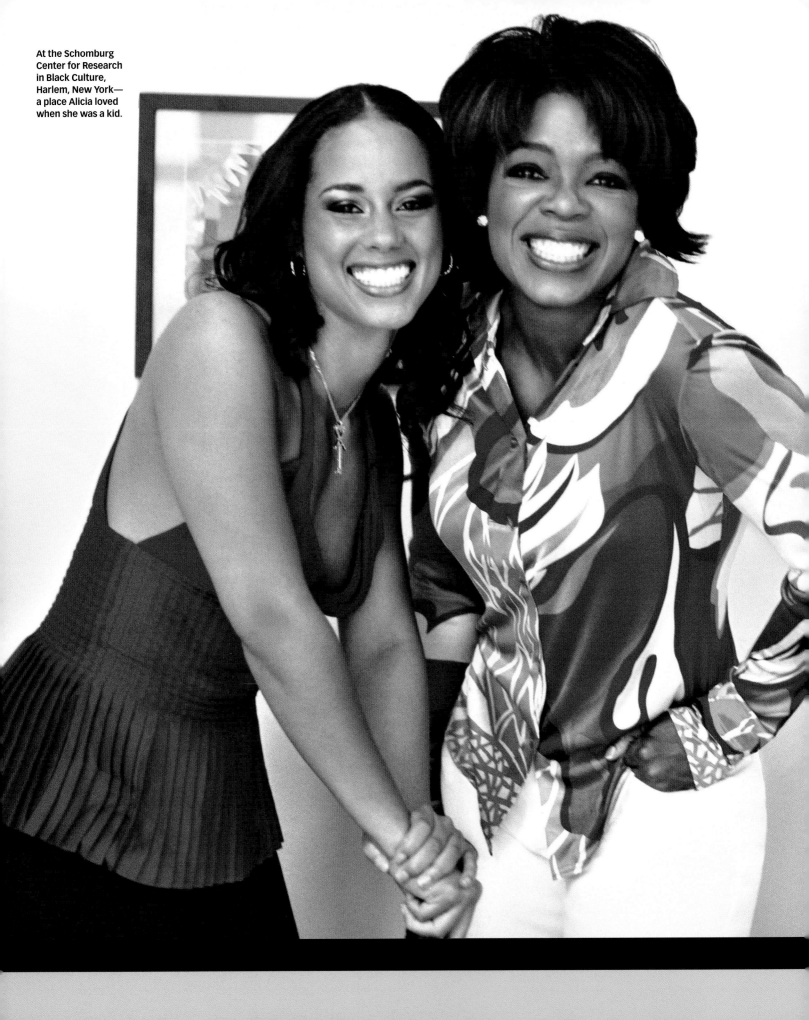

At the Schomburg Center for Research in Black Culture, Harlem, New York— a place Alicia loved when she was a kid.

Q+A

THE CLASSICALLY TRAINED FIVE-TIME GRAMMY-WINNING SENSATION—STILL ONLY 23!—OPENS UP HEART AND SOUL (AND DIARY ENTRIES) ABOUT HER LEAP FROM HELL'S KITCHEN TO SUPERSTARDOM: THE GOOD, THE BAD, AND THE UGLY OF DIVADOM; AND HOW SHE HANDLES THE QUESTION, WHY ME?

OPRAH TALKS TO ALICIA KEYS

Even before Alicia Keys belted out the first soulful notes of the lyrics that made her famous—*I keep on fallin' in and out of love with you*—I could feel the power of her presence. As she sat across from me on the stage of my show last spring, I decided that I wanted to have a real conversation with her, away from the cameras and commercial breaks. I finally do, on a Saturday morning in Harlem, at the Schomburg Center for Research in Black Culture, where writer Langston Hughes is buried.

The girl born Alicia Augello-Cook spent most of her childhood in Hell's Kitchen, one of New York's toughest neighborhoods. Though she was on decent terms with her father, Craig, she lived with her mother, Terri, who scraped by financially as a paralegal. Even with her meager means, Terri insisted that her daughter take piano lessons on a dilapidated upright a friend had given them. At 7 Alicia was learning classical piano, and by age 12, she was writing her own songs. After graduating as valedictorian from New York's Professional Performing Arts School, she was accepted at Columbia University.

Four weeks into her freshman year (at age 16), Alicia traded one Columbia for another, eager to build a career with her record label. When her deal with Columbia Records crumbled, legendary music producer Clive Davis, president of Arista, signed her. But in 2000, just as Alicia was completing her debut album, Davis was ousted from Arista and *Songs in A Minor* was put on hold. Later that year, Davis formed his own label, J Records, and promptly signed Alicia. Her first single, "Fallin'," soared to the top of the Billboard charts. She won five Grammys for the album, tying Lauryn Hill's record for the most wins for a female artist in one year. Her second album, 2003's *The Diary of Alicia Keys,* debuted at number one on the charts.

When I was working on *The Color Purple,* Quincy Jones said to me, "Your future is so bright it burns my eyes." I feel the same way about Alicia. The depth of who she'll become will startle her and the rest of the world.

OPRAH: *After this interview, you're flying to London, Cannes, and Rome—and you're a girl raised in Hell's Kitchen. Many girls never make it beyond that 12-block radius.*

ALICIA KEYS: I've often thought, *Why me?* Not in the sense that I don't believe it should be me. I've just seen how many people live on their blocks and never even go downtown. I know people who are my age—23—and already on their fourth child. That's fine....

OPRAH: *It's nice of you to say, but it isn't fine. You know why? At 23 you can't manage your own life and the lives of four other people. The 20s are about discovering who you are. Having a child changes the trajectory of your life.*

ALICIA: That's why I wonder why one of my simple, silly

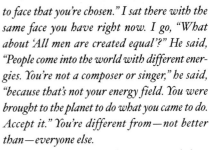

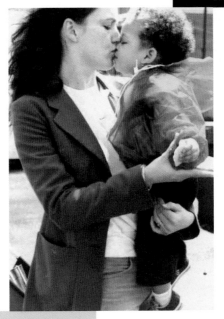

From top: Alicia and her mother post-Grammys, 2002; and 20 years earlier, when Alicia was just 1.

misjudgments didn't turn my life upside down. It's like, "Oops"—and your reality is completely different. I was blessed and, in a way, chosen to experience more of the world.

OPRAH: *I can tell that you use the word* chosen *hesitantly. Why?*

ALICIA: It's my nature to downplay.

OPRAH: *I sense you're where I was until a few months ago. I struggled with the word* chosen *until I shared a plane ride with one of my greatest mentors, Sidney Poitier. He said, "You have to face that you're chosen." I sat there with the same face you have right now. I go, "What about 'All men are created equal'?" He said, "People come into the world with different energies. You're not a composer or singer," he said, "because that's not your energy field. You were brought to the planet to do what you came to do. Accept it." You're different from—not better than—everyone else.*

ALICIA: Right. It's such a responsibility. Maybe the reason I stutter over the word *chosen* is that it's scary. I believe in the limitlessness of humans. We're capable of incredible things. At times that realization is frightening.

OPRAH: *Why not just flow with it?*

ALICIA: I do. I'm not up at night thinking about it—yet it's a vulnerable place.

OPRAH: *At 23 make peace with it. It'll be life changing.*

ALICIA: Different is great.

OPRAH: *We're a world of differences.*

ALICIA: Not enough people want to be different from me. I want people to want to be themselves.

OPRAH: *Do you think you have something others don't have?*

ALICIA: I definitely feel blessed—with heart.

OPRAH: *That heart comes through in your music.*

ALICIA: I don't take that gift lightly, especially when I look at TV. It kills me to see how some people present themselves. We're going to hell.

OPRAH: *I feel the same way. I've heard you say that music and television have become semipornographic.*

ALICIA: Absolutely. We're one step away from triple-X-rated.

OPRAH: *Years ago I saw my niece sitting mesmerized in front of the TV, watching a music video with the lyrics "Back that thing up." These women were shaking their behinds. If you live in a world where that's the behavior you see, it*

little dizzy. *I heard that so many people wanted to sing your song "Fallin'" that it was banned from* American Idol.

ALICIA: It was banned on pop idol shows all over the world. I've heard that the producers said, "You're ruining the song." I couldn't believe it.

OPRAH: *I heard that Simon Cowell said it's the most ruined song ever. Doesn't that make you feel...*

ALICIA: Crazy?

OPRAH: *No—good.*

OPRAH: *I've lived in this fame trip since 1986. I've found that unless you're rooted in something bigger than fame, you start believing your own hype. I'm so impressed with you because you seem grounded. You must've had some kind of mother!*

ALICIA: She has given me something real to hold on to. She's so strong. When I was younger, there were times when I'd look at her and think, *Wow, it's just you and me.*

OPRAH: *Didn't your parents separate when you were 2?*

"You're flying to London, Cannes, and Rome—and you're a girl raised in Hell's Kitchen. Many girls never make it beyond that 12-block radius."

"I've often thought, *Why me?*... I definitely feel blessed."

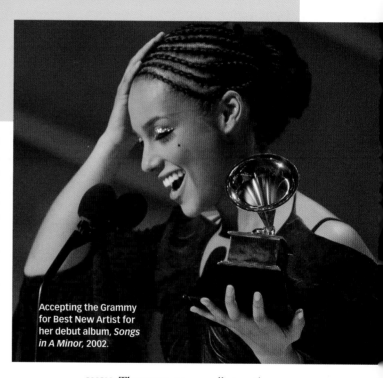

Accepting the Grammy for Best New Artist for her debut album, *Songs in A Minor*, 2002.

becomes your reality—and that's how you learn to represent yourself.

ALICIA: That's it. When I'm walking down the street, I see these 12-year-olds who look 17. Their skirts are tiny, and their shorts are as short as can be. Whoa.

OPRAH: *How did you escape that world?*

ALICIA: My neighborhood was porno hell—prostitutes everywhere. I saw women on street corners in the dead cold of December. I've seen the hard lives they live. I remember thinking, *I don't care how difficult it gets, I will never do that.*

OPRAH: *As a girl, when did you know that the music was in you and you were in the music?*

ALICIA: First I was working on classical music that didn't move me at all. I hated it. So I decided to discover the kinds of classical music that did move me—like Chopin, Satie, Beethoven, and certain Mozart songs. Mozart would play a counterpart with his left hand while using his right to mock it. It was blue, dark, shadowy—and it made me feel something. That's when I realized music was inside me.

OPRAH: *When I listen to Chopin, I just feel a*

ALICIA: It feels great that people want to perform it. When I was younger, there were songs I'd always sing, like "You Bring Me Joy," by Anita Baker, "Memories," from the show *Cats,* "The Greatest Love of All," by Whitney Houston.

OPRAH: *Everybody sang that one.*

ALICIA: Yes. "Fallin'" was a song I fought for, shook people over, and stood up and said, "I'm not changing it."

OPRAH: *When and how did you write that song?*

ALICIA: It started in 1998, when I was at Columbia Records. I wanted to write one of those incredible songs Michael Jackson sang back in the day: You could feel his passion as if he were 50 rather than 9. I messed with some ideas, then threw them to the side. Later, as I began experiencing a lot of things for the first time—I was in my first serious relationship—I continued writing what became "Fallin'."

ALICIA: They were never really together.

OPRAH: *So your father was never there.*

ALICIA: Right, and my mom had to struggle.

OPRAH: *Working two, three jobs.*

ALICIA: She worked around the clock. I don't know how she stood up from day to day. If there was a big trial, she'd come home at 3 A.M., then get up at 6 A.M. and keep going.

OPRAH: *Where were you on the food chain—poor or lower-middle-class?*

ALICIA: It fluctuated.

OPRAH: *You were robbing Peter to pay Paul.*

ALICIA: Definitely. But I realized that if everything fell apart, she'd always be there.

OPRAH: *Didn't you beg to quit piano lessons because you were so poor?*

ALICIA: Yes. A friend was getting rid of this old, brown upright piano she rarely played, and she agreed to let us have it if we'd move it from her apartment. We used the piano as a divider between our living room and my bedroom. That gift is one of the main reasons I'm playing today. God was with us. I wrote my first song—a tune about my grandfather, my Fa-Fa, who'd passed away—on that piano. I'd just returned from seeing *Philadelphia,* and it was after the movie that, for the first time, I could express how I felt through the music.

OPRAH: *How do you define yourself spiritually?*

ALICIA: I feel the presence of a higher power. I believe that what you give is what you get. It's universal law. I believe in the power of prayer and of words. I've learned that when you predict that negative things will happen, they do. And I pray about 75 times a day.

OPRAH: *Marianne Williamson writes about what she learned from* A Course in Miracles *[a self-study guide]: Rather than praying on your knees, remain in a state of being on your knees. Then your life is lived in a prayerful mode. You're open to the universe working through you instead of you trying to direct it.*

ALICIA: Right.

OPRAH: *I've read that you said, "Music is everything." Is it your peace, your therapy, your relaxation?*

ALICIA: It's my joy. A great song can pull me out of a slump and lighten my heart. For me that song is "As," by Stevie Wonder.

OPRAH: *That's my favorite song!*

ALICIA: What sign are you?

OPRAH: *Aquarius.*

ALICIA: Of course you're an Aquarius—I'm an Aquarius! I want you to know that we're one of the coolest signs on the planet. I love being an Aquarius!

OPRAH: *You don't have a choice. You're obviously a Stevie admirer. Who else did you listen to growing up?*

ALICIA: Curtis Mayfield, Sly and the Family Stone, Aretha Franklin, Nina Simone, Billie Holiday, Ella Fitzgerald.

OPRAH: *Chopin and Mozart.*

ALICIA: Nirvana and Led Zeppelin.

OPRAH: *You signed with Columbia Records when you were 15. Didn't somebody hear you when you were on the road?*

ALICIA: My manager put together these showcases so that the heads of various labels could hear me play. They were all interested, so we had a bidding war. Columbia brought me in to play in this gorgeous building that looks out over Manhattan. I was on, like, the 579th floor with this white piano. The whole room was white and glass, and I'd never seen anything like it. I was like "Wow." So I played my little songs and everyone was excited. I was in heaven. Then the exec cleared everybody out and said to me, "If you sign with us, I'll give you this piano." All I had at home was my broken-down room divider. He might as well have been offering me diamonds. The guy says, "I'll give you 15 minutes," then he walks out. It was a game.

OPRAH: *Was it a baby grand?*

ALICIA: Yes. It was a $26,000 piano—and I signed with Columbia. Life has since taught me that signing for a piano is not always the best thing to do.

OPRAH: *What happened?*

ALICIA: At first it was good, but I was a baby and had no idea how to put together an album. They plunged me into the circuit of writing with producers.

OPRAH: *What many people don't know is that record companies are marketing machines. They size you up and say, "We can fit you into this niche. If you do it our way, we'll make you a star."*

ALICIA: Exactly. I was writing with these people, and I hated it. I remember driving to the studio one day with dread in my chest. Months had passed since I'd been signed, and Columbia was asking, "Where's the music?" I was miserable. Then some of the people I worked with started saying things like "You wanna come to my house or meet me at my hotel room?" It was horrible.

OPRAH: *Wasn't Columbia trying to make you the next Whitney or Mariah?*

ALICIA: I think that's what they were hoping would happen naturally. The person who's now my collaborator, Kerry Brothers, said to me, "You wouldn't play as well as you do if you didn't have your own piano. So how do you expect to be a producer and an arranger if you don't have your own equipment?" I bought my own things.

Through the music I wrote then, I was finally able to express the turmoil I'd been feeling. My manager was ecstatic, but some people at the label were saying, "What's this? It's kind of soulful. Where are the pop smashes?" They wanted my hair blown out and flowing, my dresses shorter. And they wanted me to lose weight.

OPRAH: *You?*

ALICIA: Absolutely.

OPRAH: *Oh, Lord.*

ALICIA: I believe I'm so much more, and they wanted me to be the same as everyone else.

OPRAH: *Manufactured. Nobody has an imagination until someone like you comes along. Now they'll try to make the next person like you. When did you decide to leave Columbia?*

ALICIA: Once I saw that these people were completely disrespecting my musical creativity, I was devastated and crushed, like a blooming flower that's trampled on. Nothing hurts more. I'm fortunate that my manager was confident.

OPRAH: *Twenty-five years ago, you wouldn't have believed you had a right to your musical creativity. I think about all the people who came before—the entire Motown generation—who did what they were told.*

ALICIA: Some of our incredible legends will die with nothing. They were jerked.

OPRAH: *Yes. That's what I love about you, little girl: You'll always be a wealthy woman because you own yourself. You've become what those who came before you couldn't be. You're part of that evolution. Is it true that when you first met Clive Davis, he said, "Tell me who you want to be"?*

ALICIA: Exactly. Leaving Columbia was a hell of a fight. Out of spite, they were threatening to keep everything I'd created even though they hated it. I thought I'd have to start over again just to get out, but I didn't care.

OPRAH: *Sounds like a Prince thing.*

ALICIA: Yes. I did leave with the music, and that was nice. The gentleman who'd helped me set up those first showcases knew Clive, and he took my music to him. My first meeting with Clive was great. I'd never had anyone of his stature ask me how I saw myself, and what I wanted to do.

OPRAH: *How would you describe what you do?*

ALICIA: If I have anything to do with it, my music will never be describable. I want to keep redefining my work and trying new things. I want my music to be able to fit into any category. I want it to float wherever my heart goes. My music is heart music; giving it any other description is dangerous.

OPRAH: *It puts you in a box. How do you prepare for a meeting with Clive Davis—the man who worked with Aretha Franklin, Whitney Houston, and Bruce Springsteen?*

ALICIA: I was definitely trying to find my cutest outfit. That's why I was late.

OPRAH: *Oh, boy.*

ALICIA: The train was delayed, so I hopped in a cab and got stuck in traffic. I ran down the block and into the lobby. You can imagine my manager's face. He was like, "Do you know what the hell you're doing?" He knew my life was on the line. I was like, "I'm sorry." Fortunately, a meeting Clive was in ran over, so it worked out.

OPRAH: *How does it feel to be where you are in your life right now?*

ALICIA: It feels like the beginning of a journey. It feels like a lot of hard work and a lot more to do.

OPRAH: *Do you have a dream for yourself?*

ALICIA: I have many dreams, big ones.

OPRAH: *We watched you take home five Grammys. Was that one of your dreams?*

ALICIA: Part of the dream was to be...I don't know if *successful* and *accepted* are the right words.

OPRAH: *Those are good words, and I know where they're coming from. I know you don't mean bling or a big house.*

ALICIA: Right. I kept diaries when I was young....

OPRAH: *I've kept them since I was 15. They're among my most prized possessions.*

ALICIA: It's like, "If the house is burning down, get the diaries out." When I was 9, I was in my first music group. I wrote this stupid little thing about how this boy asked me to dance at this party, and at the end of my diary, I wrote, "Please, please, please let this group work out." It didn't, but other things did.

OPRAH: *In my first diary, I wrote, "My dad won't let me go to Shoney's with Anthony Otey. Dad doesn't understand true love."*

ALICIA: That's so cute.

OPRAH: *I'll go back and read something I've described as painful, and I can't even remember the incident. You always manage to* walk through the pain and come out on the other side.

ALICIA: Ain't that something?

OPRAH: *What other dreams do you have for yourself?*

ALICIA: I want to do the kinds of things that make a difference. Like the community-based charities I support, Keep a Child Alive [which supports kids with AIDS] and Frum tha Ground Up. They're about uplifting kids, giving them a direction.

OPRAH: *I meet a lot of celebrities with a little camp here, a little charity there, but your desire to contribute feels part of something bigger. Is it?*

ALICIA: Everything I do stems from something personal, not just because it will look good on paper or be a tax write-off. Camps are great and I want to do one, but I want to be involved, hands-on. These possibilities give my life meaning, and they give me

> **"They wanted my hair blown out and flowing, my dresses shorter. And they wanted me to lose weight."**

something other than the red carpet to look forward to.

OPRAH: *Is the red carpet fun for you?*

ALICIA: It depends. Sometimes I think, "Wow!" Other times I see how shallow it is and I ask myself, *What am I doing here?* I participated in the Billboard Latin Music Awards, my first Latin awards show, and they were the most professional, efficient, and welcoming group of people. I performed my song in Spanish. It was a magical moment.

OPRAH: *I bet. When I was growing up, I always wanted to look the way you do. Girls like you were called cupcakes. I was a brownie. When did you know you were cute?*

ALICIA: I never really had a moment when I thought, *I am cute.* Like everybody, I tried to wear things that looked good on me. But I was a lazy bum. I wasn't the girl who always had my hair and nails done. In high school, I wore my hair in the tightest bun.

OPRAH: *Did you see* The Vagina Monologues?

ALICIA: Yes, in London.

OPRAH: *There's a great passage about what your vagina is wearing. I came away thinking, Mine is wearing red patent leather boots. What is yours wearing?*

ALICIA: A hat and gloves.

OPRAH: *I thought you'd say a hat and a cane.*

ALICIA: I like that better! I have a thousand hats that change my mood and add to my personality. I love them.

OPRAH: *I have a hat room. How was it going on tour with Beyoncé and Missy Elliott.*

ALICIA: Very good. Ultimately, we did something big and special just by coming together to share a stage. I was proud of that.

OPRAH: *Is it true that there's competition between you and the other so-called pop divas?*

ALICIA: There's competition? I've never heard that. What's beautiful is that we all have different styles and thoughts to offer. That's what makes the world interesting.

OPRAH: *Do you have a significant other?*

ALICIA: He does exist. He's secure enough not to wonder why I haven't wanted to talk about him. That's part of why I love him. He understands me. We have space and togetherness. We have it all. I'll never tell who he is.

OPRAH: *You're doing a great job of not being seen publicly with him.*

ALICIA: Aren't I doing good? Neither of us is a party person.

OPRAH: *When you're onstage performing at the piano, does it become an otherworldly experience?*

ALICIA: Many times I feel as if I were away from myself.

OPRAH: *When you performed on my show, you went to that place. I'm like, "She gone!" I was surprised it could happen so early in the morning.*

ALICIA: It doesn't always happen. That was a special moment.

OPRAH: *When you look out at an audience and see your mom there—the same mom who came home from work at 3 in the morning and got up again at 6—what do you feel?*

ALICIA: I feel so proud of her—so proud of us. In a world that's so unpredictable, she is my solid foundation. Just by looking into her eyes, I can go to that place where I know I am loved and everything is all right. ●

scientists with a typical grant of $250,000, and in 2004 they divided $14 million among approximately 70 researchers. "Some of the most recent research is the most exciting," says Lauder, whose exuberance when speaking of the foundation's achievements is as pure and proud as if she were bragging about a grandchild's first steps. For example, Michael Wigler, PhD, and coworkers have identified two new genes implicated in breast cancer. One is KCNK9, an oncogene—a stretch of DNA that can turn normal cells into cancer cells. The other, DBC2, is a tumor suppressor that normally prevents cells from becoming malignant but that may allow cancer to develop when it's missing or damaged. Pinpointing these genes could help create new, effectively targeted treatments.

Other exciting developments come from the New York Breast Cancer Study—a program funded solely by the foundation since 1997. The study has been examining breast and ovarian cancer among Ashkenazi Jewish women who carry mutations in two breast cancer susceptibility genes, BRCA1 and BRCA2. One of the

"Rather than curing the disease, we plan to stop it from starting"

Ten years ago, Evelyn Lauder decided to commit her time, energy, and fund-raising savvy to help stamp out breast cancer. Seventy million dollars later, her foundation is supporting research that seems to be on the verge of cracking the mysteries of this disease. Stand by.... AMY BLUMENFELD reports.

ASK EVELYN LAUDER WHAT THE greatest surprise of the past decade has been for her, and without hesitation she'll say, "That it's really, really working."

"It" refers to the unstoppable ripple effect of her brainchild, the Breast Cancer Research Foundation (BCRF). "It" is the more than $70 million she and her team have raised over the past ten years to make prevention and cure a reality in their lifetime. "It" is a series of groundbreaking studies made possible by her foundation that are shedding light on everything from the role of nutrition in breast cancer to the 2,000 or more genes involved in the disease. And a large part of why "it" all is "really, really working" has to do with the fact that at least 85 cents of every dollar contributed to BCRF—which gets top

ratings from the American Institute of Philanthropy—goes directly to research, not administrative costs.

Lauder, senior corporate vice president of the Estée Lauder Companies, founded BCRF in 1993 after watching a video of cancer patients, who had lost their hair, undergoing cosmetic makeovers. Learning that about 40,000 women die of breast cancer every year, she created the foundation in the hopes of moving great scientific ideas from the lab to the bedside. "We want to find the seminal new hypotheses which, if evaluated and proven correct, can change the face of research," says BCRF's president, Myra J. Biblowit.

In its first year, the foundation awarded an average of $12,500 to each of eight investigators. In 2003, they funded 63

researchers' more significant findings is that for Jewish women with an inherited predisposition to breast cancer, exercising as a teenager can delay the onset of the disease.

Additional research notches in BCRF's belt include proof that retinoic acid, a derivative of vitamin A, can help stop the growth of breast cancer when combined with Herceptin or tamoxifen, and the development of a test to predict which tumors will respond to chemotherapy—the hope being to eliminate unnecessary treatment. So when do they expect a cure? "That's the $64,000 question, isn't it?" says Lauder, hedging on a time frame. But she does foresee the end of breast cancer. "Rather than curing the disease," she says, "we plan to stop it from starting." ●

O

Make a Connection

A young father is fatally shot, but his heart beats on in an older man's body. A teenage girl dies in a car crash, and four people get to live as a result. Are they grateful? Yes. Do they want to meet the donor's family? That's where it gets tricky. GRETCHEN REYNOLDS considers a new ethical question and listens in on reunions that range from deeply upsetting to mystical and life affirming.

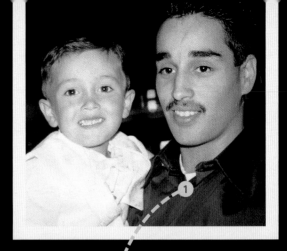

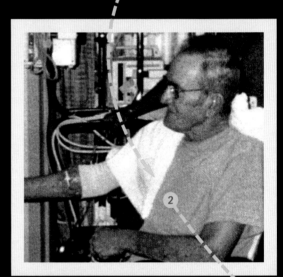

Heart to Heart
The Transplant Connection

MACK SCOGGINS IS NOT THE type to dither over his appearance, but in April 2003 he had uncharacteristic difficulty choosing what to wear to the ceremony of recognition, sponsored by the California Transplant Donor Network (CTDN). After consulting with his wife, Linda, he finally put on a brown corduroy suit jacket, an unstarched dress shirt, polished work boots, and a slightly strained smile. His palms were sheened with sweat.

Scoggins, 66, is a lean, gray-haired man, a retired electrician, quiet and courtly. Twenty years ago he had his first heart attack, and by January 2002 he was confined to a hospital cardiac unit in San Francisco, hooked to snaking coils of oxygen canisters, catheters, monitors, and IVs. Early in March, his family was told they should visit him for the last time. Although he was on the waiting list for a new heart, he was becoming too frail to remain a candidate. Then, with the dizzying suddenness of all transplants, a heart became available, and on March 23 he was rushed into surgery. His rehabilitation proceeded well, and Mack Scoggins, to his bewildered delight, was handed back his life. Eight weeks after the transplant, he danced at his eldest son's

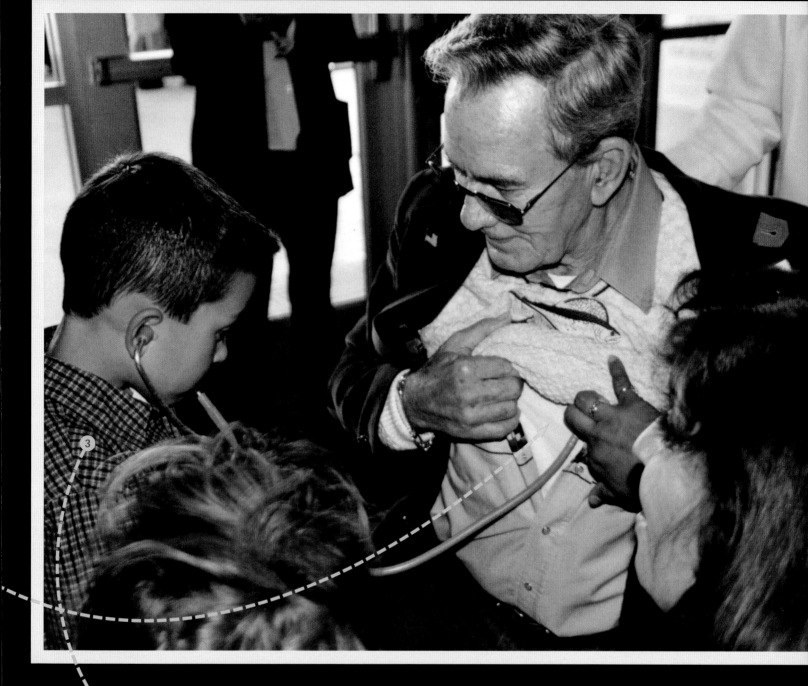

In a life-and-death match game, organ transplants are creating a whole new kind of kinship. (1) Mark Tornai Jr., with son Mark, was only 23 when he was fatally shot. His heart went to… (2) Mack Scoggins, 66, who in March 2002 was so ill, his family was told to visit for the last time. A year—and a miracle—later, Scoggins lets young Mark (3) listen to his father's heart. (4) Helen Genel, Mark's grandmother, can hear her son's vitality beating in the chest of… (5) Scoggins, in July 2004, well enough to take a fishing trip.

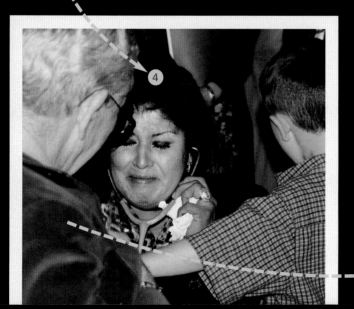

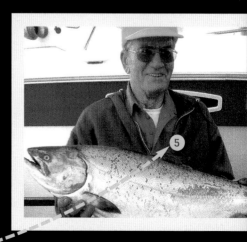

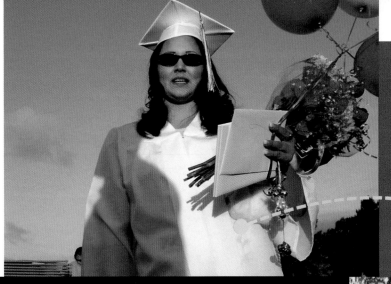

On June 13, 2002, Alica De La Grange (*left*) received her high school diploma. Six months later, she was brain dead, the victim of a car accident. Honoring her wishes, Alica's mother, Anna Kelly, donated her organs. One of them, a kidney, revived the ailing Merlando Espiritu (*below*), 55, who had been on dialysis for 15 years. When he and Anna met, he told her that after the surgery he developed a huge appetite and had so much energy. Says Anna: "It was like hearing someone describe Alica."

Merlando Espiritu fingers the scar over the kidney he got from Alica De La Grange. "I will always keep it safe," he tells her mother.

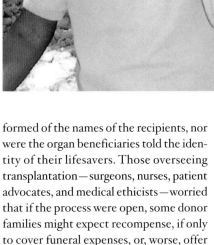

wedding. Photos from that day show him looking stalwart, flushed, and amazed.

Less than a year later, Linda, dressed in a practical cotton blouse and slacks, patted his arm as they stood in the foyer of Chabot College's Performing Arts Center in Hayward, California, watching a blonde woman approach. The woman whispered to the Scogginses and drew them toward a large group of people waiting nearby. Mack squared his shoulders and reached his hand toward the nearest person, a handsome Hispanic woman, who ignored his gesture and enveloped him in a grand, exuberant embrace. For an instant, Scoggins stiffened; then his eyes closed, his face relaxed, and he hugged her in return. Tears sparked on his cheeks. The heart of this woman's son is in Scoggins's chest.

In the past few years, meetings between organ-donor families and organ recipients have begun to increase, although such occurrences remain both rare and controversial. Some organ-transplant surgeons and advocates believe they are a mistake, prolonging grief or hindering healing. Others, although wary, accept that there might be benefits to the interactions. But by and large, the impetus for these meetings has come from the patients and relatives involved, who, like adoptees decades before them, have begun pushing for the right to understand the most hidden aspects of their family ties. In the process,

these pioneers are raising reverberant questions about what lingers of a person when he or she is gone, how expansive the notion of family can be, and what we mean by miracles.

Helen Genel released Scoggins from the hug and turned to a small boy who appeared to be 5 or 6 standing solemnly beside her, clutching a pink stethoscope. "Do you want to hear your daddy's heart now, Mark?" Genel asked. The boy nodded, his eyes wide, and watched in silence as Mack Scoggins unbuttoned his shirt. Glancing questioningly at his grandmother, Mark let her guide both the stethoscope and his ears into position, then listened, his brows knit. "Hear it?" Genel prodded. The crowd of watchers was tensely silent.

Mark looked up, his face inscrutable. He pulled away from the stethoscope and instantly placed his palm full upon Scoggins's chest, maintaining contact. "*Whoomp*," he whispered, imitating the sound he'd just heard, the beating of the heart of his 23-year-old father, Mark Tornai Jr., who'd died 13 months ago after being shot to death by an acquaintance. "It says *whoomp*."

ORGAN TRANSPLANTS FROM deceased donors first became medically possible in the 1960s, and from the onset, anonymity was central. Donor families weren't in-

formed of the names of the recipients, nor were the organ beneficiaries told the identity of their lifesavers. Those overseeing transplantation—surgeons, nurses, patient advocates, and medical ethicists—worried that if the process were open, some donor families might expect recompense, if only to cover funeral expenses, or, worse, offer organs to the highest bidder.

Then, too, there were thornier issues of human need. Grief is an abiding, unpredictable emotion. Would bereaved donor families really benefit from meeting the person whose life had been furthered as a consequence of their sorrow? Or would they be overcome by longing and despair? Would guilt consume the recipient? As Scoggins said after his encounter with

Genel, "What is the right thing to say? She lost her son. 'Thank you' isn't enough, not near enough. But what else is there?"

Such questions echo the concerns that surrounded adoptions before they were opened, says Lisa Colaianni, a donor family advocate at the Washington Regional Transplant Consortium and past chairperson of the Donor Family Services Council of the Association of Organ Procurement Organizations. "Most experts worried that the negative consequences of adopted children meeting their biological mothers would outweigh any positive results. It was the same with organ transplants." So for 30 years, if a donor wished to write to a recipient or vice versa, any identifying details, no matter how innocuous, were usually blacked out.

By the mid-1990s, however, a smattering of people began to question such high security. "Some of the donor families wondered why they'd been considered emotionally strong enough to donate their loved ones' organs but not strong enough to contact the person who'd received that gift," Colaianni says. "They thought they should have the right to decide for themselves whether it was a good idea or not."

Her agency's first attempt at breaching the wall between donors and recipients came in 1993, when a woman asked to meet the recipient of her husband's heart. Colaianni forwarded the request to the transplant center, which returned it with the terse comment that, as she remembers, "the guys didn't think it was a good idea." "The guys" were the transplant surgeons. There would be no meeting at that time.

Over the next few years, a tiny number of families in the D.C. area managed to contact one another surreptitiously—through newspaper accounts, Colaianni assumes. No dire consequences followed. When Colaianni found out, she wasn't surprised. "In my experience, people who choose to donate their loved ones' organs tend to be more spiritual on average," she says. "For them, there's something life affirming in knowing more about the recipients. Seeing them gives hope, not pain."

She pauses. "But meetings or even a written contact are not for everyone. I've seen cases in which it was not a good idea. Unfortunately, the process is completely ad hoc. There aren't any mandated or even consistent national guidelines." Meanwhile the number of meetings is slowly but inexorably increasing.

TO DATE, NO AGENCY KEEPS tabs on how many people nationwide have met because they share a connection to an organ. Transplantation as a medical procedure is tightly regulated; its aftermath is not.

The CTDN, which coordinates organ procurement in parts of California and Nevada and provides counseling and support for the affected families, is one of the few transplant organizations in the nation that officially helps willing participants meet. Many other organ procurement organizations have informally loosened their rules, passing messages to recipients'

> "I thought it could make her happy to see how good I am doing, how much her daughter has done for me."

counselors and, if both sides are interested, setting up introductions. "The process absolutely must be consensual on both sides," says Anne Paschke, spokesperson for the United Network for Organ Sharing (UNOS), the umbrella organization for all local networks, which agrees that it won't stand in the way if families want to meet. "Not everyone is ready at the same time, and some people are never ready. They cannot be forced and shouldn't even be nudged."

Overall, the donor side tends to want the meetings; the recipients and doctors are more reluctant. "I've been to support meetings for transplant patients," says Eileen Johnson, a former intensive care nurse and the Family Care Services Department manager for the CTDN. "Time after time they say, 'I just can't meet the donor family. I feel so guilty.'" In those cases, negotiations end. But if both sides do express a wish to interact, says Johnson, "we'll try to make things happen."

FOR ANNA KELLY, 40, THE possibility of meeting the recipients of her daughter's organs became a way to sustain herself through her grief. A former corporate buyer who is now a full-time mother to her two surviving children, she sits in the living room of her airy stone home in affluent Cupertino, California, while golden retrievers bound in the backyard. The house is filled with family photos and the construction detritus of an ongoing renovation. Despite the comfy, idyllic setting, normalcy ended a few days before Christmas 2002, when Kelly's eldest daughter, Alica, 19, was in an automobile accident outside San Francisco. "We knew she was brain dead," Kelly says. "I watched the doctors do the tests. I knew that she would never wake up. But her heart was still beating. I could put my hand on her chest and feel it. To think that my beautiful girl was leaving me…" Kelly's voice cracks, but she regains a practiced calm. "She had just gotten her own place, and on Friday we were going to go shopping for her first Christmas tree. Then Friday came, and we're in the emergency room."

Complying with Alica's wishes, Kelly donated her daughter's organs. Her kidneys, pancreas, liver, lungs, and heart were transplanted successfully.

Within weeks, Kelly began to think about the possibility of contacting the recipients. "We usually advise donor families to wait at least a year," says Cherry Wise, PhD, a clinical psychologist in Kentfield, California, and a consultant to the CTDN and UNOS. "The Victorians were onto something," she continues, referring to their prescribed period of formal mourning, which lasted more than a year. "It takes that long for most people to begin to come to terms with the depth and finality of their loss."

But Kelly's desire was so heartfelt and her grief unalloyed with any apparent hope of her child somehow reappearing that her counselors at the CTDN agreed she might be ready. Cautioning that those who received the organs might not be, they agreed to pass her request to the recipient networks. (The original communications must be forwarded from the center, since the two families don't exchange names and addresses unless both agree.)

Kelly immediately set about writing each of the recipients a three-page letter describing Alica in loving, wrenching detail and ending: "I don't want you ever to feel guilty about my daughter. She gave you a second chance to live. Cherish this and please enjoy a longer, healthier life with your families and live on to fulfill your dreams." The intention of the letter, Kelly says, was to let them know "how lucky they were to have that person in them."

Almost immediately, a reply came from one of the recipients, Merlando Espiritu, 55, of nearby Milpitas, California. In a coincidence that struck Kelly as wondrous and eerie, he was also a corporate buyer and had a daughter who worked as a clerk at a JCPenney store Kelly frequented. He'd been on kidney dialysis for 15 years, he wrote her. But since the surgery, he'd felt reborn. His entire extended family was so grateful. Separately, his elderly mother e-mailed Kelly her own fervid thanks. In his response, Espiritu begged to meet Kelly, despite how recent his surgery and her loss were.

Letter in hand, she went to her coordinator at the transplant network and said, in essence, please.

LISA COLAIANNI OF THE Washington, D.C., transplant network estimates that her agency oversees fewer than ten introductions a year. At CTDN's donor recognition ceremony in 2004, only three meetings took place—down from six in 2002, when of the 227 families donating that year, only 50 even got letters or other acknowledgments from their organ recipients.

This attitude confounds Espiritu, who was eager to meet the mother of the girl whose kidney he now carries. "I thought it could maybe make her happy to see how good I am doing, how much good her daughter has done for me," he says. Voluble and insistent, with an energy partly fueled by despair—his daughter suffers from the same hereditary, kidney-destroying polycystic kidney disease he has—Espiritu harried the patient advocates at his transplant center until they sent his reply to Kelly's letter.

THE INTRODUCTION OF Kelly and Espiritu at CTDN's ceremony of recognition in April 2003 was stirring, if almost wordless. She wore a drapey white silk blouse, her hair fussed into a neat ponytail. "Most of the time, people treat these meetings like a blind date," says

> Inevitably, there's a story of how the donor loved cheesecake or okra, which the recipient never did—until after the surgery.

Colaianni. "They get nervous. They get all dressed up. They want to look their best." He had dragged out his finest suit for the occasion. Both sides had brought along small entourages, and the two groups, guided together by a CTDN coordinator at the Performing Arts Center's theater—where Scoggins and Genel embraced nearby—were as tentative as shy teenagers. Kelly cleared her throat. Espiritu started to speak, then changed his mind and, without preamble, hugged her. His wife and mother hugged her. He hugged her mother.

The whole crew, grouped in a tight circle, passed photos of Alica and of Espiritu looking wan and neurasthenic before surgery and ruddy now. At one point, he pulled up his shirt and fingered his scar, telling Kelly how he holds a hand protectively over the kidney while he drives. "I will always keep it safe," he declared.

Later Kelly marvels at their easy camaraderie and at the connection that she felt, through him, with her daughter. "Merlando told me that after the surgery he developed a big appetite and had so much energy," she says. "It was like hearing someone describe Alica. She loved to eat, and she had so much energy." Kelly sniffs and smiles. "Something of her still exists on this earth, thanks to Merlando. I am so grateful to him."

THE HUMAN URGE TO rationalize tragedy, to give it meaning and weight, is potent. So, too, is the longing to connect, as a poet or two have pointed out. What gives exceptional resonance to the meetings between those who've lost someone they love and those who harbor a piece of the departed is that, there, these needs seem to mesh and in some portion be answered. Time and again, the two groups speak afterward of their sense of "reunion," of "familiarity," of "meeting a long-lost family member." They reverently mention the portentous-seeming parallels between the donor and recipient: Both like fishing, say, or the color red. Inevitably, there's a story of how the donor loved cheesecake or okra, which the recipient never did—until after the surgery.

"These encounters can be quite beautiful," says Cherry Wise. "They provide a validation of the sense that the loved one's life had a purpose." The organ donation enabled someone else to go on with life. "That idea," she continues, "becomes more solid when you see the person. It can be fortifying for the organ recipients as well, to see that their health, their life, isn't resented, that it can give joy."

Not all meetings end with such transporting emotion, though, even with good intentions all around. Last year, after a 20-something man in Oakland lost his mother, he asked to meet the woman who'd inherited her heart. With the assistance of the CTDN, he did, and soon started telephoning her, insinuating himself into her life. "It seemed as if he wanted Mom back," Eileen Johnson says. "We'd worried beforehand that he wasn't really ready, that he hadn't come to terms with the reality of his mother's death. But he assured us he was fine, and he's a grown-up, so we made the arrangements. It was a mistake." The woman eventually sat him down and kindly but firmly discussed boundaries.

"For those of us working with the families, our biggest concerns are when someone is overwhelmed by their grief," Wise says, "or when they don't seem to have come to terms with the irrevocability of their loss. If they are looking for a replacement, that raises a red flag. No one can be that, and certainly not an organ recipient."

Johnson recalls a mother from Northern California whose teenage son was killed two years ago. When she was introduced to the boy's heart recipient a year later, she reached toward him and was undone by grief. At least that's what it seemed like. "Afterward," Johnson remembers with a slight, bemused smile, "she told me that the experience had been wonderful."

If it's difficult to predict and assess the emotional reaction to a meeting, almost as troubling is the disappointment of people who feel ready to meet but are turned down by the recipients. "When stories start coming out about families meeting, we get a spike of interest from others," Colaianni says. "They always say, 'I didn't know this was even possible. Can I do it?' But not everyone is willing."

COLLEEN BAPTISTA, A HOUSE-wife and mother in Millbrae, California, knows what it's like to be rejected. When her 20-year-old son, Tim, died three and a half years ago after slipping from a cliff in Santa Barbara (he and some college friends had been drinking and playing around), she donated his organs and soon afterward wrote to the recipients. "I told the wife of the heart recipient, who I knew was an older man, to be patient with him if he started flirting with 20-year-olds. That would be Tim." The kidney and pancreas recipients responded with gentle missives saying thank you. But from the heart recipient, there was silence. "I know it must be hard [for the recipients]. They must feel guilt for surviving," Baptista said in the spring of 2003. "But I don't begrudge them their life. I am so happy for their families. It's just that I would give anything," she choked slightly, "anything to feel that heart one more time."

Johnson says they will never make someone participate. "And we will never forbid someone, even when we think it's a bad idea. We can only offer strong advice. What I hope is that as we do this more often, we'll understand better who will benefit and who won't."

As it turned out, Baptista found a reprieve from her grief when, in June 2004, the recipient of her son's heart agreed to meet. "I was able to hug him and feel the heart beat," she says. "It was unbelievable." The man even played in a golf tournament honoring Tim.

> ## "I was able to hug him and feel the heart beat. It was unbelievable."

The word that comes to mind for me is *acceptance,*" says Vicente Agor, who received a kidney and pancreas from Mark Tornai Jr., the same young father who provided Mack Scoggins's heart. Agor's severe diabetes disappeared with the surgery, but his anxiety didn't. "So much of the process of transplant surgery is about organ rejection," he says. "You take pills against rejection. You worry about it. But it's such a negative concept. I hated thinking about it. I wanted to be surrounded by acceptance. And from the minute I met Helen and her family, that's what I felt."

Agor, 42, was introduced to Helen Genel, little Mark, and 24 other members of their extended family at the donor ceremony, where he also shook hands with Scoggins. "I was a little worried beforehand," Agor admits, "thinking it might be awkward. But it could not have been easier. In 30 seconds, we were chattering away, gossiping about *American Idol.* Me and my partner; my minister, Mack, and his wife; Helen and her huge group—it felt like family, an odd family, maybe, but family." Formerly a financial adviser, Agor had quit his job when he became ill and begun his own jewelry-design business. At the ceremony, he gave Genel a necklace he'd created featuring a dove-shaped pearl. She exclaimed and became teary, saying the first gift Mark Jr. ever bought her, as a child, was a necklace. And at his funeral, they'd released doves. "Maybe those signs don't mean anything," Agor says today. "But I choose to believe they do. There's something so big in all of this."

ARE THE BONDS FORMED during these interactions lasting? No one knows. The process is too new. Many of those involved profess a hope that the connections will be "lifelong," in the words of Anna Kelly. But Eileen Johnson is skeptical. "In my experience, most families only meet the one time," she says. "They think there will be more, but they wind up getting what they hoped for from that single encounter, and that's fine. The donor families just want to see the person once and make some type of connection, maybe even touch them and feel where the organ is, especially if it's the heart."

Back at the donor ceremony, Genel waited patiently for young Mark to finish with the stethoscope before moving almost greedily into his place. The knobs in her ears, she appeared incandescent with wonder. "As a mother, you know that sound so well," she'll say later. "I heard it when he was inside me, and I felt it when he was a little boy sleeping. And then I felt it on his deathbed. It was the last thing I felt, before he was taken away from me. And now to hear it again, as strong as ever. It's a miracle."

Mack Scoggins rebuttoned his shirt and turned to Genel. "Your son must have had a great heart," he said quietly, "to have had so many people love him. I am so very sorry for your loss. And I, uh, I thank you." By nature reserved, he hesitated for an instant, then wrapped her in another sturdy embrace. It was, she would later say, exactly the way Mark used to hug. ●

Nancy Pelosi's Aha! Moment

She was the only female in a room full of men. So why did the veteran congresswoman find herself flanked by so many cheering women?

IN OCTOBER 2001, I BECAME the first woman elected to the top leadership of either house of Congress. I'd been involved in politics my entire life and in Congress, at that point, for 14 years. I ran for Democratic whip, the second-highest-ranking Democrat in the House of Representatives (now I'm the Democratic leader). When I won, I was flooded with congratulations from all over the country, many of them from women who were excited that we'd broken through this marble ceiling into the highest reaches of government. I was honored.

Shortly after my election, the top congressional leaders were invited to the White House for a meeting with the president to talk about the agenda for the next session of Congress. I'd been there on many occasions, so I wasn't particularly apprehensive. But when the door closed behind us, I saw that there were very few other people at the table with the president, and of course they were all men. It occurred to me that this was unlike any meeting that I'd ever attended at the White House. In fact, because a woman was there as a top elected leader and not as staff, it was unlike any meeting ever held at the White House.

It was really quite profound. I realized the opportunity that I had, and it was poignant because it made me think, *Why did it take this long?* It sounds strange, but as I sat down, I felt that I was not alone. For an instant, I felt as though Susan B. Anthony, Lucretia Mott, Elizabeth Cady Stanton—everyone who'd fought for women's right to vote and for the empowerment of women in politics, in their professions, and in their lives—were there with me in the room. Those women were the ones who had done the heavy lifting, and it was as if they were saying, *At last we have a seat at the table.*

The president welcomed me and congratulated me on my election, but no one at the meeting said anything about the historical significance of the occasion. And I didn't make the point because I thought it would be appropriate for everything to be as normal as possible. But my thought was, *We want more.* I felt uplifted, as if I were seeing over the top of a mountain. And to tell you the truth, we can handle it: Women can breathe the air at these altitudes, we can do the job that needs to be done, and the day will come when we'll have a woman president of the United States. I'm sure it will happen soon.

Then the meeting began, and we got down to business. ●

Pelosi: The top-ranking Democrat in Congress broke through the marble ceiling.

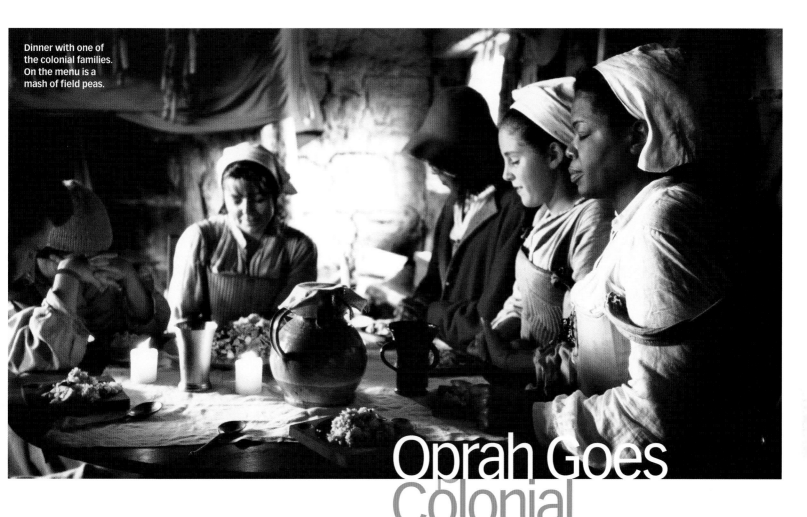

Dinner with one of the colonial families. On the menu is a mash of field peas.

Oprah Goes Colonial

Oprah and her best friend, Gayle King, spent two days roughing it in the phoneless, braless, plumbing-free 17th century on *Colonial House,* PBS's answer to reality shows. How'd they like it? OPRAH tells it like it was.

NO TOILET PAPER, NO TELEPHONE, NO shower—no problem? At a simulated colony in Maine, 26 people braved 17th-century life for five months. In September 2003, I joined them for a day and a half.

The year reenacted: 1628, when settlers arrived to eke out an existence in New England. The participants: men, women, and children—selected from nearly 10,000 applicants willing to give up beepers for bonnets—who would eventually appear in the PBS series *Colonial House.* The first Puritan African sojourners to pass through the colony: my (reluctant) best friend, Gayle King, and yours truly.

For me, the road back to 1628 is a familiar one—it runs parallel to the outhouses, smokehouses, and farmlands of my hometown in Kosciusko, Mississippi. My grandmother and I lived on a small plot of land, in a house with no running water or toilet. I don't care how many bathrooms I've had since, I've never forgotten the outhouse. With no TV, I tried entertaining myself by making speeches to the cows and playing with my homemade corncob doll, whose hair I'd comb while longing for one with real, pretty hair. We grew everything we ate, and each morning my job was to get water from the well and feed the hogs. *So how different,* I thought, *could* Colonial House *be from my own childhood?* If your name is Gayle King, stunningly different. "I grew up with a toilet—*and* a maid," she reminds me as we land in Maine.

Aha moment number one: Hand over the panties

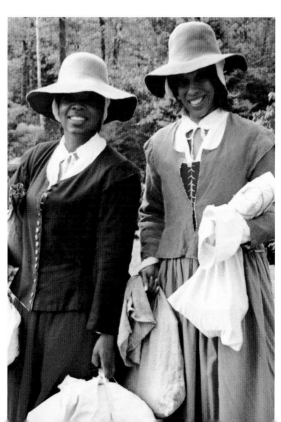

Oprah and Gayle arrive with gifts of ham, sugar, and cheese.

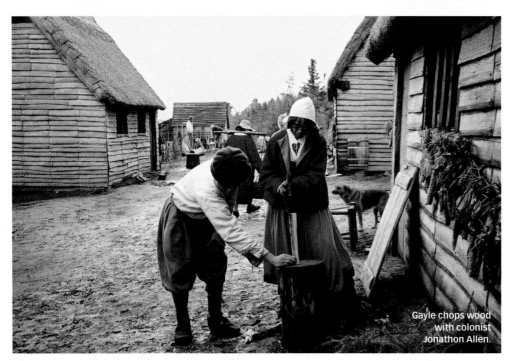

Gayle chops wood with colonist Jonathon Allen.

As our hosts show us to their one-room cabin, they fill us in on the daily challenges: Endless wood chopping. Sparse food. Isolation. Filthy clothing.

and bras. Seventeenth-century women didn't wear them. As we exchange our clothes for authentic garments (including uncomfortable corsets), the PBS producers present us with the settlers' codes of conduct. The Sabbath was to be strictly observed. Profanity, infidelity, promiscuity, and insurrection were punishable by whipping. Women were to obey their husbands, stay silent in public meetings, and keep their heads covered as a sign of submission. If a woman was spotted outside without her cap, she could receive a scarlet letter from the governor, then be tied to a stake for two hours. "Nobody better tie me to a stake," I whisper to Gayle, "or they are gonna see a real African Puritan." Gayle, still adjusting to pantielessness, tries not to crack up.

Gayle and I are given shoes that feel like they're made for two left feet ("Your feet will form to them," a producer says) as well as our roles in the story. I'm the wife of a governor, and Gayle is my widowed sister; we're passing through the colony to get herbs to take back to our ill shipmates. In exchange for the goods and a place to lodge, we bear gifts—a huge ham, some sugar, and a wheel of cheese. We're to stay

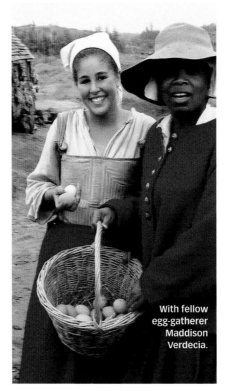

With fellow egg-gatherer Maddison Verdecia.

with John Voorhees (in real life, a carpet salesman); his wife, Michelle Rossi-Voorhees (a seamstress who runs her own business); their 11-year-old son, Giacomo;

and their dog, Chloe. In 1628 the Voorhees represent a middle-class family who sailed here from England to create a new life.

AS THE VOORHEES THANK US profusely for the ham, sugar, and cheese ("You saved us!" they keep saying) and show us to their one-room cabin, they fill us in on the daily challenges: Endless wood chopping. Sparse food. Isolation. Fear of wild animals. Filthy clothing.

"It's amazing how what may initially seem like an utterly desperate existence can seamlessly morph into a surprisingly tolerable way of life," Julia Friese, who took a leave from her job at a children's museum in Philadelphia, later says of her role as an indentured servant. "Bathing once a week, at most, and sanitation standards that would make even a fraternity boy blush all become just normal."

Each day the women cook with a fistful of scarce ingredients: eggs, flour, sugar, rice, and vegetables they've planted. Over an open fire that has been burning since daybreak (in the 1600s, it was a woman's job to keep the fire going), we roast the fresh green beans and carrots we picked. I chop wood and gather eggs from the henhouse (did I say I'd done this before?), and Gayle milks a goat—the perfect job for someone who, having never been a drinker, is known to ask a bartender, "Got milk?" Later we eat our meal with crudely shaped spoons. In 1628 commoners didn't use forks.

Nighttime brings a "colonial jamboree"—yippee yi yo. To kick things off, the women line up across from the men for a dance—two steps up, two steps back, then lift and swing your partner. Have you ever tried to lift and swing a braless, 5'10" black woman? Apparently, Gayle's partner hadn't, either. He hoisted her into the air and landed her on her backside, feet heavenward.

As for our accommodations, I wasn't anticipating the Four Seasons, but I also had no idea that I'd be sharing a loft with Gayle *and* Giacomo. After the three of us mount the rickety ladder to our individual mattresses, we're in for the night—a night so dark that I can close my eyes and open them again to see the same pitch-black.

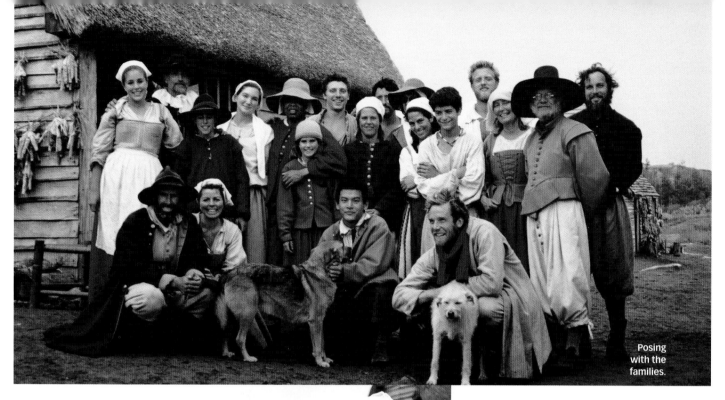

Posing with the families.

Without a watch, my only reference to time is my body's internal clock: For years I've always awakened to use the bathroom between 3:15 and 3:30 A.M. When I get up for my early morning squat in the bushes, Gayle—who has been holding it for hours because she's too scared to make her way down that ladder alone in the dark—braves the climb and the rain with me. Back in the loft, I whisper to Gayle, "Don't you just love the sound of the rain?" "No, I don't," she groans, still annoyed because she forgot to take her "toilet paper"—a big leaf—with her. "Did you hear little feet scurrying?" she asks. "That's just Chloe, the dog," I say. "So Chloe is up on the roof?" she shoots back. "If a mouse drops in from the ceiling," I say, "it's over for me." We snicker, trying not to wake up Mom and Dad Voorhees below, and give in to restless sleep again...until the cockle-doodle-dooing begins.

T'S SUNDAY MORNING, AND GAYLE and I arrive at church (in the same clothes) for a service filled with traditional hymns and a brief sermon about the spirit of community. There's been trouble in the colony surrounding the church requirement: One family resisted being forced to go and was verbally reprimanded by the minister—a punishment surely less harsh than a real settler would have received.

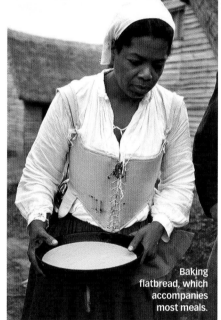

Baking flatbread, which accompanies most meals.

For five months, the lay preacher's wife, Carolyn Heinz—whose real job is anthropology professor—had the challenge of avoiding upsets over the strict codes that made women voiceless. "Being a 17th-century colonist was possibly the hardest time of my life," she said after filming ended. "It will always be a part of me—a brief, tough stretching of my imagination back to my ancestors' experience of the New World." Dominic Muir, a private tutor from London who served as a quartermaster, said, "I witnessed the resilience of the human spirit in the face of adversity, the power of prayer, being so happy with such little stuff—and finding log fires better to watch than television. I felt close to God—and close to peas and oats. It was humbling and fantastic, and I miss it." Back home in California, Carolyn, the preacher's wife, can't quite use the word *miss*. She says, "I'm glad I did it—and I'm glad it's over."

Me, too, Carolyn—after even less than two days. "We don't have to stay another night, do we?" Gayle asks after church. Our hair still smelling of smoke, we head home, more appreciative than ever of all the luxuries we sometimes overlook—and giving thanks for all the shoulders we stand upon. None of us can store food in a freezer, turn on a stove, fill up a gas tank, or soak in a bathtub without that recognition. We are who we are because someone brave walked before us.

Could you and I have survived in 1628? Sure. But the miracle is that we don't have to. Some other courageous woman already did. It is on that woman's behalf—a woman silenced by the edicts of her time—that we can speak. We can disagree. We can build, we can choose, we can own ourselves. And more than 300 years after the first colonists sailed in, we can choose whether to go to church or not, we can worship as we please—or we can lounge in bed on a Sunday morning, wearing the very cutest underwear. ●

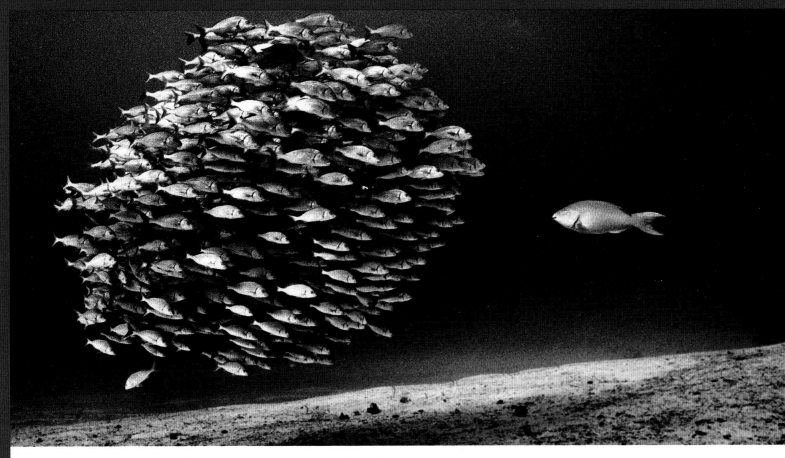

FEELING ADRIFT?

You say you'd love to have closer friendships, stronger (less stressful) family ties, deeper roots in the community, a significant other who could read your mind? Join the crowd. Here, nine ways to reach out and connect to your world. **Gretchen Reynolds** reports.

MOST OF US KNOW THE EMPTY, tinny, sometimes unbearable feeling of being alone or left out. Maybe our spouse has grown distant. Or no one seems to invite us to lunch or parties. Perhaps we are socially inept, shy, lonely, spiritually adrift, purposeless. One way or another, we're disconnected, unplugged from the sources that nourish us.

It goes without saying that connection is essential to happiness, and science has confirmed its importance to our physical health. But what can we do when the lines of communication fray? How does one go about feeling closer to others or reclaiming a sense of belonging? To find out, *O* approached experts in psychology, medicine, religion, linguistics, ethics—even a political scientist who's studied the power of picnics—and asked them to lead us through some of the more common trouble spots. Here is their guide.

■ You're single and you've met someone intriguing, but you don't feel an immediate "click." Should you get romantically involved anyway?

THE CLICK IS TRICKY. MORE THAN sexual attraction, it involves a lightning-strike sense of familiarity and an uncanny feeling of being understood. Unfortunately, it can be illusory. And while many a successful marriage has started with "we just clicked," this is not a reliable way to forecast lasting romance.

Often the sudden, flooding sense of completion results because we may be unconsciously "trying to make up for a deficiency we feel within ourselves," says Lisa Firestone, PhD, a clinical psychologist, lecturer, and coauthor of *Creating a Life of Meaning and Compassion: The Wisdom of Psychotherapy* and *Conquer Your Critical Inner Voice*. "A quiet man may be powerfully

drawn to a talkative, gregarious woman. The sexual chemistry can be incredibly strong." But later the very characteristics that attracted us may gradually start to repel us because they are, in their way, a reminder of what we (at least in some small corner of our minds) fear that we lack. For some people, the quest to find a lasting passion whose urgency never abates is an excuse to stay single. This "is a common and very effective means of protecting yourself from intimacy," Firestone says: No relationship can measure up.

A better guide to the potential of a new relationship is to ask yourself whether being with the other person is more enjoyable than not. Was your original conversation amusing, intellectually stimulating, challenging, even memorably adversarial or odd? Then it is worth pursuing. Physical intimacy differentiates our central, partnered relationship from all others, but the desire needn't be instantaneous. It can grow, often from the most mundane contact. How many women have noted how sexy a man is when he's doing laundry.

"My grandparents met at the altar," says Rachel Naomi Remen, MD, clinical professor of family and community medicine at the University of California–San Francisco School of Medicine and author of *Kitchen Table Wisdom* and *My Grandfather's Blessings.* But over the course of a 50-plus-year marriage and four children, they fell passionately in love. "Everyone who knew them describes them as inseparable," Remen says. "Their love was the foundation of all their children's families."

You feel attached to your immediate family and friends but not to your community, the nation, the broader human family. Does that matter?

WELCOME TO THE CLUB. IN THE past 30 years, the number of Americans who've become members of a group, any group—the PTA, the Elks club, the NAACP, church congregations, Girl Scouts, bowling leagues—has plummeted. "We rarely gather anymore," says Robert D. Putnam, PhD, the Malkin professor of public policy at Harvard University and author of *Bowling Alone,* a landmark book that examined 30 years of data about American civic involvement, and coauthor of *Better Together: Restoring the American Community.* Voting participation is also way down. We invite neighbors over for dinner 45 percent less often than in the 1970s.

Such disengagement does matter. "The best predictor of a low crime rate in a neighborhood is when most of the people know their neighbors' first names," Putnam says. Health suffers, too, when we cut ourselves off from others. "Your chances of dying in the next 12 months are halved by joining a group," he says. "Social isolation is as big a risk factor for death as smoking."

Happily, societal alienation is tractable; each of us can tackle it. If you have children, just attend your local school's next PTA meeting, Putnam says. Invite your friends to a cookout or lunch in the park. "There's a relatively new scientific discipline about happiness," he says. "It shows

that money can increase happiness, but not by much. By far the strongest component of happiness is how connected you are." Merely going on picnics has been found to increase a person's contentment by about 15 percent over those who never dine alfresco at all.

Turn off the television, too. The drop in American civic participation is closely tied to the period in the early 1960s when household TV ownership reached 90 percent. Participation in youth sports is also down dramatically across the country. "Instead of watching the football game on Sunday, go outside and play football with your kids," Putnam says. "This isn't like telling you to eat your broccoli. It's more like 'take two parties and call me in the morning.' America would be a happier, healthier, more prosperous place if we connected—one to another. That's a scientific fact." (For lots of specific suggestions about participating in your community, school, neighborhood, and nation, see bettertogether.org, run by the Saguaro Seminar on Civic Engagement in America at Harvard University.)

But you don't enjoy groups. In fact, you'd rather be by yourself most of the time. Should you try to make yourself more social? How?

THE GOOD NEWS ABOUT THE SCI- ence of connections is that "some people just don't need very many," says Peter D. Kramer, MD, a clinical professor of psychiatry at Brown University and the author of *Listening to Prozac* and *Should You Leave?* In many cases, one or two close relationships can be sustaining and sufficient.

"Psychiatry has come back to an interest in innate temperament," says Kramer, and experts believe that certain people are born shy or introverted. This doesn't mean they're stunted or socially maladroit. In *Solitude: A Return to the Self,* the late British psychiatrist Anthony Storr points out that creativity is often linked to seclusion. Henry James, Beatrix Potter, Franz Kafka, Beethoven—all were loners (though not all were content; Kafka claimed to want to marry but couldn't bear the thought of a wife actually watching him write).

The notion that aloneness entails loneliness is particularly American, says

Rachel Naomi Remen. "In many other cultures, silence and solitude are accepted and built into the days." Not only does imagination thrive but contemplation is easier when the mind is uninterrupted by the activity of others. Perhaps, Remen suggests, we should wonder about the person who can never be alone: "We all need time to hear ourselves."

That said, if you're cloistered in your home, day in and day out, or just too drained to see anyone, those could be signs that you may be depressed and should talk to a therapist. Sometimes just making yourself get out to meet a friend or attend an event can help your mood. For any introvert who decides to brave a party, Kramer says, "start small. Find one person to talk to." Introduce yourself. Ask innocuous questions about family and work. Ask follow-up questions. Even within the hubbub, you can remain focused and centered and enjoy the company of another.

"Social isolation is as big a risk factor for death as smoking."

Your partner has grown emotionally distant. Or you've come to take each other for granted. There's no hostility, but not much intimacy either. How to draw closer?

THANKFULLY, EMOTIONAL SPACE is relative and any distance may have more to do with how the two of you define intimacy than the way you feel. "Some people believe that the closer you are, the more you can be together without talking," says Deborah Tannen, PhD, professor of linguistics at Georgetown University and author of the groundbreaking 1990 work on male-female communication *You Just Don't Understand.* "Other people, often women, think that the closer you are, the more you talk." Both camps desire intimacy, but in a different fashion. "He may want to come home and not speak, since home is his refuge. She feels he's being withdrawn and uncommunicative," Tannen says. She asks questions. He feels pressed. She feels rebuffed. The schism grows.

"In therapy, we talk about relational currencies," says Kathleen Galvin, PhD, professor of communication studies at Northwestern University and a family therapist. "Those are the ways people have learned to express affection, whether by saying 'I love you' or giving gifts or going for a drive to spend time together." If, like bordering nations, two parties employ different currencies, transactions tangle, skirmishes erupt, cold wars set in. When one

writing a book about morality and child rearing. "In my opinion, there are no childless people," she says. "We all have responsibility for children." No one, even if he or she wishes it, can be disconnected from the next generation. We leave our marks, direct or subtle, on our children, our neighbors' children, and our nation's children.

"But there are other ways to leave something behind," says Galvin. "The wish to project oneself into the unseen future, to outlast mortality, is fundamental to human nature and prompts many of our most

forces our own harsh internal judgments and distances us from people who might offer a more positive opinion. The voice whispers that your coworkers would never enjoy your company anyway.

"When I have a patient who complains about being snubbed," Firestone says, "I ask her to look back to the moment just before. Did she do anything to provoke the other person?" For instance, when the women at the office were gathering to go out for lunch, were you hunched over your desk, looking defensive? Or if a neighbor passes you on the street, do you barely just nod before hurrying on your way?

To change the dynamics, you must be active, courageous, and willing to risk rejection. Go up and talk to a neighbor or colleague, says Firestone. "Your inner voice may scream at you to stop, but you have to persevere." Invite the very person who seemed to reject you to lunch, to a party, on a walk. People are generally kinder than we suppose.

And if not, shrug, smile, and move on, remembering that rude people have intimacy issues, too—there are plenty of others who would definitely appreciate your company.

> The way to experience spirituality is through the heart. Look around and ask, "Who needs me?"

person says, "I love you," and the other responds, "Let's go for a drive," "neither person is likely to feel satisfied."

To close the distance, try becoming an in-home anthropologist. Note when you most long to talk. Is it in the evenings, when the children are finally in bed? Is that when he's most apt to be mute? Are the silences between you tense or contented? "If you need to have conversations with your partner to feel connected, tell him," Tannen says. But listen, too. Recognizing that he might have a separate approach to intimacy can be, in its way, intimate. Ask whether you could sit quietly together, maybe listening to music (a different communion than conversation, but also valid) for half an hour or so; then take the next half hour to just talk to each other.

▣ You have no children and feel left out of the regenerative circle of life.

"CHILDREN ARE OUR ENTRÉE INTO the future," says therapist Kathleen Galvin, who is a mother of three. They're also a way to extend our youth, as anyone who has played hide-and-seek or shared Goldfish crackers with a toddler knows.

The urge to connect to a child meshes nicely with what is, fundamentally, a duty, according to Rebekah Miles, PhD, an associate professor of ethics at Southern Methodist University in Dallas, who is

lasting endeavors. Artists are often motivated by this impulse. Those who command the building of skyscrapers—especially those who attach their own names to them—know the feeling of generativity."

So take up painting, woodworking, or quilting. Or get involved with other people's children. "You can volunteer at a library or the Boys and Girls Club," says Galvin. "Or tutor. I have students who have remained a part of my life for decades." And if, after all of this, you still need more interaction with children, Miles, the mother of two young girls, has a suggestion. "Call me," she says. "I can always use babysitting help."

▣ You're in high school, the girl with no date to the prom. Only it's now and the neighbors are the ones having parties and not inviting you. Or your colleagues are going to lunch while you sit alone at your desk. You feel excluded.

IT DOESN'T TAKE MUCH FOR MOST women to start fretting about being unlikable. "There's a little voice inside each of us that is constantly judging and finding us inadequate," says psychologist Lisa Firestone, who has spent her career studying that phenomenon. This self-hectoring tape, your hypercritical inner parent, is extremely difficult to ignore, she says. It guides many of us into behavior that rein-

▣ You're forced to spend time with someone who irritates or bores you: a stepfather, your brother's new wife, your boss. How do you find common ground?

FIRST THE PRACTICAL SOLUTION. When you're confronted with a person you're connected to but feel no connection with, try this simple tactic: Pretend you're a talk show host or reporter and interview her. Ask questions. Listen. Ask more. Let your questions slide from the general to the gently personal. "It's sometimes astonishing what you will learn when you let people talk about themselves," says Deborah Tannen. "They become more animated, more interesting, when they're bathed in the spotlight of your interest." We all want to be heard, to be seen, and for ourselves, not as the boss or sister-in-law or whatever role the other person knows us in. "When you learn about people's struggles—what their hopes are, their dreams—this allows you to find the common ground," says Remen.

It's also worth considering, says Lisa Firestone, whether your original assessment of this person—boring, annoying, grating—is based on your own anxieties. Perhaps a part of you worries that your brother, now engaged, will have less time for you. Your resentment colors your opinion of his fiancée, even before you ever meet her.

This expectation of dislike can develop its own self-fulfilling momentum. When she first introduces herself, you may react a little coolly. She rightly reads your response as scorn and draws back. You find her even more unpleasant. The underlying issue, meanwhile, has nothing at all to do with her. Next time, Firestone suggests, "look at her directly, make eye contact." Try to see her as an individual, not an impediment to your desires.

If all of this querying—of the other person, of yourself—fails to improve the connection, there's a philosophical stance, a certain perspective you can adopt. Remen recalls a psychiatrist who when asked how he could work with someone he didn't like, said, "Ah, everyone, at depth, is beautiful. Remembering this can soften your judgment." Though we've heard it before, Firestone urges us to have compassion—even toward people who seem very different. "It's hard to hurt those with whom we feel we share something," she says. "If nothing else, we all have our imperfect humanity in common."

You aren't a member of an organized religion but yearn for spirituality in your life.
VIRTUALLY EVERYONE AT SOME point feels a need to be connected to something larger. This doesn't mean you've got to rush out to the nearest religious service. "There are so many definitions of the sacred," says Rabbi Tirzah Firestone (no relation to Lisa), a psychotherapist, counselor, and author of *The Receiving: Reclaiming Jewish Women's Wisdom*. "Some people can feel part of the infinite when they are in nature. Some people feel it doing yoga or meditation or listening to music."

Rachel Naomi Remen agrees. "One of the most profound ways to experience spirituality," she says, "is through the heart." Look around and ask, "Who needs me?"

Give of your time and kindness. Some of the cancer patients Remen treats, perhaps newly awakened to a sense of life's fragility as well as its value, begin doing things like reading to sick children in the hospital. "Most often it is through love that we experience the great spirit that binds us," she says.

And don't automatically discount the church—or temple, or mosque—even if you're a skeptic or haven't attended one in years. There is grace in sharing a room with others who are seeking spiritual union.

"Most cities have churches that offer ecumenical, informal services, if you're uncomfortable with sermons and such," says Rebekah Miles, who is not only an ethics professor but also an ordained Methodist minister. Or you may find, like millions before you, that you can be transported by the sacraments of a high service. "I often attend the Episcopal church near me," says Miles, despite her position in her own church. "The liturgy is really beautiful. It sounds holy"—which is why the language, and the longing for it, have endured.

You wish you had a stronger connection with tradition, ancestry—something to anchor you.
TAPPING INTO YOUR PAST, TO WHAT is bred in your bones, can be a labyrinthine journey. "Nowadays we're all a blend of ethnic backgrounds," says Kathleen Galvin. Americans can have multiple family ancestries: European, African, Hispanic, Asian, Filipino, Maori, you name it—often generations removed. Several Web sites provide access to lineage information (family search.org is the online version of the Family History Library, the largest genealogy library in the world). Beware of companies that promise you an authentic history and a "family crest" for a fee. Many of these enterprises are fraudulent.

A more immediate way to connect to your past is directly through family mem-

bers. Sit down with your grandmother or grandfather, suggests Remen. Bring a notepad. A family's past resides in its stories, not its begettings, which is all that genealogy can tell you. Send out an e-mail to far-flung uncles and cousins and ask if they'll share anecdotes, photos, or even a memento. Holding your great-grandmother's faded daguerreotype can be stirring. "You begin to understand that why you're the way you are may be related to who you came from," Remen says. "You realize, 'Oh, that's where I got my

> "Ah, everyone, at depth, is beautiful. Remembering this can **soften your judgment.**"

stubbornness, from my grandmother, who stood up to everyone.'"

Revive, too, some of the traditions and occasions that may have faded as you've grown up. If you spent every Christmas as a child at Uncle Harry's house with all your first cousins running around like banshees, invite everyone—including the next generation of banshees—for a rousing holiday feast at your home. Or throw a family reunion and include all the relatives (the great-aunts and great-uncles, the second and first cousins once removed). Sharing experiences as well as memories grounds you with a sense of belonging.

The one caveat is not to go overboard on the genealogy research, says Joyce Catlett, author, child mental health specialist, and frequent collaborator with Lisa Firestone on books and lectures. "I've seen people become obsessed. It's isolating. They spend months on the Internet," using the past to avoid engaging in the present. Instead of squirreling away what you learn, then, pass it along. "It's wonderful to claim a piece of the past for yourself, to find out that you're, say, part Irish," Galvin says. "But it's not much fun to be part Irish alone."

So read to your children about St. Paddy; wear goofy green hats together. Traditions and memories that are carried on into the future link the next generation not only to the past but also to you. •

The Charm of You

It's frothy, elusive, and leaves its subjects feeling lighter than air (and a little bit in love). PETER SMITH explains what makes some people so darned irresistible.

YOU SHOW UP AT AN ENORMOUS dinner party, a buffet for 75. Your hostess greets you at the door with effusive warmth, inquires about a mutual acquaintance she met years earlier (now, how in the world did she remember the guy's name?), then makes an offhandedly witty remark that immediately puts you at ease. Her intimate, conspiratorial manner seems to promise: Now that you're here, the fun can *really* begin.

You start doing your party thing. But no matter where you are, your attention is drawn back to your hostess. She seems to possess a heightened sensitivity to the currents in the room—a wandering but exact emotional pitch. She coaxes out the wallflowers, notices when drinks need refilling, steers a risky political discussion back to safe ground, flirts with an elderly man, engages a 5-year-old boy in animated conversation. And here's the amazing thing: When you and she are talking one on one, the other 74 people in the room turn into extras. You're the effervescent center of the universe. Her eyes never leave yours. Her words seem meant exclusively for your ears. Moreover, everything coming out of your mouth sounds fresh, riveting. Compared to

Cary Grant turns his sly magnetism on Ingrid Bergman in *Indiscreet*.

you, Stephen Hawking's a half-wit, Fred Astaire a klutz.

You leave the party feeling flattered, a little bit divine, a little bit in love. Then you realize: You've just been in the presence of what Jane Austen referred to as "easy manners" and what's more commonly known as charm.

Charm. Trying to define it is like trying to imprison fog in a cup or toss a net over a faraway sound. "The capacity to please or delight," dictionaries attempt falteringly. Though charm strongly dislikes calling attention to itself, most of us know when we're in its proximity, even when we're not entirely sure what we're responding to. The

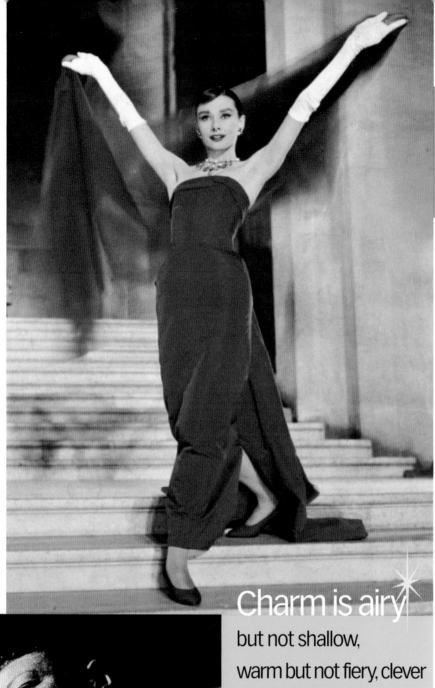

Charm is airy

but not shallow, warm but not fiery, clever but not snide. It can take effort, but in time it becomes a reflex.

holder? Though there are many different varieties of charm (ethereal, rough-hewn, winsome, etc.), its essence can be distilled into this: a natural and rippling responsiveness to other people, an alive attentiveness to what they want, what they're thinking, feeling, saying, or not saying. Whether their charm derives from a desire to be adored or to put other people at ease or both, charming people manage to make others who venture into their sphere leave feeling like their ideal selves.

In its lowest form, charm wants something—money, sex, a promotion—and knows precisely how to get it. At its middling level, charm is a social and professional lubricant, an undeniably useful quality that helps you, and not the other person, land the job or the attention of the Brazilian stranger at the end of the bar. At its best, highest form, charm is a show of generosity and moral goodness, an extension of the self toward others that permits them to shine. By helping others relax and unfold, charm allows you to shine, too. Unlike any other quality I can think of, it's self-effacing, self-protective, and attention-getting at the same time.

Growing up with parents locally legendary for their hospitality, I was a student of charm on an everyday level and in quick order picked up some of its underground characteristics: Pay attention to what's going on around you. Keep your spirits light (never to be confused with being flip), and don't take yourself too seriously. Be well informed. Learn to think quickly and to talk about a broad, weird range of subjects (the stock market, lizards, antidepressants, foam, Roman history, bad movies). And wit is a plus, preferably on the outlandish or self-deprecating side. My Boston-born father treated all people graciously, no matter who they were or what their background was. My southern-born mother would deflect attention from herself, never letting on if she was put out or bored or annoyed.

"You are absolutely fantastic," my mother would say to the telemarketer whose phone call had rudely interrupted

early Beatles. Nat King Cole singing "Unforgettable." Audrey Hepburn in *Funny Face*. Diane Keaton in *Annie Hall*. Cary Grant in everything. In real life, it's the breezily self-deprecating guy at work, or your grandmother, the one who always wants to hear what *you've* been up to.

So what exactly is this ephemeral, mysterious quality, this force that makes it nearly impossible to turn away from its

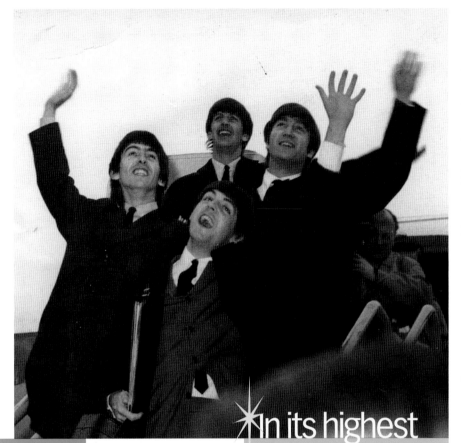

In its highest form, charm is a show of generosity, an extension of the self toward others that permits them to shine.

dinner, "and I would leap at your wondrous dental plan if I felt my teeth were remotely worth saving." (Her teeth were fine.) But it was during intimate, candlelit gatherings that her charm reached its height. She would lower her voice to a near inaudible pitch, causing listeners to pull their chairs a few inches closer, as if they were being lured inside a gilded force field, even if my mother was merely asking people whether they knew that when lobsters lose a claw, it's gone for good.

From observing my parents and others, it became abundantly clear to me that charming people have an uncanny, almost architectural sense of harmony. They're able to pick out subtle energies in a room—the silences, hesitations, miscues, awkwardnesses—and if they perceive that something's wrong, or off, they'll step in to fill the missing beat. But it's not merely attending to others and drawing them out; it's also caring enough to remember what people say. (People often remarked that one of ex-president Bill Clinton's most famous political gifts was his remarkable memory for names, faces, and facts about people he'd met years earlier.)

CHARM, I'VE DISCOVERED over the years, has little to do with background or social class—the Beatles and Cary Grant, for instance, were all from working-class English families—though sometimes it appears inseparable from breeding and good manners. There's an apocryphal story about Queen Elizabeth II and a dinner guest who, never having seen a finger bowl before, proceeded to drink from it. Without missing a beat, the queen immediately followed suit. Is that charming or what? As for the opposite of charm? Narcissism. People who talk about themselves incessantly. People with a stormy, heavy presence. People who don't *notice,* or who can't be bothered.

Charm, then, manages to be superaware but never conspicuously vigilant. It's airy but not shallow, warm but not fiery, clever but not snide. It's original, unexpected, seemingly improvisatory—well, at least until you overhear your hostess repeating the same enchanting story she's just regaled you with to the couple in the corner. Ultimately, charm has to do with something basic: a genuine desire to make other people feel their lives are interesting and worthy, even intriguing. Because of its indirection, and because women are typically trained to pick up on things more than men are, charm has always seemed to me more female than male, though men, of course, can be just as good at it as women. (Male charm, however, is sometimes associated with slyness, the sort of seductive ne'er-do-well legerdemain that coaxes women easily into bed—*oops*—or rooks them out of their last $50.)

Do charming people know they're charming? Yes, typically they've been told it enough times that they do. Does charm take effort? Yes, often it does, though over time it becomes a reflex. Can anybody be charming? The simple answer is that charm can't be taught; you're born with it or you're not. Which isn't to say that with practice you can't learn how to simulate hyperattentiveness or adopt an easy manner. But you can't really learn to be witty. Or light. And most people can't be bothered to pretend to care if they don't.

A few months ago, I rented and rescreened the 1951 film version of Tennessee Williams's *A Streetcar Named Desire.* There's a famous scene toward the end in which Blanche DuBois's suitor, Mitch, rips the paper lantern off a lightbulb and accuses Blanche of deceiving him with "malarkey." In a way, he's also forcing charm to confront the wear and tear of its own incandescence. "Get real," Mitch seems to be saying.

So what, I wondered as I watched, if charm is only an embroidery on the burlap of life? So what if, compared to curing cancer or obliterating starvation, charm ranks fairly low? So what if charm's innocent ambition is only to bring some joy to a scary, harried world? Though I knew how it all turns out, I found myself rooting for Blanche all the way. •

The sign on her desk was modest, the words deceptively simple. Fifteen years and 100 temp jobs later, DEBORAHANN SMITH tells what she's learned from her excellent adventures.

BE EXCELLENT TO EACH OTHER

IT BEGAN 15 YEARS AGO WITH A sign reading BE EXCELLENT TO EACH OTHER, which I printed from my computer in Gothic type and taped to my workspace. I was about to launch into a series of temporary jobs to supplement my freelance writing income. My plan was to temp for a few months, save enough money so I could stay home and write for a while, back and forth, my intention being eventually to write full-time. As is often the case with best-laid plans, however, I soon discovered an unexpected goal within my temporary career: the pursuit of excellence as a way of life.

The phrase on the sign was borrowed from the silly eighties movie *Bill & Ted's Excellent Adventure.* I hoped it would remind me to be helpful, apply myself fully to every task, and be kind to even the most unpleasant individuals. I also secretly wished people would see the slogan and take the words to heart. My fellow temps were skeptical. "People treat temps like dirt," they scoffed. "You'll be lucky if you can maintain excellence through your first assignment." They had a point: I was likely to meet challenges. Nevertheless, I rolled up my sleeves and went to work.

The sign made its debut at a corporation that designed robots (affectionately called "the girls") for the food-packaging industry. Dubbing myself Robo Temp, I typed, filed, and amused my coworkers by invariably responding "I'll tell your fans" when they announced their departures for lunch. No one seemed to notice the sign until several days into the job, when I set up a videotape for a troubleshooting meeting. The tape showed "the girls" malfunctioning—throwing chocolate chip cookies at each other instead of neatly filing them into their respective boxes. "Hey," I heard a software engineer exclaim as I left the room. "They aren't being excellent to each other!" "Yeah!" someone else shouted. "Be excellent to each other!" Later someone left a box of the girls' cookies in the break room, accompanied by a note: "For the team. Thanks for your excellent help."

Not everyone embraced excellence with such enthusiasm. Some people ignored the sign (and the intention). Others were short-tempered, despite my best efforts. But, for the most part, my colleagues responded positively to kindness. They grew radiant when I told them their jade earrings made their eyes look beautiful or when I complimented them on a haircut. They took pride in their work when I admired the brilliant organization of a paper they'd written. They opened up more to others when I inquired about their weekend and actually listened to their responses. When I smiled, they smiled back.

On one occasion, being excellent even helped redirect the career of an unhappy administrative assistant. After overhearing her on the phone with her daughter, I asked if she had majored in child psychology, since she seemed especially gifted at dealing with children. Several weeks later, she came to thank me for my observation and to say goodbye: She was leaving to open her own day-care center.

As a longtime Zen student, I had been taught to appreciate small, mundane moments—moments opportune for practicing excellence in the workplace. For example, seemingly endless sit-at-the-receptionist-desk moments prompted me to be aware of when someone needed a sympathetic ear. Humdrum xeroxing moments were great for noticing harried coworkers who might appreciate assistance in meeting a deadline. Oh-so-yawnish envelope-stuffing projects were ideal times for spotting bottles to be carried to the recycling bin and spiders that needed to be taken outside in paper cups.

During mundane moments, I came to understand that excellence wasn't about being perfect or about being nice so people would like me. On the contrary, sometimes it meant defending someone against vicious gossip or saying no to a colleague who asked me to lie about his overtime hours. I also realized that there were some people I couldn't be excellent to, like the account manager who regularly screamed at his staff. There were other people no amount of excellence could save, like the typist who would rather be treated as a victim than receive any kind of help.

Eventually, I would carry my sign to more than 100 jobs in Boston and Boulder, Colorado, at universities, high-tech companies, museums, manufacturers, publishers, environmental research organizations, and even a wildlife rehab center. My tasks included FedExing socks and underwear to a corporate spy whose business trip was unexpectedly extended and feeding warm milk from eyedroppers to newborn squirrels. After a few years of temping, I branched out. First I wrote two books on what Buddhists call right livelihood—earning a living without doing harm—hoping that others might benefit from what I had learned. Next I offered employment workshops through university extension programs and community centers, where I intended to present practical information but somehow ended up teaching excellence as well. Meanwhile, in my personal life, I attended to my relationships with renewed commitment. I listened more fully and was more readily available to friends and family than I'd ever been before. I was given the opportunity to test this commitment when my best friend and my father died within the same year and I was called upon to devote full-time hospice care to them both. I was there until their very last breaths—my most profound experience with excellence yet.

I finally met my writing goal and am no longer temping, though we are all temps in one form or another, since nothing really lasts forever. Still, my practice of excellence endures. Now, instead of a sign, I carry excellence within me as a mantra, as a presence. Excellence has the most impact when I first focus on my own peace and happiness, and then send it out into the world. ●

About the Contributors

AIMEE LEE BALL is the coauthor of several books, including *Changing the Rules* with Muriel Siebert.

CHRISTINE BARANSKI, a Tony- and Emmy-winning actress (*The Real Thing, Cybill*), has appeared on television, in movies, and on Broadway.

MARTHA BECK is a life coach and author of *The Joy Diet, Leaving the Saints,* and other books. She writes a monthly column for *O.*

MARGIT BISZTRAY has written for *Gourmet* and *Vogue,* and is the author of *The Complete Key West Dining Guide.*

AMY BLOOM has written for *The New Yorker, The Atlantic Monthly,* and *The New York Times.* She is the author of numerous books, including *A Blind Man Can See How Much I Love You.*

AMY BLUMENFELD's articles have appeared in *Self, Fitness,* and *People.*

LIZ BRODY is *O*'s health and news director.

MICHELLE BURFORD, *O* contributing features writer, teaches at the Columbia University Publishing Course.

CANDACE BUSHNELL wrote the *Sex and the City* column that became the book that inspired the HBO series. She is also the author of *Trading Up,* among other novels.

BO CALDWELL is the author of the novel *The Distant Land of My Father.*

HARRY CONNICK JR., a three-time Grammy winner, is a pianist, singer, songwriter, and actor who has appeared on NBC's *Will & Grace.*

RAPHAEL CUSHNIR is the author of *Setting Your Heart on Fire* and *Unconditional Bliss: Finding Happiness in the Face of Hardship.* He leads workshops throughout the country.

SARA DAVIDSON is a contributing editor/writer at *O.* Her books include *Loose Change* and *Cowboy: A Novel.*

ISABEL DAVIS is a writer and English professor.

AMY DICKINSON writes *Ask Amy,* the *Chicago Tribune*'s replacement for Ann Landers's advice column.

BEVERLY DONOFRIO is the author of *Riding in Cars with Boys* and *Looking for Mary: or, the Blessed Mother and Me.*

LESLEY DORMEN is the coauthor of *How To Survive Your Boyfriend's Divorce* and *The Secret Life of Girls.*

JANCEE DUNN is a contributing editor at *Rolling Stone.*

SAMANTHA DUNN has written for the *Los Angeles Times, In Style,* and *Shape.* She is the author of the memoir *Not by Accident: Reconstructing a Careless Life.*

SEAN ELDER has written for *The New Yorker, Vogue, National Geographic,* and *The New York Times Magazine.*

JONI EVANS is a senior vice president at a literary agency in New York City.

TINA FEY became the first woman to hold a top writing spot in *Saturday Night Live*'s history. She wrote the screenplay for and appeared in the movie *Mean Girls.*

SUZANNE FINNAMORE is the author of the novels *The Zygote Chronicles* and *Otherwise Engaged.*

VALERIE FRANKEL is the author of *The Not-So-Perfect Man* and coauthor of *The Best You'll Ever Have: What Every Woman Should Know About Getting and Giving Knock-Your-Socks-Off Sex.*

WENDY KING FREDELL works for the Beaufort, South Carolina, Chamber of Commerce. She is currently writing a memoir.

LISE FUNDERBURG is a journalist and author of *Black, White, Other: Biracial Americans Talk about Race and Identity.*

CHEE GATES is an editorial assistant at *O.*

CYNTHIA GORNEY writes for *The New Yorker, Harper's,* and *The Washington Post.* She teaches at the graduate school of journalism, University of California, Berkeley. Her most recent book is *The Business of News: A Challenge for Journalism's Next Generation.*

LAUREN GRAVITZ is *O*'s associate health editor.

BOB GREENE is Oprah's trainer and the author of several books, including *Get with the Program!* and *Bob Greene's Total Body Makeover.*

HARVILLE HENDRIX and **HELEN LaKELLY HUNT** are marital therapists who teach workshops nationwide. Hendrix is the author of *Getting the Love You Want;* he and Hunt have coauthored several books, including *Giving The Love That Heals.*

PAM HOUSTON, director of creative writing at the University of California, Davis, is the author of several books, including *Cowboys Are My Weakness* and *Sight Hound.*

BETH JANES was the associate beauty editor at *O.*

ROBERT KAREN, PhD, a clinical psychologist in Manhattan, is the author of *The Forgiving Self: The Road from Resentment to Connection.*

DAVID L. KATZ, MD, is a professor at Yale University School of Medicine and the author of *The Way to Eat.*

JULIE KLAM is a freelance writer.

LISA KOGAN is *O*'s writer at large.

CLAUDIA KOLKER has written for *The Boston Globe* and *Salon.com,* and is the former Houston bureau chief for the *Los Angeles Times.*

RONNA LICHTENBERG is the president of Clear Peak Communications, a management consulting firm. Her most recent book is *Pitch Like a Girl: How a Woman Can Be Herself and Still Succeed.*

ANN MARSH, a former *Forbes* staff writer, has written for the *Los Angeles Times, Red Herring,* and *Salon.com.*

MARK MATOUSEK is the author of a memoir, *The Boy He Left Behind,* and other books.

PHILLIP C. McGRAW, PHD, hosts a daily television show, *Dr. Phil,* and is the author of several books, including *The Ultimate Weight Solution* and *Family First.* He writes a monthly column for *O.*

CATHLEEN MEDWICK is the author of *Teresa of Avila: The Progress of a Soul.*

J.J. MILLER is director, Executive Offices/Harpo liaison at *O.*

VALERIE MONROE, *O*'s beauty director, is the author of *In the Weather of the Heart,* a memoir.

JULIE MORGENSTERN is a time management coach and founder of Taskmasters, a consulting firm that helps companies and individuals get organized. Her many books include *Organizing from the Inside Out* and *Making Work Work.* She's a contributing editor at *O.*

KATHLEEN NORRIS contributes to *The Christian Century* and *Ruminator Review* magazines. She has written several books, including *The Cloister Walk* and *Amazing Grace.*

SUZE ORMAN, host of CNBC's *The Suze Orman Show,* is the author of several books on personal finance, including *The Laws of Money, The Lessons of Life.* She writes a monthly column for *O.*

ANN PATCHETT is the author of *The Patron Saint of Liars, The Magician's Assistant, Bel Canto,* and *Truth and Beauty: A Friendship.*

BARBARA PAULSEN is an articles editor at *National Geographic.*

HOLLY ROBINSON PEETE is an actress and cofounder of the HollyRod Foundation, which provides financial, physical, and emotional support for patients living with Parkinson's disease.

NANCY PELOSI represents California's Eighth District in the House of Representatives. She is the first woman in American history to lead a major party in the U.S. Congress.

LYNN SNOWDEN PICKET is a freelance writer and the author of *Looking for a Fight: A Memoir.*

FRANCINE PROSE is the author of numerous books, most recently *A Changed Man, Blue Angel,* and *The Lives of the Muses.*

MARY LOU QUINLAN, founder of Just Ask a Woman, which helps corporations understand what female consumers want, is the author of *Time Off for Good Behavior: How Hard-Working Women Can Take a Break and Change Their Lives.*

DAWN RAFFEL is executive articles editor of *O.* Her most recent novel is *Carrying the Body.*

RACHEL NAOMI REMEN, MD, a clinical professor of medicine at the University of California, San Francisco, School of Medicine, is the author of *Kitchen Table Wisdom* and *My Grandfather's Blessings.* She is the founder and Director of the Institute for the Study of Health and Illness at Commonwealth.

GRETCHEN REYNOLDS writes about infectious diseases for *The New York Times Magazine.* She is also a contributing editor for *National Geographic Adventure.*

AMANDA ROBB is working on a book about the murder of her uncle, Dr. Bart Slepian, who was killed by an antiabortionist in 1998.

ROSEMARY ROGERS is the coauthor of several books, including *Mother-Daughter Movies: 101 Films to See Together.*

M.J. ROSE is the author of several novels, including *The Halo Effect* and *Sheet Music.* Her work has appeared in *Poets & Writers* and *Book* magazines, and on *Salon.com.*

JEFFREY B. RUBIN, PHD, a psychoanalyst, is the author of *The Good Life: Psychoanalytic Reflections on Love, Ethics, Creativity, and Spirituality.*

SUSANNE RUPPERT is a senior copy editor at *O.*

SHARON SALZBERG is the author of *Faith: Trusting Your Own Deepest Experience,* among other books. She has been teaching meditation for 30 years.

JUDITH SILLS, PHD, a clinical psychologist, is the author of *The Comfort Trap or, What If You're Riding a Dead Horse?* and other books.

GARY SINISE is an actor, director, and producer who stars in *CSI: NY.*

DEBORAHANN SMITH is the author of *Temp: How to Survive and Thrive in the World of Temporary Employment* and *Work with What You Have: Ways to Creative & Meaningful Livelihood.*

PETER SMITH has written for *The New York Times Magazine, Travel + Leisure, The New Yorker,* and *Self.* He is the author of *Two of Us: The Story of a Father, a Son and the Beatles.*

MICHELLE STACEY is the author of *The Fasting Girl: A True Victorian Medical Mystery.*

JUDITH STONE is a contributing writer/editor at *O* and is working on *When I Was White,* a book about South Africa during apartheid.

MAIA SZALAVITZ has written for *The New York Times, The Washington Post,* and *Newsweek.* She is the coauthor of *Recovery Options: The Complete Guide.*

PATRICIA VOLK is the author of *Stuffed: Adventures of a Restaurant Family* and other books. She has written for *The New York Times* and *The New York Times Magazine.*

HANNAH WALLACE is an associate editor at *Travel + Leisure* and has written for *Elle* and *Alternative Medicine* magazines.

SARAH WILDMAN has written for *The New York Times Book Review, The Washington Post,* and *The Christian Science Monitor.*

MARION WINIK, a commentator for NPR's *All Things Considered,* is the author of *The Lunch-Box Chronicles: Notes from the Parenting Underground* and other books.

LAUREN F. WINNER is the author of *Girl Meets God,* a memoir, and several other books.

LISA WOLFE, a freelance writer, is working on a novel.

Photography & Art Credits

161 Courtesy of Miiko and Herbert Horikawa; **162** Courtesy of Georgia and Jerry Carter; **163 top** Courtesy of Dee Ito and Marshall Arisman; **163 bottom** Courtesy of Beth and Martin Johnson; **165** Karen Hirshan photograph, courtesy of Craig Krull Gallery, Santa Monica, California; **167** Stephen Swintek/The Image Bank/Getty Images; **169–170** Chris Bartlett; **171–173** Brian L. Velenchenko; **174** Fitzroy Barrett/GLOBE Photos, Inc.; **178** Art Streiber; **179** Thomas: Debra M. Gussin; Kraus-Bell and Stewart: Paramount Pictures; **181** Howard Schatz; **182** Alberto Rizzo; **184** Art Streiber; **188** and **190** John Lund/Stone/Getty Images; **189** Martin Barraud/Stone/Getty; **191** Brian L. Velenchenko; **194** Art Streiber; **196** The Kobal Collection; **198** Everett Collection; **203** photograph: Everett Collection; mosaic: Robert Silvers/Photomosaic.com; **206–207** Courtesy of M.J. Rose; **208–209** David Lewis Taylor; **210** Brian L. Velenchenko; **214** Dana Gallagher; **217** Greg Kesseler; **220–223** Rob Howard; **225** Johannes Labusch; **226** Linda Farwell; **228** Reuters/Corbis; **229** Sam Jones/Corbis Outline; **230 left** Noah Greenberg; **230 right** Brown W. Cannon III; **232 left** Brown W. Cannon III; **232 right** Noah Greenberg; **234–235** Courtesy of Lisa Wolfe; **237** The Image Bank/Getty Images; **240** *The Dance, I* ©2005 Succession H. Matisse, Paris/Artists Rights Society (ARS), New York; **242 and 244** Joshua Paul; **246** Noah Greenberg; **249** Ann Stratton; **250** M. Courtney-Clarke; **254** Livia Corona; **255 top right** David Sutton/MPTV.net; **255 middle right** Mike Theiler/Reuters/Corbis; **255 bottom left** NBC/GLOBE Photos, Inc.; **255 middle left** PHOTOFEST; **257** Susanna Howe; **259** Dennis Cook/AP/Wide World Photos; **262** Ryan McVay/Photodisc Red/Getty Images; **263 top** Kirk Aeder/Icon SMI/Corbis; **263 middle** Courtesy of MacArthur Foundation; **263 bottom** Jeff Gross/Getty Images; **264 top** Jeff Nicholson; **264 bottom** Courtesy of Fadya Resho O'Neill; **265 top** Steve Groer; **266 top** Lynn Goldsmith; **266 bottom left** Annie Musselman; **266 bottom right** Michael Branscom; **267** Carla Frank; **268–271** Brian Doben; **272** photographs: Courtesy of The Rudisill Regional Library, Tulsa; collage: Clifford Alejandro; **274** Michael Stravato; **275** Clifford Alejandro; **276–277** Avigail Schimmel; **278** Courtesy of Erika Schneider; **280–287** Benny Gool; **289** Marc Royce; **290** Spencer Platt/Getty Images; **291 top** Marc Royce; **291 bottom** Courtesy of Barak Obama; **295** Peter Kramer/Getty Images; **296** Benny Gool; **298 left** Carlo Allegri/Getty Images; **298 right** Frank Trapper/Corbis; **299** Reuters/Corbis; **301 top** Courtesy of U.S. soldiers and operationiraqichildren.org; **301 bottom** Charlie Riedel/AP/Wide World Photos; **302** Rob Howard; **304** Courtesy of Alicia Keys; **305** Reuters/Corbis; **308** Photograph by Jennifer Livingston; **310–312** Courtesy of families; **316** Gary Hershorn/Reuters/Corbis; **317–319** Debra Falk/Thirteen/WNET New York; **320–323** David Doubilet; **324** The Kobal Collection; **325 top** PHOTOFEST; **325 bottom** Bettmann/Corbis; **326** Getty Images

Index

Abandonment, 206–207
Abbey of Regina Laudis, 108–114
  Benedictine Rule, 114
Activism
  and grief, 261
  helping organizations, 261
Acupuncture, as headache treatment, 48
Addiction, 13, 73
  drug, 56
  food, 13
  and relationships, 151
Aging, 42
  Age: The Real Tip-Offs, 42
Aha! Moments
  Baranski, Christine, 228
  Bushnell, Candace, 85
  Connick, Harry, Jr., 229
  Fey, Tina, 91
  Peete, Holly Robinson, 295
  Pelosi, Nancy, 316
Alcohol, drinking, 18
  driving age for, 259
  quitting, 18
  risk factors of, 44
  Science's Best New Strategies, 18
American soldiers
  helping in Iraq, 301
  and Operation Iraqi Children, 301
Apology, 198–200
  elements of an, 199
  and forgiveness, 200
Arguing
  breaking the cycle of, 192
  over finances, 191–193
  winning vs. understanding, 191–193

Baggage, emotional, 137
Balance, 53–66, 269
  Getting a Life, 61
Beauty, therapeutic properties of
  pretty things, 69, 76–77
Beauty treatments, 40–42
  laser hair removal, 41
  makeup, 41
  professional teeth whitening, 40–41
  salon hair conditioning, 42
  spa facials, 42
  toners, 42
Behavior
  annoying, 143–145
  changing your partner's, 143–145,
    146–148
  responsibility for bad, 200
  rewarding favorable, 143–145
Biofeedback, for managing pain, 49
Blood pressure, 29
  effects of being overweight on, 29–30
Bone density testing, 43
Botox, as treatment for migraine, 49

Breaking up
  dating after, 156
  figuring out why, 155

Caffeine, avoiding, 55
Calcium, 45–46
Cancer, 254, 256, 308
  Breast Cancer Research Foundation
    (BCRF), 308
  fighting, 266
  fighting with comedy, 254, 256
  support groups for, 52
  treatment for, 247, 308
  vaccine for cervical, 266
  and volunteering, 323
Career
  changing, 102, 111–114, 269
  dreams in, 97–98
  fears in, 97–98
  path, 91
  transitions in, 97
Caretakers, 56, 61, 170, 204, 327
  and excellence, 327
  letting others be, 61
Charm, 324–326
Citta, organization of, 277
Civil rights movement, 293
Commitments
  to finances, 71
  to friends, 247
  keeping, 61
  to others, 62
  to work, 62
Communication, 194–195
  feedback in, 194, 241
  honesty in, 241
  one-way, 194
Community
  art in the, 270
  becoming part of a, 320–323
Confidence, 81–94
  after a breakup, 156
  sexual, 178–180
Confrontation, 190
Coping mechanisms, 47, 170
Criticism
  in conversation, 195
  of men by women, 139–141
  in stepfamilies, 196
  of yourself, 88–90, 320
Currency
  expressing feelings through, 132–133
  what matters to people, 132–133

Dating, 121–130
  after a breakup, 156
  after divorce, 124–125
  and being yourself, 122–124

  blind dates, 130
  online, 122–124
  Personal Ads: The Dos, the Don'ts, and
    the Absolute Musts, 124
  younger men, 136–138
Depression, 68, 73, 79, 156, 181, 321
  and not having friends, 245
  and seasonal affective disorder (SAD), 68
  and sex, 181
  and support groups, 52
  treatment of, 73, 320–323
Divorce, 137, 148, 154, 156, 170
  and living together before marriage, 167
  and stepfamilies, 196–197
Dr. Phil's MENtors, 132–135. See also
  McGraw, Phillip C. (Dr. Phil).
Dreams, 95–102
  achieving your, 263
  Big-Dream contest, 277–278
  in career, 97–98
  following through with, 97–98

Education, 264
  pursuing an, 265
  in South Africa, 286
  What One Person—You—Can Do, 286
Ego, 139–141, 147
Emotions, 133
Empathy
  deficit, 291, 293
  in society, 293, 294
Empowerment, 180
  for mothers, 224
  of women in politics, 316
Energy, 54–55, 59, 73, 97
  amount spent on relationships, 65–66
  negative, 55
  positive, 55
  and praying, 59
  reiki, 105
  and rescheduling, 59
  restoring, 54–55
  and self-promotion, 83, 84
  sexual, 182–183
  of the spirit, 105
  and too much activity, 59
Entertaining, 93–94
Exercise, 13, 16, 59, 61, 63, 68, 75
  accompanied by music, 33
  away from the gym, 32–34
  ball workout, 37
  But I Love to..., 34
  dance as, 33
  extra activity, 24, 25
  to lose weight, 13, 23
  making it fun, 32–34
  making time for, 35–38, 57
  Oprah's Boot Camp, 30
  and osteoporosis, 45

relapse, 16
specific exercises, 28–31
staying interested in, 27
in swimming pool, 24
varying, 27

Faith, 104, 107, 113, 128, 135, 150, 151, 263
in the face of fear, 107
in friends, 248
Family, 201–218. *See also* Fathers,
Grandmothers, Mothers.
Family-to-Family, 267
role reversal in, 217–218
Fathers
Men Behaving Dadly, 231
stay-at-home dads, 230–233
Fears, 106–107
of abandonment, 207
in career, 97–98
and illness, 295
in love, 148
overcoming, 102, 106–107, 263
and rebellion, 291–292
of rejection, 133–134
Feedback, in communication, 194, 241
Fidelity, 135, 138
Finances, 142. *See also* Money.
arguing over, 191–193
debt, 70
Finances: The Spring Cleanup, 71
financial stability, 142
and prenuptial agreements, 168
separate, 168
in stepfamilies, 197
Food
addiction, 13
bingeing on, 14, 15, 17
as comfort, 12, 18–19, 29, 70, 76
eating properly, 57, 80
Food Pyramid, 26
and jet lag, 74
journal (or diary), 23, 27
labels, reading, 22, 23, 80
Michelle's Menus, 16
mini-meals, 16
and time of day, 15, 17, 55, 74
Forgiveness, 210–212, 213
parents and, 210–212
of perpetrators, 260
Friendship, 239–249, 320–323
annoyances in, 189–190
conflicts in, 188–190
and depression, 245
and effect on health, 245, 320–323
fixed roles of friends, 241
reconnecting with, 242, 245
and staying connected, 249
Talking Cure, The, 245
trust in, 241

Gaining weight, 18, 26
due to smoking, 18
Gender, 85, 155. *See also* Men, Women.
being a person first, 85

and blame for breakup, 155
differences, 140
and division of labor, 137
and feelings, 140
roles, 137
and words, 140
words vs. feelings, 140
Goals, 241
in arguments, 192
and attitude in relationships, 134
in communicating, 241
in living life, 97–98
for weight loss, 12–13
Grandmothers, 217–218
Greene, Bob, 8–19, 28–31
Grief, 116
and activism, 258, 261
after, 258
dealing with, 116
Growing up, 211, 215–216, 226–227
and letting go, 216

Happiness, 67–80, 180, 320
in friendship, 320–323
in partnership, 164–166
and sex, 180
Hatred, 189–190
Headaches, 47–49
chronic, 47–49
diary of, 48
Latest Treatments, The, 49
Types of Headaches, 48, 49
Health, 39–52
and balance, 269
effect of having friends on, 245
Real Health Clubs, The, 52
HIV/AIDS
crises in South Africa, 297–298
Keep a Child Alive, 307
World AIDS Day concert, 298
Honesty, 123, 134
among friends, 241
and betrayal, 134
in communication, 241
and dating, 122–124
and happiness, 71
in raising children, 238
in relationships, 155
truth is beauty, 300
Hormones
during sex, 181
HRT (hormone replacement
therapy), 44
Hostility, 189–190, 196
from acquaintances, 189–190
how to handle, 189–190
Humor
finding in tragedy, 256
sense of in marriage, 159, 160, 161

Infatuation, 148
Interpretation of events, 146–148, 150
Intimacy, 132, 151, 184, 185, 186
among friends, 241

avoiding, 320–323
and charm, 324–326
male, 139–141
in stepfamilies, 197
Intuition, 150, 151, 156
Iraq, 264–265, 269, 301
American soldiers' goodwill in, 301
Operation Iraqi Children, 301
working as a translator in, 264–265

Jealousy in stepfamilies, 197
Jersey Girls, 257–258
activists after September 11, 2001,
257–261
Journal (or diary), 61
food, 23, 27
headache, 48
leisure log, 61
Joy Diet, 74–77
feasts, 74–77
and ritual, 75
Jujube doll, 140–141
and a man's self-esteem, 140–141

Keeping weight off, 12–13, 20–26, 27.
See also Losing Weight.
Keeping It Off Forever: The 10 Rules, 23
long-term losers, 22–26
National Weight Control Registry, 22

Laser hair removal, 41
Laughter, 68, 255
Laugh-A-Thons, 256
as treatment for illness, 254–256
Leadership
in American society, 290
in politics, 290–294
Letting go, 227
of children, 216
of houses, 216
Lifestyle, 78–80
changing, 13, 15, 16, 19, 25, 31, 36–38,
56–57, 61, 111–114
monastic, 110–114
Listening, 187–200, 240, 322
actively, 195
compassionate, 192–193
during arguments, 192–193
filters, 195
rules of, 194–195
Win-Win at Home, 192
Losing weight, 12–13, 15. *See also* Keeping
Weight Off.
Are You Ready to Change?, 19
falling off weight loss program, 17, 18–19, 23
getting back on track for, 16, 26
Give Us This Day Our Daily Motto, 17
and muscle, 27
programming yourself for, 13
protein and, 27
reasons for, 28, 29–31
support for, 13, 17, 27
Words to Lose By, 17

Love, 77, 107, 111, 114, 145, 146–148, 170, 211, 226–227
  changing your thoughts on, 146–148
  distinguishing counterfeit love from the real thing, 148
  infatuation or, 148
  a mother's, 228, 291
  from parents, 211
  romantic, 148, 170, 181
  spiritual, 147
  unconditional, 105, 211
  your body, 14
  for your children, 226–227

Mandela, Nelson, 283, 285, 286, 298
Manipulation, 190
Marriage, 157–174
  4 Steps to a Better Marriage, 170
  confrontation in, 191–193
  going your own way in, 174
  Imago partner in, 169
  patience in, 160
  Program, The, 129–130
  respect in, 159
  sense of humor in, 159, 160, 161
  and separate dwellings, 167–168
  sex in, 160, 163
  successful, 174
Martyr, in relationships, 197
McGraw, Phillip C. (Dr. Phil), 12–13, 66, 132–135, 178–180, 184–186, 194–195. See also Dr. Phil's MENtors.
Medical care, 51
  getting a second opinion, 51
  strategies for the best, 51
  taking notes, 51
  Who's the Boss? How to Ensure You Get A-Plus Medical Care, 51
Medications, 49, 78–79, 80
Meditation, 106–107, 111
Men
  demystifying, 134
  how they think, 132–135
  How to Find the Good Ones, 135
  How to Recognize a Good Guy When You See Him, 128
  and intimacy, 134
  male characteristics, 132
  and potential, 140–141
  understanding, 132–135
  What Men Want from Women, 133
  women's expectations of, 132
  word-oriented, 140
  younger men, 136–138
Menopause, 30–31
  adjusting diet for, 30
  and muscle and bone loss, 31
  Wisdom of Menopause, The, 30
Metabolism, 24, 30
  basal metabolic rate (BMR), 27
  and protein, 27
Migraines, 47–49. See also Headaches.
  Latest Treatments, The, 49
  medications for, 49
Million Mom March, 265

Money, 70. See also Finances.
  and emotional state, 70–71
  managing, 70–71
  and spending, 70–71
Mothers, 202–205, 208–209, 213, 228, 234–236, 237–238
  as foundation of the family, 305–307
  How Not to Turn into Your Mother, 205
  and letting go, 227
  the mind-mother, 204
  and mommy time, 225
  patchwork mom, 204–205
  as sole support, 305
  and sons, 238
  and spirituality, 222, 223, 224
  and untold stories, 206–207
Mothers Against Drunk Driving (MADD), 257, 259, 261
Motivation, 32–34
  in business, 97
  currency of, 132–133
  for exercising, 36
  health as, 26, 31
  for losing weight, 13, 18–19
Muscle
  and basal metabolic rate (BMR), 27
  building, 27
  loss after menopause, 31
Music, 77, 298–300, 304–307
  accompanying exercise, 33
  Bono, 296–300
  Keys, Alicia, 302–307
  U2, 298

Nagging, 140
Native American community theater, 277–278
NORA (National Osteoporosis Risk Assessment) study, 43, 46
Notes from parents to their grown children, 208–209

Obama, Barack, 288–294
Obesity, 14, 15, 16, 22, 33
Online dating, 122–124
Optimism, 88–90
  "learned optimism," 88
Organ transplant, 310–315
  and acceptance, 315
  donor families, 310–315
  and grief, 312
  recipients, 310–315
Orman, Suze, 70–71, 142
Osteopenia, 43–46
  and menopause, 45
Osteoporosis, 43–46, 79
  Ann Richards Bones Up, 43
  Bare Bones, The, 44
  drugs that fight, 46
  dual energy X-ray absorptiometry (DXA or DEXA), 44, 46
  high-risk categories, 44
  National Osteoporosis Risk Assessment (NORA) study, 43, 46

  and post menopause, 46
  screening for, 43–46
  susceptibility to, 46
  T score, 44
  when to get tested for, 46
  why get tested for, 46
Overweight, effect on health, 29–31

Pain
  growing up, 212
  management, 47–49, 114
  from relationships, 152–156
  and visualization, 47, 48
Parenting, 98, 196, 219–238
  and commitment to children, 229
  and forgiveness, 210–212
  sending clippings to grown children, 208–209
  stepparenting, 196–197
Parkinson's disease, 295
  HollyRod Foundation, 295
Partners/partnership, 158–163, 164–166. See also Marriage, Relationships.
  to avoid, 126–128
  How to Recognize a Good Guy When You See Him, 128
  making your partner happy, 164–168
  in marriage, 159, 164–166
  parents, 224
  respect in, 159, 160, 161
  sense of humor in, 159, 160, 161
  sex in, 163
  traditional, 166
Passion, 193
  for a cause, 263
  in relationships, 184, 185
Patience, 115–116
  in compassionate listening, 192
  in marriage, 160
  true patience, 116
Patient
  advocacy, 50–52
  being a, 256
Personal ads, 124, 154
  creating, 124
  for dating, 124
Personal trainer, 25, 36
  hiring, 16, 17, 18
Pessimism, 90
Pet ownership
  and depression, 68
  health benefits of, 68
Plateau of weight loss, 27
  explanation of, 27
  getting past, 27
Politics, 288–294, 316
Positive thinking, 91, 180
  saying yes, 91
Prayer, 59, 117
  and giving thanks, 117
  Gregorian chant as, 113
  and positive outcome, 306
  and success, 293
Putting yourself first, 54–66
  Instant Restoratives, 57

Raising children, 228, 230–233, 237–238
    a father's role, 230
    sons, 234–236, 237–238
Relationships, 85, 118–238. *See also*
        Friendship, Marriage, Parenting.
    and apologies, 198–200
    arguing in, 191–193
    breaking up, 152–156
    changing behavior in, 143–145
    destructive, 151
    emotional baggage of, 125
    expectations in, 146–148
    feeling wanted in, 185, 320–323
    financial compatabilities in, 142
    going your own way in, 174
    How to Recognize a Good Guy When
        You See Him, 128
    living together, 167
    maintaining, 65–66
    maintaining your identity, 168
    men to avoid, 126–128
    Moment I Knew It Was Over, The, 150
    with parents, 210–212
    passion in, 184
    and self-esteem, 85
    and separation, 167–168
    sharing responsibilities at home, 168
    staying together, 149–151
    What Never to Do, 134
Religion
    nuns, 110–114
    monks, 105
    religious life, 111–114
Respect, 190
    in marriage, 159
Resting
    and guilt, 63
    permission to, 59
Retreat, 58–59, 114
Risk taking, 99–101
Rituals, 75, 117
    saying grace, 117
Role reversal, 217
Romance, 154

Safety, 106–107
    from terror threats, 107
Salon hair conditioning, 42
    cost of, 42
    determining worth of, 42
Segregation, overcoming, 273–275
Self-doubt, 88–90
    overcoming, 88–90
Self-esteem, 85, 92–94, 139–141
    in children, 222
    job related, 193
    and jujube doll, 140–141
    male, 139–141
    and potential, 141
    and relationships, 85
    robbing a man's, 141
Self-image, 185, 92–94
Self-promotion, 82–84
    differences of between men and women,
        82–83

    and discounting, 83–84
    Friendly Feedback, 84
    Panic Room, The, 83
    preparing for, 83
    Tooting 101, 84
September 11, 2001
    assisting relief workers, 256
    and findings of independent
        investigation, 257
    grief after, 258
    Jersey Girls, 257–261
    lobbying for answers after, 258
    National Commission on Terrorist
        Attacks on the United States, 258
    support groups after, 258
Sex, 135, 175–186
    biological clock and, 190
    and body image, 178–180
    Chemistry Notes, 185
    confidence, 178–180, 183
    and desirability, 183
    and expectations, 183
    experience, 179
    frequency of, 181, 184
    health benefits of, 181
    men's view of, 135
    in marriage, 160, 163
    and power, 179
    priority of having, 184, 186
    satisfaction, 178–180
    and self-consciousness, 180
    Sex Experts vs. the Shy Girl, The, 177
    shyness, 176–177
    women's view of, 135
    youth vs. experience, 138
Sleep, 58–59, 68, 77
    deprivation of, 77
    insomnia, 77
    maps, 77
    and sunlight, 68
Smoking cigarettes
    quitting, 18
    risk factors of, 44, 46
    Science's Best New Strategies, 18
South Africa, 280–287, 297, 298
    What One Person—You—Can
        Do, 286
Spirituality, 103–117, 222, 223, 224
Spiritual refueling, 55, 58–59
    overconnected and disconnecting,
        64–66
    and rest, 59, 63
    and sleeping, 58–59
Stepfamilies, 196–197
    criticism in, 196
    finances in, 197
    intimacy in, 197
    jealousy in, 197
    stepmothers, 196–197
Sunlight, 68
    and sleep, 68
Support groups, 52, 56, 154
    after September 11, 2001, 258
    effect on health, 52
    family as a, 154
    friends as a, 154

    searching Internet for, 17
    social, 68
    types of, 52
    for weight loss, 17, 18

Talking, 187–200
    changing how you are, 88–90
    gossip, 188–190
    positively, 88–90
    rules of, 194–195
    Talking Cure, The, 245
    Talking Cures: A Crib Sheet, 195
    verbal attack, 189–190
Terrorism, fighting, 266
Theater
    and Big-Dream contest, 277–278
    community, 277–278
    Yankton Sioux reservation, 277–278
Time, 247
    the greatest gift, 256
    mommy time, 225
    for yourself, 223–224
Traditions, 215, 323
Travel, 86–87, 96–98
    alone, 86–87, 96–98, 228
    and eating, 74
    in a foreign country, 86–87

Values, 291, 292
Verbal attack, 189–190
    countering, 189–190
Visualization, 47, 48
Vitamin supplements, 46, 80
Volunteering, 61, 68, 323
    health benefits of, 68, 323

Walking, 23, 24, 34, 36, 38, 61
Weddings, second, 171–173
    and gift alternatives, 171–173
Weight training, 16, 27, 31, 38, 45
    getting started, 45
    routines for, 31
Women
    being verbal, 140
    expressing emotions, 133
    and feelings, 140
    and their influence over men,
        139–141
Working, 61
    and disconnecting, 64–66
    Getting a Life, 61
    and overconnection, 64–66
    starting a business, 63, 97
    starting a new job, 102, 111–114
    workaholic, 60–61, 62–63
    work ethic, 61

Yankton Sioux reservation, 277–278
    Big-Dream contest and, 277–278
    community theater, 277–278
Yes, saying, 91, 98, 101, 105
Yoga, 269

Published by Oxmoor House, Inc.
Book Division of Southern Progress Corporation
P.O. Box 2262, Birmingham, Alabama 35201-2262

ISBN: 0-8487-3105-0
Library of Congress Control Number: 2005929033

Printed in the United States of America
Second printing 2005

To order additional publications, call 1-800-765-6400.

O, The Oprah Magazine
FOUNDER AND EDITORIAL DIRECTOR: Oprah Winfrey
EDITOR IN CHIEF: Amy Gross
EDITOR AT LARGE: Gayle King
DESIGN DIRECTOR: Carla Frank
EXECUTIVE ARTICLES EDITOR: Dawn Raffel
DIRECTOR, EXECUTIVE OFFICES/HARPO LIAISON: J.J. Miller
EDITORIAL ASSISTANT: Rachel Bertsche
ASSISTANT PHOTO EDITOR: Jordan Barnes

HEARST BOOKS
VP, PUBLISHER: Jacqueline Deval

OXMOOR HOUSE, INC.
VP, PUBLISHER: Brian Carnahan
EDITOR IN CHIEF: Nancy Fitzpatrick Wyatt
COPY CHIEF: Allison Long Lowery

Live Your Best Life
COPY EDITOR: L. Amanda Owens
EDITORIAL ASSISTANTS: Julie Boston and Terri Laschober
DIRECTOR OF PRODUCTION: Laura Lockhart
PRODUCTION MANAGER: Greg A. Amason
PRODUCTION ASSISTANT: Faye Porter Bonner
PUBLISHING SYSTEMS ADMINISTRATOR: Rick Tucker

CONTRIBUTORS
EDITOR: Susan Randol
DESIGNER: Deborah Kerner
GRAPHIC ARTIST: Carol Damsky
INDEXER: Mary Ann Laurens
INTERN: Mary Catherine Shamblin